T0362211

Hypogonadism

Editors

SHALENDER BHASIN
CHANNA N. JAYASENA

ENDOCRINOLOGY AND METABOLISM CLINICS OF NORTH AMERICA

www.endo.theclinics.com

Consulting Editor
ADRIANA G. IOACHIMESCU

March 2022 • Volume 51 • Number 1

ELSEVIER

1600 John F. Kennedy Boulevard • Suite 1800 • Philadelphia, Pennsylvania, 19103-2899

http://www.theclinics.com

ENDOCRINOLOGY AND METABOLISM CLINICS OF NORTH AMERICA Volume 51, Number 1
March 2022 ISSN 0889-8529, ISBN 13: 978-0-323-89678-8

Editor: Katerina Heidhausen
Developmental Editor: Jessica Cañaberal

Endocrinology and Metabolism Clinics of North America (ISSN 0889-8529) is published quarterly by Elsevier Inc., 360 Park Avenue South, New York, NY 10010-1710. Months of issue are March, June, September, and December. Periodicals postage paid at New York, NY and additional mailing offices. Subscription prices are USD 394.00 per year for US Individuals, USD 1058.00 per year for US institutions, USD 100.00 per year for US students and residents, USD 467.00 per year for Canadian individuals, USD 1079.00 per year for Canadian institutions, USD 512.00 per year for international individuals, USD 1079.00 per year for international institutions, USD 100.00 per year for Canadian students/residents, and USD 245.00 per year for international students/residents. To receive student/resident rate, orders must be accompanied by name of affiliated institution, date of term, and the signature of program/residency coordinator on institution letterhead. Orders will be billed at individual rate until proof of status is received. Foreign air speed delivery is included in all *Clinics* subscription prices. All prices are subject to change without notice. **POSTMASTER:** Send address changes to *Endocrinology and Metabolism Clinics of North America*, Elsevier Health Sciences Division, Subscription Customer Service, 3251 Riverport Lane, Maryland Heights, MO 63043. **Customer Service: Telephone: 1-800-654-2452** (U.S. and Canada). **Fax: 1-314-447-8029.** E-mail: **journalscustomerservice-u-sa@elsevier.com (for print support);** journalsonlinesupport-usa@elsevier.com **(for online support).**

Reprints. For copies of 100 or more, of articles in this publication, please contact the Commercial Rights Department, Elsevier Inc., 360 Park Avenue South, New York, NY 10010-1710; phone: +1-212-633-3874; fax: +1-212-633-3820; E-mail: reprints@elsevier.com.

Endocrinology and Metabolism Clinics of North America is covered in *MEDLINE/PubMed (Index Medicus), EMBASE/Excerpta Medica, Current Contents/Clinical Medicine, Current Contents/Life Sciences, Science Citation Index, ISI/BIOMED, BIOSIS,* and *Chemical Abstracts*.

Contributors

CONSULTING EDITOR

ADRIANA G. IOACHIMESCU, MD, PhD
Emory University School of Medicine, Atlanta, Georgia, USA

EDITORS

SHALENDER BHASIN, MB, BS
Professor of Medicine, Harvard Medical School, Director, Research Program in Men's Health: Aging and Metabolism, Director, Boston Claude D. Pepper Older Americans Independence Center for Function Promoting Therapies, Brigham and Women's Hospital, Boston, Massachusetts, USA

CHANNA N. JAYASENA, MA, PhD, MRCP, FRCPath
Section of Endocrinology and Investigative Medicine, Reader, Imperial College London, Consultant in Reproductive Endocrinology and Andrology, Hammersmith Hospital, London, United Kingdom

AUTHORS

BRADLEY D. ANAWALT, MD
Professor and Vice Chair, Department of Medicine, University of Washington School of Medicine, Seattle, Washington, USA

SHALENDER BHASIN, MB, BS
Professor of Medicine, Harvard Medical School, Director, Research Program in Men's Health: Aging and Metabolism, Director, Boston Claude D. Pepper Older Americans Independence Center for Function Promoting Therapies, Brigham and Women's Hospital, Boston, Massachusetts, USA

ARTHUR L. BURNETT, MD, MBA, FACS
Patrick C. Walsh Distinguished Professor of Urology, Professor, Oncology Center, Johns Hopkins School of Medicine, Brady Urological Institute, Baltimore, Maryland, USA

WALJIT S. DHILLO, FRCP, FRCPath, PhD
Section of Investigative Medicine, Imperial College London, Hammersmith Hospital, London, United Kingdom

ADRIAN S. DOBS, MD, MHS
Director, Johns Hopkins Clinical Research Network, Baltimore, Maryland, USA

MARCELO RODRIGUES DOS SANTOS, PhD
Instituto do Coração (InCor), Hospital das Clínicas HCFMUSP, |Faculdade de Medicina, Universidade de São Paulo, Sao Paulo, Brazil

ANGEL ELENKOV, MD, PhD
Department of Translational Medicine, Lund University, Reproductive Medicine Centre, Skane University Hospital, Malmö, Sweden

ALEKSANDER GIWERCMAN, MD
Professor, Department of Translational Medicine, Lund University, Reproductive Medicine Centre, Skane University Hospital, Malmö, Sweden

ANNA GOLDMAN, MD
Associate Program Director, Endocrinology Fellowship, Division of Endocrinology, Diabetes and Hypertension, Instructor in Medicine, Harvard Medical School, Brigham and Women's Hospital, Boston, Massachusetts, USA

FRANCES J. HAYES, MB, BCh, BAO, FRCPI
Reproductive Endocrine Unit, Associate Professor of Medicine, Harvard Medical School, Associate Clinical Chief of Endocrinology, Massachusetts General Hospital, Boston, Massachusetts, USA

CARMEN LOK TUNG HO, BSc
Section of Endocrinology and Investigative Medicine, Imperial College London, United Kingdom

RAVI JASUJA, PhD
Director, Preclinical Discovery Core, Research Program in Men's Health: Aging and Metabolism, Boston Claude D. Pepper Older Americans Independence Center, Brigham and Women's Hospital, Harvard Medical School, Boston, Massachusetts, USA

CHANNA N. JAYASENA, MA, PhD, MRCP, FRCPath
Section of Endocrinology and Investigative Medicine, Reader, Imperial College London, Consultant in Reproductive Endocrinology and Andrology, Hammersmith Hospital, London, United Kingdom

GEN KANAYAMA, MD, PhD
Associate Director, Substance Abuse Research, Biological Psychiatry Laboratory, McLean Hospital, Belmont, Massachusetts, USA; Research Associate, Harvard Medical School, Boston, Massachusetts, USA

MARTIN KATHRINS, MD
Assistant Professor of Surgery, Division of Urology, Harvard Medical School, Brigham and Women's Hospital, Boston, Massachusetts, USA

JASON A. LEVY, DO, MS
Clinical Instructor of Urology, Johns Hopkins School of Medicine, Brady Urological Institute, Baltimore, Maryland, USA

RONG LUO, MBBS
Section of Investigative Medicine, Imperial College London, Hammersmith Hospital, London, United Kingdom

ALVIN M. MATSUMOTO, MD
Professor Emeritus, Division of Gerontology and Geriatric Medicine, Department of Medicine, University of Washington School of Medicine, Clinical Investigator, Geriatric Research, Education and Clinical Center, V.A. Puget Sound Health Care System, Seattle, Washington, USA

NIKOLETA PAPANIKOLAOU, MBBS, MRCP
Section of Investigative Medicine, Imperial College London, Hammersmith Hospital, London, United Kingdom

KAROL M. PENCINA, PhD
Chief Biostatistician, Research Program in Men's Health: Aging and Metabolism, Boston Claude D. Pepper Older Americans Independence Center, Brigham and Women's Hospital, Harvard Medical School, Boston, Massachusetts, USA

LIMING PENG, MSc
Manager, Brigham Research Assay Core Laboratory, Research Program in Men's Health: Aging and Metabolism, Boston Claude D. Pepper Older Americans Independence Center, Brigham and Women's Hospital, Harvard Medical School, Boston, Massachusetts, USA

HARRISON G. POPE, Jr., MD
Director, Biological Psychiatry Laboratory, McLean Hospital, Belmont, Massachusetts, USA; Professor of Psychiatry, Harvard Medical School, Boston, Massachusetts, USA

ADITI SHARMA, MBBCh, MRCP
Section of Investigative Medicine, Imperial College London, Hammersmith Hospital, London, United Kingdom

PETER J. SNYDER, MD
Professor of Medicine, Perelman School of Medicine, University of Pennsylvania, Smilow Center for Clinical Research, Philadelphia, Pennsylvania, USA

THOMAS W. STORER, PhD
Research Program in Men's Health, Aging, and Metabolism, Brigham and Women's Hospital, Boston, Massachusetts, USA

RONALD S. SWERDLOFF, MD
Chief, Division of Endocrinology, The Lundquist Institute and Harbor-UCLA Medical Center, Torrance, California, USA

ARTHI THIRUMALAI, MBBS
Associate Professor, Department of Medicine, University of Washington School of Medicine, Seattle, Washington, USA

CHRISTINA WANG, MD
Division of Endocrinology, Site Director, Clinical and Translational Science Institute, The Lundquist Institute at Harbor-UCLA Medical Center, Harbor-UCLA Medical Center, Torrance, California, USA

GARY A. WITTERT, MBBCh, MD
Freemasons Centre for Men's Health and Wellbeing, Medical School, University of Adelaide, Department of Endocrinology, Royal Adelaide Hospital, South Australian Health and Medical Research Institute, Adelaide, South Australia, Australia

BU B. YEAP, MBBS, PhD
Medical School, University of Western Australia, Department of Endocrinology and Diabetes, Fiona Stanley Hospital, Perth, Western Australia, Australia

Contents

The epidemiology of male hypogonadism has been understudied. Of the known causes of endogenous androgen deficiency, only Klinefelter syndrome is common with a likely population prevalence of greater than 5:10,000 men (possibly as high as 10–25:10,000). Mild traumatic injury might also be a common cause of androgen deficiency (prevalence 5–10:10,000 men), but large, long-term studies must be completed to confirm this prevalence estimation that might be too high. The classic causes of male androgen deficiency—hyperprolactinemia, pituitary macroadenoma, endogenous Cushing syndrome, and iron overload syndrome—are rare (prevalence < 10,000 men).

Male hypogonadism is a clinical syndrome characterized by the diminished functional activity of the testis resulting in low levels of testosterone and/or spermatozoa. Defects at one or more levels of the hypothalamic-pituitary-testicular (HPT) axis can result in either primary or secondary hypogonadism. The changes that occur in the HPT axis from fetal to adult life are fundamental to understanding the pathophysiology of hypogonadism. In this article, we summarize the maturation and neuroendocrine regulation of the HPT axis and discuss the major congenital and acquired causes of male hypogonadism both at the (1) hypothalamic-pituitary (secondary hypogonadism) and (2) testicular (primary hypogonadism) levels.

A systematic approach to diagnose hypogonadism initially establishes the presence of symptoms/signs of testosterone deficiency, considers other potential causes of manifestations, and excludes conditions that transiently suppress testosterone. Hypogonadism is confirmed by measuring fasting serum total testosterone in the morning on at least 2 separate days, or free testosterone by equilibrium dialysis or calculated free testosterone in men with conditions that alter sex hormone–binding globulin or serum total testosterone near lower limit of normal. To guide management, further evaluation is performed to identify the specific cause of hypogonadism and whether it is potentially reversible or an irreversible pathologic disorder.

Diagnosing testosterone deficiency requires accurate and precise measurement of total testosterone levels by an accurate method, such as liquid chromatography–tandem mass spectrometry in a laboratory certified by an accuracy-based program (eg, Centers for Disease Control and Prevention's Hormone Standardization (HoST) Program), and, if needed, free testosterone level. Free testosterone level should ideally be measured by equilibrium dialysis method. Testosterone levels should be measured in 2 or more fasting samples obtained in the morning. Harmonized reference ranges for total testosterone can be applied to laboratories that certified by the HoST Program.

All approved testosterone replacement methods, when used according to recommendations, can restore normal serum testosterone concentrations, and relieve symptoms in most hypogonadal men. Selection of the method depends on the patient's preference with advice from the physician. Dose adjustment is possible with most delivery methods but may not be necessary in all hypogonadal men. The use of hepatotoxic androgens must be avoided. Testosterone treatment induces reversible suppression of spermatogenesis; if fertility is desired in the near future, human chronic gonadotropin, selective estrogen receptor modulator, estrogen antagonist, or an aromatase inhibitor that stimulates endogenous testosterone production may be used.

For hypogonadal men treated with testosterone, the goal is to ensure that benefits are optimized, risks are minimized, and any adverse effects are identified early and managed appropriately. This can best be achieved by careful patient selection, excluding men with contraindications and addressing any modifiable risk factors in those at increased risk. A standardized plan should be used for monitoring that includes evaluation of symptoms, side effects, adherence, and measurement of testosterone and hematocrit. Shared decision making should be used to determine whether to screen for prostate cancer and informed by age, baseline cancer risk, and patient preference.

substances are widely used illicitly by AAS users at the end of a course of AAS as so-called postcycle therapy. Many endocrinologists still have only limited experience in diagnosing and treating AAS-induced hypogonadism.

Anna Goldman and Martin Kathrins

Electronic health records (EHRs) have enabled electronic documentation of a tremendous amount of clinical data. EHRs have the potential to improve communication between patients and their providers, facilitate quality improvement and outcomes research, and reduce medical errors. Conversely, EHRs have also increased clinician burnout, information clutter, and depersonalization of the interactions between patients and their providers. Increasing clinician input into EHR design, providing access to technical help, streamlining of workflow, and the use of custom templates that have fewer requirements for evaluation and management coding can reduce this burnout and increase the utility of this advancing technology.

ENDOCRINOLOGY AND METABOLISM CLINICS OF NORTH AMERICA

SERIES OF RELATED INTEREST

Medical Clinics
https://www.medical.theclinics.com
Primary Care: Clinics in Office Practice
https://www.primarycare.theclinics.com/

VISIT THE CLINICS ONLINE!
Access your subscription at:
www.theclinics.com

Foreword

Updates in Male Hypogonadism

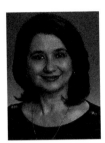

Adriana G. Ioachimescu, MD, PhD
Consulting Editor

The "Hypogonadism" issue of the *Endocrinology and Metabolism Clinics of North America* offers a comprehensive update on a topic that is of great interest to primary care physicians, internists, and many specialists (endocrinologists, geriatricians, urologists). We chose this topic due to developments in recent years, such as publication of clinical trials and updated practice guidelines.

First, I would like to thank our two guest editors, who brought together a large group of experts to author 15 outstanding review articles. Professor Shalender Bhasin, MB, BS from the Harvard Medical School is the Director of the Research Program in Men's Health at Brigham and Women's Hospital in Boston. Dr Channa N. Jayasena, MD, PhD is a Reader at the Imperial College in London and Consultant in Reproductive Endocrinology and Andrology at Hammersmith Hospital in London, UK.

I would also like to thank the authors for their contributions, which provide state-of-the-art updates in epidemiology, pathophysiology, diagnosis, and management of male hypogonadism. The collection of articles addresses many clinical practice aspects that are actively developing, such as assays and interpretation of total and free testosterone levels and cardiovascular impact of hypogonadism and testosterone replacement. Other articles focus on special patient categories that are at risk for low testosterone, such as those with diabetes mellitus, cancer survivors, and those experiencing anabolic steroid withdrawal. Fertility in patients with hypogonadism and the multifaceted effects of testosterone replacement in the elderly are also discussed.

Last but not least, I would like to acknowledge the Elsevier editorial staff for their support.

Endocrinol Metab Clin N Am 51 (2022) xiii–xiv
https://doi.org/10.1016/j.ecl.2021.12.001
0889-8529/22/© 2021 Published by Elsevier Inc.

endo.theclinics.com

I hope you will find the "Hypogonadism" issue of the *Endocrinology and Metabolism Clinics of North America* both interesting and meaningful for your practice.

Adriana G. Ioachimescu, MD, PhD
Emory University School of Medicine
1365 B Clifton Road, Northeast, B6209
Atlanta, GA 30322, USA

E-mail address:
aioachi@emory.edu

Preface

Hypogonadism

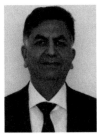
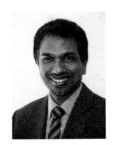

Shalender Bhasin, MB, BS   Channa N. Jayasena, MA, PhD, MRCP, FRCPath
Editors

This special issue of the *Endocrinology and Metabolism Clinics of North America* offers a compendium of articles authored by the leading experts on the epidemiology, diagnosis, and treatment of hypogonadism in men. A confluence of historical factors renders this compendium on Hypogonadism in Men timely. The growing public interest in men's health, particularly in men's sexual health, is reflected in the extraordinary increase over the past 20 years in testosterone's prescription sales in the United States and some other Western countries, combined with the opening of large numbers of men's health clinics across the United States. Testosterone prescription sales in the United States increased from less than 100 million dollars at the turn of the millennium to more than 2 billion dollars in 2013. The issuance of an advisory by the Food and Drug Administration in 2013 about the potential risk of cardiovascular events during testosterone treatment was followed by a short period of decline in testosterone prescription sales; however, testosterone prescriptions in the United States have since resumed their growth trajectory. Women's health clinics have long existed in academic medical centers all around the world; however, the emergence of men's health as a distinct discipline in medicine is a welcome recent development.

Testosterone deficiency is an important reason that motivates men to seek medical attention. Several well-conducted randomized trials, including two of the largest trials of testosterone treatment: the Testosterone Trials and the T4DM Trial, have provided a large body of information about testosterone's efficacy and safety. Wide availability of liquid chromatography tandem mass spectrometry assays for testosterone in laboratories certified by the Centers for Disease Control and Prevention's Hormone Standardization Program and the publication of harmonized reference ranges for testosterone have greatly enhanced the accuracy and interpretability of testosterone measurements in clinical practice.

This special issue comprehensively addresses nearly all aspects of testosterone deficiency: its epidemiology, diagnosis, treatment, and monitoring. Two separate

Endocrinol Metab Clin N Am 51 (2022) xv–xvi
https://doi.org/10.1016/j.ecl.2021.11.015
0889-8529/22/© 2021 Published by Elsevier Inc.

articles describe strategies for enhancing the accuracy of diagnostic evaluation. Several articles provide detailed guidance on the indications for testosterone replacement, how to administer testosterone replacement therapy, and how to monitor testosterone treatment. The potential adverse effects of testosterone, especially the risks of cardiovascular and prostate events, are covered extensively in multiple articles. As middle-aged and older men are the most frequent recipients of testosterone prescriptions, most clinicians would find valuable the articles on benefits and risks of testosterone treatment in men with age-related decline. Another article covers the emerging dual epidemics of anabolic-androgen steroid use and body image disorders in young men.

The authors and the editors have prioritized clinically relevant content, strived to include evidence-based guidance whenever possible, and attempted to strike the right balance between being concise as well as being comprehensive. We hope the practicing clinicians, trainees as well as researchers in men's health find the compendium's state-of-the art content valuable in their clinical practice, education, and research.

Shalender Bhasin, MB, BS
Harvard Medical School
Brigham and Women's Hospital
221 Longwood Avenue
Boston, MA 02115, USA

Channa N. Jayasena, MA, PhD, MRCP, FRCPath
Imperial College London
Hammersmith Hospital
Du Cane Road
London W12 0NN, UK

E-mail addresses:
sbhasin@bwh.harvard.edu (S. Bhasin)
c.jayasena@imperial.ac.uk (C.N. Jayasena)

Epidemiology of Male Hypogonadism

Arthi Thirumalai, MBBS, Bradley D. Anawalt, MD*

KEYWORDS

- Androgen deficiency • Male hypogonadism • Prevalence • Incidence rate
- Epidemiology

KEY POINTS

- Of the known pathologic causes of hypogonadism, Klinefelter syndrome is the most common cause of male hypogonadism, and it is often undiagnosed (50-75% undiagnosed).
- Iatrogenic causes are the most common causes of male hypogonadism.
- Common iatrogenic causes include oncotherapy, with the most important of these being the following: androgen deprivation therapy for prostate cancer; systemic chemotherapy and radiation for testicular cancer, leukemia, and lymphoma; and radiation therapy for head and neck cancers.
- Medication-induced hyperprolactinemia, exogenous corticosteroids, and opioids might also be common causes of iatrogenic hypogonadism in certain populations.
- Classic causes of hypogonadism including pituitary nonfunctional adenomas, prolactinomas, iron overload syndromes, and Cushing syndrome are uncommon or rare.

INTRODUCTION

There are many benefits to understanding the epidemiology of male hypogonadism. The benefits include determining the merits of screening for androgen deficiency in large populations, the predictive value of diagnostic testing for male hypogonadism in specific patients, and the calculation of the potential socioeconomic cost of the disorder to the society. This information is useful to clinicians providing care for patients, researchers developing and recruiting for clinical and translations studies, biomedical research and industry leaders making decisions about financial investments in research and development, and government officials making public health decisions around the world.

In the past 3 decades, testosterone therapy prescription and use has greatly expanded in some countries, and it has become a topic of great public and

Drs A. Thirumalai and B.D. Anawalt report no commercial or financial conflicts of interest.
Drs A. Thirumalai and B.D. Anawalt receive funding from the NIH-NICHD (HHSN275000251), and Dr B.D. Anawalt is the site PI on NIH-RO1HL1343653 (Kanias, PI).
Department of Medicine, University of Washington School of Medicine, Box 356420, 1959 Northeast Pacific Avenue, Seattle, WA 98195, USA
* Corresponding author.
E-mail address: banawalt@medicine.washington.edu

government interest. There have been developments in the diagnostic tools (eg, chromatography-tandem mass spectrometry assays and methods for accurate assessment for free, unbound testosterone) and therapies (eg, transdermal and long-acting testosterone formulations) during that period. However, despite this broad fascination with a hormone that has multiple systemic effects, there is relatively little known about the global epidemiology of male hypogonadism.

The testes have 2 primary functions: production of sperm and androgens (and estrogens via aromatization of androgens). Male hypogonadism encompasses abnormal sperm production (in quantity and/or quality) and androgen deficiency. The prevalence of male infertility is generally quoted to be 10% to 15%, and most of these men have dysspermatogenesis.[1] However, a 2017 systematic review commissioned by the World Health Organization concluded that due to the very low quality of evidence, "it is not possible to determine an unbiased prevalence of male infertility within global, regional or national populations."[2] Dysspermatogenesis is consistently present in men with male hypogonadism, but most infertile men have normal Leydig cell function and normal serum testosterone concentrations. In this article, the authors focus on the epidemiology of androgen deficiency and use the terms "male hypogonadism" and "androgen deficiency" interchangeably. They use the standard epidemiologic definitions for "prevalence" and "incidence rate"; note that prevalence and incidence rate often do not correlate.

As with male infertility, there are many barriers to understanding the global epidemiology of male hypogonadism. First, there are many pathophysiological processes that lead to suppression of the hypothalamic-pituitary gonadal axis and lead to symptoms, signs, biochemical findings, and clinical outcomes that are similar to or overlap with male hypogonadism. Any severe chronic or acute systemic illness or disorder including malnutrition, infections, cancer, inflammatory diseases, sleep apnea, and uncontrolled metabolic disorders (eg, diabetes mellitus) may suppress the gonadal axis.[3] Second, aging is associated with declines in serum testosterone in men starting their fourth and fifth decades. Although testosterone therapy might be beneficial to some or even many older men with low serum testosterone concentrations and no identifiable cause of hypogonadism, age-related declines in serum androgen should not be considered a disorder or a disease and therefore should not be described as hypogonadism per se. Third, the definition of low serum total testosterone concentrations in epidemiologic studies has been fraught with problems because of the use of inaccurate total and free testosterone assays and inconsistent and nonuniform normal ranges in serum testosterone assays. Furthermore, the lower limit of the normal serum testosterone concentration has not been agreed on (even in national and international guidelines including the 2 guidelines that used systematic review and systematic analysis in their methodology) or connected to clinical outcomes.[3–5] In addition, there has been no harmonization and standardization of testosterone assays (although there has been a recent effort to do so).[6] Unlike the epidemiologic studies of diabetes mellitus that are based on serum hemoglobin A1c and glucose concentrations that have low variability between assays and laboratories in different geographic areas, there has been significant interassay variability of serum testosterone measurements in published epidemiologic studies. A fourth impediment to the accurate determination of the prevalence and incidence rate of male hypogonadism is the variability of iatrogenic causes. Drugs that cause hyperprolactinemia (eg, psychotropic drugs), exogenous corticosteroids, and opioids may cause hypogonadism, and the use of these drugs fluctuates by geographic region and over time. Furthermore, there is no clear dosage threshold for these drug-induced causes of hypogonadism, and the documentation of dose and duration is problematic. A fifth barrier to understanding the epidemiology of male hypogonadism has been the lack of large, systematic studies of the prevalence of male hypogonadism in younger and older men in large areas of Africa, Asia, and South America.

This final limitation is very important because it precludes the accurate assessment of the global and the locoregional epidemiology of male hypogonadism. For example, sickle cell disease is cited as a cause of hypogonadism in endocrinology textbooks and review articles, but it has only been reported as a cause of hypogonadism in small case series, and the prevalence of hypogonadism in sickle disease is not known.[7–9] However, 300,000 to 400,000 children are born each year with sickle cell disease, and approximately two-thirds are born in sub-Saharan Africa.[10] Immigration patterns have increased the prevalence of sickle disease in certain regions including in India, Europe, and North America. The incidence rate of sickle cell disease in men born in Africa or from ancestors from Africa is approximately 1:500 male births. Thus, sickle cell disease could be a significant, but unidentified, contributor to the incidence and prevalence of male hypogonadism in many areas of the world.

There is controversy about the diagnosis of male hypogonadism in the large number of men with nonspecific symptoms and signs of androgen deficiency, slightly low to low-normal serum testosterone concentrations who do not have an identifiable cause of dysfunction of the hypothalamus pituitary or testes. This constellation is more common in older men, men with diabetes mellitus, and men with high body mass indices. These men are not identified as hypogonadal in this review, but are included as "possible hypogonadism."

There have been several approaches to estimating the prevalence or incidence rate of male hypogonadism. Most investigators have used a definition of hypogonadism of an arbitrary threshold based on a low serum testosterone concentrations or symptoms of male hypogonadism and a low serum testosterone concentration. A second approach would be to define hypogonadism based on testosterone replacement therapy prescriptions in large population databases, but that method overestimates the prevalence of male hypogonadism (due to secular trends of androgen therapy for indications other than male hypogonadism) and underestimates the prevalence of bona fide hypogonadism (due to underrecognition of causes such as Klinefelter syndrome; see the discussion in the section on Congenital and genetic causes of primary hypogonadism). In a third approach, the authors also attempt in this review to estimate the prevalence and incidence rate of male hypogonadism based on the epidemiology of known causes of primary and secondary causes.

EPIDEMIOLOGY OF MALE HYPOGONADISM BASED ON LOW SERUM TESTOSTERONE CONCENTRATIONS

Early epidemiologic studies focused on middle-aged and older men and defined male hypogonadism based on low serum testosterone concentrations without or with symptoms and signs of androgen deficiency (**Table 1**). The Baltimore Aging Longitudinal Study demonstrated a prevalence of low serum total testosterone concentrations of ~10% in men aged 50 to 59 years, 20% in men aged 60 to 69 years, and 70% in men aged 70 to 80 years.[11] Other studies of American, European, and Asian men (Framingham, European Male Aging Study [EMAS], and Osteoporotic Fractures in Men) have confirmed age-related decreases in serum total testosterone concentrations with a prevalence of low serum total testosterone in ~10% in men with a mean age of 40 years and ~24% and 40% in men with mean ages of ~60 and 73 years, respectively.[12–14] A more recent (2015) large study of Australia confirmed the age-related decline in serum testosterone.[15]

Table 1		
Epidemiology of causes of possible male hypogonadism		
Causes of Possible Hypogonadism[a]	**Comments**	**Prevalence of hypogonadism due to this possible cause**
Aging	Additional research must be done to determine if this is a cause of androgen deficiency and if the benefit of androgen replacement therapy exceeds the risk.	Unknown– 2%–8%? References:[13,15–18]
Obesity	Mean BMI has continually increased in countries and regions that have adopted diets with more processed foods and more sedentary lifestyles. The possible association of obesity and male hypogonadism has been inadequately studied. No definitive comments can be made about the possible prevalence of male hypogonadism due to obesity.	Unknown
Diabetes mellitus	The incidence and prevalence of diabetes mellitus has increased in parallel to global obesity. As with obesity, no definitive comments can be made about the possible prevalence of male hypogonadism due to obesity.	Unknown

Abbreviation: BMI, body mass index.
[a] Possible hypogonadism indicates a disorder associated with low serum testosterone concentrations without clear evidence that there is evidence of end-organ androgen deficiency.

The prevalence of hypogonadism is much lower in older men when low serum testosterone concentrations are coupled with symptoms that suggest hypogonadism. For example, the EMAS study of more than 3000 men aged 40 to 79 years demonstrated an overall prevalence of 2.1% when using a combination of 3 sexual symptoms (erectile and decreased frequency of morning erections and sexual thoughts) and a low total testosterone concentration.[13] There was an age-related increase in male hypogonadism (0.1% for 40–49 years, 0.6% for 50–59 years, 3.2% for 60–69 years, and 5.1% for 70–79 years). Similarly, 2 smaller cohort studies in Massachusetts (United States) demonstrated a baseline prevalence of hypogonadism of ~6% in men aged 30 to 79 years and 40 to 69 years, respectively, based on a definition of hypogonadism that included a low serum testosterone and symptoms or signs of hypogonadism. In these studies, the prevalence increased with age.[16,17] Finally, a 2021 cohort study of more than 6000 Chinese men aged 40 to 79 years (mean age 57 years) demonstrated similar findings with an ~8% prevalence of hypogonadism based on a low serum testosterone concentration and sexual symptoms that suggest androgen deficiency.[18]

There are important limitations to the aforementioned epidemiologic studies. Men with known causes of hypogonadism were excluded. Thus, these epidemiologic studies form the basis for the estimation of "possible hypogonadism" due to the effects of aging (with attendant obesity and comorbidities). The studies used different testosterone assays and different (and somewhat arbitrary) thresholds to define a low serum testosterone concentration. Furthermore, no men who were 18 to 30 years old and few men younger than 40 years were included in these studies.

EPIDEMIOLOGY OF MALE HYPOGONADISM BASED ON THE EPIDEMIOLOGY OF SPECIFIC CAUSES

The epidemiology of androgen deficiency might also be estimated based on the prevalence and incidence rate of known causes of primary and secondary male hypogonadism (**Table 2**). This estimation is confounded by the variation in the expression

Table 2
Incidence rate and prevalence of known causes of male hypogonadism

	Incidence Rate of the Disorder	Prevalence of Androgen Deficiency[b]
Congenital and genetic causes of primary hypogonadism		
Klinefelter syndrome	9–22;10,000 births	> 5:10,000 Possibly 0.2%–0.3% prevalence in men
Congenital bilateral anorchia	0.5:10,000 births	Rare[a]
Down syndrome (trisomy 21)	10–30:10,000 births	Unknown
Noonan syndrome	4–10:10,000 births	Rare
Myotonic dystrophy	1–4:10,000 births	Rare
Autoimmune polyglandular syndromes	<5:100,000 births	Rare
46 XY disorders of sexual development with male genitalia	<1:10,000 births	Rare
Wolfram syndrome	<1:10,000 births	Rare
Ataxia-telangiectasia	<1:10,000 births	Rare
Prader Willi syndrome	<1:10,000 births	Rare
Noniatrogenic acquired causes of primary hypogonadism		
Bilateral testicular trauma	<<1:10,000 patient-years	Likely rare
Testicular torsion	<<1:10,000 patient-years	Rare
Bilateral orchidectomy (for causes other than testicular cancer)	Likely < 1:10,000 patient-years	Likely rare
Infectious orchitis	Likely < 1:10,000 patient-years	Likely rare
Congenital and genetic causes of secondary hypogonadism		
Kallmann syndrome/ congenital hypogonadotropic hypogonadism	1:4000–1:30,000 male births	Likely rare
Holoprosencephalopathy	1:10,000 births	Likely rare
Septo-optic dysplasia	1:10,000 births	Likely rare
Congenital hypopituitarism	1–3:10,000 births	Likely rare
Congenital hypogonadotropic hypogonadism with adrenal hypoplasia	<1:10,000 births	Likely rare
CHARGE syndrome	<1:10,000 births	Likely rare
Bardet-Biedl syndrome	<1:10,000 births	Likely rare

(continued on next page)

Table 2
(continued)

	Incidence Rate of the Disorder	Prevalence of Androgen Deficiency[b]
Selective defects in synthesis of luteinizing hormone	<1:10,000 births	Likely rare
Noniatrogenic acquired causes of secondary hypogonadism		
Non–prolactin-producing macroadenoma	< 1:10,000 patient-years	Rare
Traumatic brain injury	40:10,000 patient-years	Unknown Possibly > 5:10,000
Subarachnoid hemorrhage	0.6–1:10,000 patient-years	Likely rare
Pituitary apoplexy	<1:10,000 patient-years	Rare
Primary empty sella syndrome	Unknown; much higher in women	Likely rare
Iron overload syndromes	Rare; see text	Rare; see text
Endogenous Cushing syndrome	<1:1,000,000 male patient-years	Rare
Iatrogenic causes of hypogonadism		
Prostate cancer treatment	See text	Up to 2%–3% interval prevalence for men 55–70 years old
Testicular cancer treatment	See text	Up to 0.06% lifetime prevalence in men
Systemic chemotherapy	See text	Likely rare
Radiation therapy of pelvic area for nontesticular cancers	Rare	Likely rare
Radiation therapy of benign brain tumor		
Pituitary adenoma	<1:10,000 patient-years	Rare
Benign nonpituitary brain tumor	1:10,000 patient-years	Rare
Radiation therapy of malignant brain tumor	Unknown	Unknown
Radiation therapy of brain metastasis	10–30:10,000 patient-years	Unknown
Total body irradiation for bone marrow transplantation	Rare	Rare
Radiation therapy for head and neck cancer	Unknown	Unknown
Iatrogenic Cushing syndrome	Unknown	Unknown
(Iatrogenic) opioid abuse	Unknown	Unknown
Iatrogenic medication-induced hyperprolactinemia	Unknown	Unknown

[a] A prevalence less than 5:10,000 is considered rare.[19]
[b] Prevalence = percentage of men in general population with hypogonadism due to this cause.

of androgen deficiency with known causes of male hypogonadism, the implausibility of including all causes of primary and secondary hypogonadism, the imperfect knowledge of the epidemiology of these causes, and the secular and geographic variation in acquired causes of primary hypogonadism and secondary hypogonadism. Acquired causes of primary hypogonadism and secondary hypogonadism vary across regions and over time due to a broad range of factors such as genetic clustering, differences in environmental exposure (eg, infections), and differences in use of therapeutic drugs or drugs of abuse. Nonetheless, this approach is a useful exercise to describe the epidemiology of male hypogonadism due to known pathologic causes.

In this section, a prevalence of 5:10,000 is considered a rare disease (the United States definition is closer to 8–9:10,000), and incidence rate of less than 1:10,000 per live birth or patient-years is considered low frequency.[19] The prevalence of androgen deficiency will be estimated when possible. The authors err on the side of overestimation of hypogonadism to highlight that most of the causes of male hypogonadism affect a very small percentage of the overall male population. Their estimations are often crude and imprecise, but they provide a reasonable assessment of the overall prevalence of male hypogonadism.

Congenital and Genetic Causes of Primary Hypogonadism

Primary hypogonadism with low serum testosterone concentrations and high serum gonadotropins is generally accepted as incontrovertible evidence of androgen deficiency. By far, the most common cause is Klinefelter syndrome. The incidence rate of Klinefelter syndrome is ~9 to 22:10,000 male births (0.09%–0.22%) and only 25% to 50% are diagnosed during their lifetimes.[20–24] The prevalence of Klinefelter syndrome is likely to be slightly lower in older men because the average longevity of men with Klinefelter syndrome seems to be reduced by 5 to 6 years; the prevalence is still likely to exceed 5:10,000 overall.[23,24] Although it is generally assumed that virtually all men with Klinefelter syndrome will eventually develop androgen deficiency, this assumption has not been proved.

In addition to Klinefelter syndrome, there are several structural and genetic causes of congenital primary hypogonadism. Men with congenital bilateral anorchia have severe androgen deficiency. This condition is found in only 0.5:10,000 male births, and the cause is unknown.[25] There are several genetic syndromes that occasionally present with androgen deficiency. Down syndrome (trisomy 21) affects 10 to 30:10,000 births (1214 in the United States because of 50% elective abortion rate), and the prevalence in the United States and Europe is ~6-14:10,000.[26,27] Most men with Down syndrome have hypospermatogenesis, and many have elevated serum follicle-stimulating hormone (FSH) and luteinizing hormone (LH) concentrations, but the majority of adolescent boys and men with Down syndrome have normal serum testosterone concentrations and go through puberty normally.[28–32] The incidence rate and prevalence of androgen deficiency in this supernumerary chromosomal syndrome is not known, but it is likely much rarer in older men because the life expectancy is shorter by 10-15 years compared with men without Down syndrome.[32] Men with Noonan syndrome and myotonic dystrophy commonly have isolated defects in spermatogenesis and have normal serum testosterone concentrations. For example, Noonan syndrome is found in 4:10,000 to 10:10,000 births, but men with Noonan syndrome commonly have cryptorchidism but typically have normal serum testosterone concentrations after puberty.[33–36] Myotonic dystrophy occurs in ~1:10,000-1.4:10,000 male births of European ancestry but even less common in other populations with different gene pools.[37–39] About 80% of men with myotonic dystrophy have spermatogenic defects, but only ~20% to 40% have low testosterone concentrations.[38,39] Autoimmune polyglandular syndrome type 1 and type 2 are rare (<5:100,000 births) and may cause primary hypogonadism in women, but seldom in men.[40–42] Men with 46, XY disorders of sexual development (DSD) due to partial androgen insensitivity syndrome or gonadal dysgenesis (eg, congenital abnormalities in androgen production) may rarely present with incomplete or small male genitalia and primary hypogonadism. There are no comprehensive epidemiologic studies for these rare clinical syndromes, but the prevalence and incidence rate of men with male genitalia and primary hypogonadism due to any 46, XY DSD seems to be much lower than 1:10,000.[43] Finally, there are many complex genetic syndromes that are associated multiple congenital anomalies and disorders that may include primary hypogonadism as a manifestation. These disorders include Wolfram syndrome, ataxia-telangiectasia (with gonadal dysfunction more common in women), Prader-Willi syndrome (that is associated with mixed primary and secondary hypogonadism), and other very rare disorders.[44–46] The incidence rate of these complex genetic syndromes is 0.25:10,000 to less than 0.1:10,000 births worldwide, and many of the patients with these syndromes are infertile but may not have primary hypogonadism. Overall, only Klinefelter syndrome is a common cause of congenital primary hypogonadism, but Down syndrome might be a more common cause of male hypogonadism than recognized (**Box 1**).

Noniatrogenic Acquired Causes of Primary Hypogonadism

Noniatrogenic acquired causes of primary hypogonadism with androgen deficiency include severe bilateral testicular trauma, testicular torsion, bilateral orchidectomy, and infectious orchitis. The epidemiology of acquired primary hypogonadism varies significantly due to secular trends, temporal changes in medical therapies, and differences related to geography, cultural mores, and other factors.

Hypogonadism due to severe bilateral testicular trauma (blunt or penetrating) is rare.[47,48] In a national database analysis, only ~8000 of 3.5 million men who had trauma requiring evaluation at a US trauma center had scrotal or testicular trauma between 2007 and 2016.[49] Of these, ~45% had blunt trauma, and ~55% had penetrating trauma. Only 1% to 2% of men with blunt testicular trauma and ~30% of men with penetrating testicular trauma have bilateral testicular trauma that might result in sufficient loss of Leydig cells to cause androgen deficiency. Thus, the incidence rate of androgen deficiency of severe bilateral testicular trauma is less than 1:10,000 patient-years, and the lifetime prevalence of androgen deficiency due to testicular trauma can be inferred to be less than 5:10,000. Hypogonadism due to testicular torsion is even rarer. Testicular torsion typically occurs in men younger than 25 years, and the annual incidence rate is 4:100,000 with an estimated lifetime prevalence of 3 to 7:10,000 by age 25 years.[50,51] Unilateral orchidectomy may be required in 25% to 45%.[50,51] Although decreased spermatogenesis may occur as a

---

Box 1
Klinefelter syndrome is the only common cause of congenital primary hypogonadism

Of the known congenital causes of primary hypogonadism, Klinefelter syndrome is the only common cause of hypogonadism with an incidence rate of 9-22:10,000 men. The prevalence of Klinefelter syndrome in adult men is not known, but it is likely greater than 5:10,000. All other congenital causes of hypogonadism seem to be rare, but none of these congenital causes have accurate assessments of prevalence of hypogonadism. Karyotyping for Klinefelter syndrome should be considered in a man who presents with primary hypogonadism. Perinatal screening for Klinefelter might be considered too.

long-term consequence, androgen deficiency seldom, if ever, occurs as a result of testicular torsion or its treatment.[52]

Mumps orchitis commonly causes dysspermatogenesis, particularly when there is postpubertal infection.[53,54] Androgen deficiency due to Leydig cell dysfunction only occurs with severe bilateral orchitis in postpubertal men. Mumps causes bilateral orchitis in ~30% of postpubertal adolescents and men, and few cases are severe. The mumps vaccine effectively prevents bilateral mumps orchitis. Thus, despite a recent increase in mumps infections in regions of the world where there are barriers to vaccination, mumps orchitis is now a very rare cause of primary hypogonadism with androgen deficiency. Other, even rarer, infectious causes of androgen deficiency due to orchitis include toxoplasma gondii, mycobacteria, brucella, echovirus, (undertreated) human immunodeficiency virus, and arbovirus infections.

Overall, the noniatrogenic causes of acquired primary hypogonadism seem to be very uncommon (**Box 2**).

Congenital and genetic causes of secondary hypogonadism
There are various uncommon congenital/genetic causes of secondary hypogonadism. These include congenital developmental disorders that are variably associated with hypogonadotropic hypogonadism such as holoprosencephaly and septo-optic dysplasia that both have incidence rates of 1:10,000 births and Kallmann syndrome.[55,56] There is a genetic overlap between holoprosencephaly and Kallmann syndrome that has a quoted incidence rate of approximately 1:10,000 male births (1:4000–1:30,000).[55,57–59] Congenital hypopituitarism with multiple pituitary deficiencies (including gonadotropin deficiency) occurs in 1.25:10,000 to 2.5:10.000 births.[55] There are very rare causes (<1;10,000 births) of congenital/genetic hypogonadotropic hypogonadism including congenital hypogonadotropic hypogonadism with adrenal hypoplasia, CHARGE syndrome (that may overlap genetically with Kallmann syndrome), Bardet-Biedl syndrome (a ciliopathy that also overlaps with Kallmann syndrome), and selective defects in synthesis of luteinizing hormone.[60–65]

Acknowledging that some of these syndromes might overlap, the overall incidence rate of congenital causes of secondary hypogonadism is quite low, but the prevalence of these syndromes is unknown (**Box 3**).

Non-iatrogenic acquired causes of secondary hypogonadism
Acquired causes of secondary hypogonadism include macroadenomas and other pituitary masses, traumatic brain injury (TBI), intracranial hemorrhage, empty sella syndrome, hyperprolactinemia, iron overload syndromes, and endogenous Cushing syndrome.

Pituitary Macroadenomas and Sellar Masses and Empty Sella Syndrome
The overall incidence rate of pituitary adenomas is ~0.3-0.7:10,000 patient-years, but the prevalence is ~8-12:10,000.[66–69] About 40%-60% of these adenomas are macroadenomas with a higher percentage of macroadenomas reported in men; the remainder are mostly small pituitary microadenomas that do not cause secondary

---

Box 2
Noniatrogenic causes of acquired primary hypogonadism are rare

The prevalence of noniatrogenic causes of acquired primary hypogonadism is not well described, but causes such as traumatic testicular injury and infectious orchitis seem to be rare (lifetime prevalence likely ≤ 5:10,000) and does not significantly affect the overall incidence rate and prevalence of hypogonadism.

Box 3
Congenital causes of secondary hypogonadism are rare but should be considered in infants with micropenis or boys with failure to go through puberty

The incidence rate of congenital causes of secondary hypogonadism is very low. The prevalence rate of these congenital causes is unknown, but they collectively are rare (<5:10,000 men). Congenital causes of hypogonadotropic hypogonadism should be considered in infant boys with micropenis or boys who fail to go through puberty and have low serum testosterone and gonadotropins. Boys and young men with secondary hypogonadism with extragonadal symptoms or signs such as impairment of hearing or sense of smell, coloboma, polydactyly, or cerebellar findings (eg, synkinesis) suggest rare genetic syndromes associated with congenital secondary hypogonadism.

---

hypogonadism. About 50% of the macroadenomas are prolactinomas, and most of the remainder are nonfunctional (gonadotrope or corticotrope) macroadenomas. (The macroprolactinomas are also discussed in the *Hyperprolactinemia* section.) Of the men with nonfunctional macroadenomas, 25%-50% will present with hypogonadism.[70–73] Based on limited data, large sellar masses (eg, large Rathke cysts) other than pituitary macroadenomas are rare (prevalence likely <1:10,000 people), but they seem to have similar associations with secondary hypogonadism (10%–60%).[73,74] Thus, the prevalence of hypogonadism due to non–prolactin-producing macroadenomas and other benign sellar masses is very low (rare; ~1–1.5:10,000 men; **Box 4**).

Traumatic Brain Injury, Subarachnoid Hemorrhage, and Pituitary Apoplexy

The incidence rate of TBI is approximately 40:10,000 patient-years in men, and it is more common in younger men.[75] There is some modest geographic variation in the incidence rates. Most (80%–90%) of the TBIs worldwide are classified as mild (ie, a brain injury leading to a concussion with transient loss of consciousness without focal neurologic deficits or injury on brain imaging).[75] Although chronic pituitary dysfunction including secondary hypogonadism (28%–32%, with some reports as high as 55%–70% with more severe trauma) has been reported after moderate-to-severe TBI, mild TBI is associated with much lower rates (<10%), with growth hormone deficiency being the most common deficit.[76–79] Minor TBI commonly causes a biochemical pattern consistent with secondary hypogonadism early after the traumatic event, but the hypothalamus-pituitary-testicular axis typically returns to normal within 1 year of mild TBI.[80] Based on these data, the incidence rate of hypogonadism due to all TBI might be 6.0 to 8.2:10,000 patient-years (**Box 5**). This estimated incidence rate is probably too high.[76,77,79]

Subarachnoid hemorrhage is associated with similar rates of panhypopituitarism (25%–35%), but only ~5%–20% patients with incident subarachnoid hemorrhage have secondary hypogonadism after 6 months to 5 years of follow-up.[81,82] The annual

---

Box 4
The estimated prevalence of hypogonadism due to nonfunctional macroadenomas and benign sellar masses is low

Calculation: the estimated prevalence of male hypogonadism due to pituitary nonfunctional macroadenomas and benign (non-adenoma) sellar masses is the prevalence of adenomas (8-12:10,000) plus benign (non-adenoma) sellar masses (<1:10,000) in men times the percentage of adenomas in men that are macroadenomas (50%) times the percentage that are nonfunctional (50%) times the percentage of male patients with nonfunctional macroadenomas who have secondary hypogonadism (50%) equals 1-2 :10,000 men.

> **Box 5**
> **Hypogonadism due to traumatic brain injury is potentially common**
>
> Calculation: the incidence rate of secondary hypogonadism due to mild traumatic brain injury (TBI) is the incidence rate of TBI in men (40:10,000 patient-years) times the percentage that is mild TBI (80%–90%) times the percentage of hypogonadism due to mild TBI (10%) plus the incidence rate of TBI in men (40:10,000 patient-years) times the percentage that is moderate to severe TBI (10%–20%) times the incidence rate of hypogonadism due to moderate-to-severe TBI (70%) equals 6.0 to 8.2:10,000 patient-years. This estimate is probably too high.

incidence rate of subarachnoid hemorrhage is only 0.6 to 1:10,000 patient-years and has a high mortality (~35% mortality at a median of 4 years); the prevalence of secondary hypogonadism due to subarachnoid hemorrhage is likely to be very low.[82–84] Pituitary apoplexy has a similarly very low incidence rate (0.2:10,000 patient-years) and lifetime prevalence (~0.6:10,000 people).[85,86] Despite a reported association with secondary hypogonadism in up to 70% of men, pituitary apoplexy—similar to subarachnoid hemorrhage—is a rare cause of acquired secondary hypogonadism.[85–87]

A primary empty sella is a highly prevalent anatomic finding (2%–20%) in autopsy and radiology series. The clinical incidence rate and prevalence of primary empty sella syndrome (characterized by the anatomic finding plus headaches and/or pituitary hormone deficiency) seems to be much lower, and it is much more common in women than men (4–6:1).[88–90] The prevalence of hypogonadism has been reported to be 10% to 55% in patients with primary empty sella syndrome. The overall prevalence of some form of hypopituitarism due to primary empty sella syndrome has been estimated to be approximately 5:10,000 people, but it is likely lower in men.[90] There could be a significant underestimation of empty sella syndrome due to underdetection, but the best (albeit weak) evidence indicates that empty sella syndrome is probably found primarily in women and is a rare cause of secondary male hypogonadism.[90]

Iron Overload Syndromes: Hereditary Hemochromatosis and Blood Dyscrasias

Iron deposition due to any iron overload syndrome may cause secondary hypogonadism. The most well-known iron overload syndrome is hereditary hemochromatosis, but any disorder that is associated with chronic and frequent blood transfusions might result in an iron overload syndrome.

The incidence rate of homozygosity for hereditary hemochromatosis is common (up to 25:10,000–50:10,000 births) with significant variation among populations, but the penetrance of this disorder is much lower.[91–93] In one long-term Irish retrospective study over 20 years, only 6% (9/141) developed secondary hypogonadism.[91] Hypogonadism due to overload has been reported in men with beta thalassemia major and other congenital anemias who receive frequent transfusions.[94,95] However, this complication of iron overload occurs in only uncommon, severe blood dyscrasias and is fully preventable (and treatable with iron chelation therapy). Overall, iron overload syndromes are associated with a low incidence rate of secondary hypogonadism that is preventable, and these syndromes likely do not contribute significantly to the overall lifetime prevalence of hypogonadism.

Hyperprolactinemia

A 2017 Scottish study demonstrated that the prevalence of hyperprolactinemia in men increased from 0.6:10,000 in 1993 to 9.4:10,000 in 2012.[96] This study defined hyperprolactinemia as greater than 1000mU/L (> ~50 ng/mL), a threshold that is often used clinically to trigger further evaluation. The increased prevalence of hyperprolactinemia was attributable primarily to the increased prescription of antipsychotics and antidepressants that increase serum prolactin concentrations. The most common cause was medication-induced hyperprolactinemia that accounted for almost 50% of the cases followed by pituitary causes (eg, adenomas) that accounted for ~25% of the cases. (Hypogonadism due to drug-induced hyperprolactinemia is discussed in the *Iatrogenic causes* section.). The incidence rate of pituitary causes of hyperprolactinemia remained ~0.1-0.2:10,000 patient-years for men over the 20-year period except a slight increase to 0.26:10,000 patient-years in the last 5-year interval that the investigators attributed to increased testing. In this study, 45% of pituitary causes of hyperprolactinemia in men were due to a macroadenoma, and case series of prolactinomas generally report that 50%-75% of men with prolactin-producing adenomas have macroadenomas. About 75%-90% men are hypogonadal at the time of presentation with a macroprolactinoma, a rate that is higher than nonfunctional gonadotrope or corticotrope adenomas.[97–99] About 35% to 40% will remain hypogonadal after surgery and ~30% to 50% after medical therapy.[97–99]

Based on the 2017 Scottish study, the prevalence on male hypogonadism due to noniatrogenic hyperprolactinemia (ie, all causes of hyperprolactinemia minus drug-induced hyperprolactinemia) is likely low enough to qualify as a "rare disease" (<5:10,000 men; **Box 6**).

Cushing syndrome due to endogenous causes

It has been well known for decades that corticosteroids suppress pituitary secretion of LH and FSH and may cause secondary hypogonadism in men.[100] However, there seems to be variation between individuals, as not all men with endogenous Cushing syndrome have secondary hypogonadism.[100,101] Remarkably little is published about the effects of endogenous Cushing syndrome (ie, the degree of hypercortisolism) on the gonadal axis or the dose-response of exogenous corticosteroids on the male gonadal axis.[98,99] This lack of knowledge is in part due to epidemiology of this syndrome. The incidence rate is only 0.7-2.4:1,000,000 patient-years (0.0024:10,000 patient-years), and it is much more common in women than men.[102–104] Because it has a very low incidence rate in men and it is associated reduced longevity, endogenous Cushing syndrome is likely to be a very rare cause of male hypogonadism.[105,106]

SUMMARY OF THE CONGENITAL SECONDARY AND NONIATROGENIC ACQUIRED SECONDARY CAUSES OF HYPOGONADISM

Of the known congenital and noniatrogenic acquired causes of secondary hypogonadism, TBI is likely the most common cause (estimated incidence rate 6.0–8.2:10,000 patient-years). Congenital causes and noniatrogenic acquired secondary causes of hypogonadism other than trauma are likely to be rare (**Box 7**). Important gaps in

---

Box 6
The prevalence of hypogonadism due to noniatrogenic hyperprolactinemia is low

Calculation: according to a 2017 Scottish study,[93] the prevalence of male hypogonadism due to noniatrogenic hyperprolactinemia is the overall male prevalence of hyperprolactinemia (9.4:10,000 in 2012) minus the portion attributed to medications and macroprolactin (~50% or 4.7:10,000) times the percentage of men who developed hyperprolactinemia-induced secondary hypogonadism. Assuming that 100% of all men with hyperprolactinemia not due to medications become hypogonadal (clearly an assumption that is too high; see text), the male prevalence of hypogonadism due to noniatrogenic hyperprolactinemia is still rare (<5:10,000).

> **Box 7**
> **Moderate-to-severe traumatic brain injury is the most common noniatrogenic causes of secondary hypogonadism**
>
> The most common noniatrogenic cause of secondary hypogonadism is likely to be moderate-to-severe traumatic brain injury; mild traumatic brain injury infrequently causes hypogonadism that persists beyond 1 year. Congenital secondary causes are rare although there are no high-quality data on prevalence. Classic causes of noniatrogenic acquired causes of hypogonadism such as nonfunctional macroadenomas, prolactinomas, iron overload syndromes, and endogenous Cushing syndrome are also rare.

knowledge include the lack of high-quality studies on the incidence rate and prevalence of persistent androgen deficiency in men with TBI, primary empty sella syndrome, and who are taking drugs that raise serum prolactin concentrations, chronic corticosteroids, or opioids.

Iatrogenic Causes of Male Hypogonadism

Treatment of prostate cancer

Androgen deprivation therapy is commonly prescribed for men with prostate cancer. Androgen deprivation therapy may cause primary hypogonadism (eg, surgical castration or medical therapy that inhibits androgen synthesis such as abiraterone), secondary hypogonadism (eg, suppression of gonadotropin secretion by a gonadotropin-releasing hormone analogue), or decreased androgen effect (eg, an androgen receptor blockade with enzalutamide).

Prostate cancer is the second most commonly diagnosed cancer in men worldwide.[107,108] In 2020, the cumulative risk of prostate cancer between birth and age 75 years was 3.86%, and the cumulative risk of death by age 75 years was 0.63%.[108] There are 3 categories of men with prostate cancer who might benefit from androgen deprivation therapy. First, men with intermediate- or high-risk prostate cancer treated with radiation therapy benefit with adjuvant androgen therapy (for 4–36 months depending on the perceived risk of recurrent disease).[109–112] Second, men with high-risk prostate cancer treated with radical prostatectomy might benefit from neoadjuvant and/or adjuvant androgen therapy; there is no consensus on the recommended duration of androgen deprivation therapy for this group of men.[109–112] Third, men with metastatic or recurrent prostate cancer after primary therapy are considered candidates for life-long androgen deprivation therapy.[109,112] Thus, androgen deprivation therapy for prostate cancer represents a major potential cause of hypogonadism.

Although there are no data on the incidence rate and prevalence of this potential cause of hypogonadism, we can estimate a range of the upper limit of the potential use of androgen deprivation therapy for prostate cancer based on current evidence. The authors use the data obtained from the core age group of the ERSCP study, the best long-term study of active prostate cancer screening.[113–116] The core-age group of this multisite study consisted of more than 240,000 European men aged 55 to 69 years who were randomized to no study intervention or active prostate cancer screening with serum prostate–specific antigen measurement at regular intervals. After up to 16 years of follow-up, 13.3% of the men who were enrolled in the active screening group were diagnosed with prostate cancer. In the control group, 10.3% of men were diagnosed with prostate cancer during the same time of follow-up. In the active screen group, 79% of the men who were diagnosed with prostate cancer had low-risk or intermediate-risk prostate cancer (low risk = stage $\leq$T2a, PSA $\leq$10 ng/mL, and Gleason score $\leq$6; intermediate-risk = stage T2b, a Gleason score of 7, or a PSA level of $\geq$10 and $\leq$20 ng/mL) and 21% had high-risk prostate cancer. Current evidence and guidelines support the use of long-term androgen deprivation therapy only for patients with high-risk prostate cancer.[109,111,112] Thus, in men (aged 55–69 years) who are offered prostate-cancer screening at regular intervals for up to 16 years, there is approximately a 2.8% screening-interval incidence rate of androgen deprivation therapy for aggressive prostate cancer. Assuming that prostate cancer screening was widely offered to men between ages 55 and 69 years, uniformly accepted, and performed, the lifetime prevalence of hypogonadism due to androgen deprivation therapy could be as high as 2% to 3% in men between ages 55 and 70 years (**Box 8**).

Treatment of testicular cancer
Global data indicate that the risk of development of testicular cancer is 0.14% between birth and 79 years.[108] Testicular cancer can be treated with orchidectomy, but only 0.5% to 1.0% of testicular cancers include both testes.[117] Testicular cancer is often treated with alkylating chemotherapy. Patients with testicular cancer are often treated with chemotherapy (for nonseminomas) or irradiation (for seminomas), and these therapies may result in androgen deficiency. The definition of androgen deficiency (and therefore prevalence) varies greatly in the studies of long-term of survivors, but a prevalence of 20% to 40% seems to be a reasonable estimation of the upper limit of androgen deficiency due to chemotherapy and/or radiation therapy for testicular cancer.[118–125] Thus, the upper limit of the lifetime prevalence of androgen deficiency due to treatment of testicular cancer is 6:10,000 (**Box 9**).

Systemic chemotherapy for nonprostatic and nontesticular cancers
Long-term survivors of cancer treated with systemic chemotherapy may develop androgen deficiency due to primary, secondary hypogonadism, or combined primary and secondary hypogonadism. Pelvic and cranial irradiation may cause androgen deficiency due to primary and secondary hypogonadism, respectively.

Systemic chemotherapy (particularly alkylating agents) commonly causes damage to germ cells and dysspermatogenesis, but few long-term male survivors of nonprostatic, nontesticular cancer develop primary or secondary hypogonadism with androgen deficiency due to systemic chemotherapy. About 10% to 11% of all male childhood survivors develop secondary hypogonadism with androgen deficiency.[126–131] However, male survivors of childhood (or early adulthood) cancer treated with systemic chemotherapy and radiation for lymphoma or leukemia develop androgen deficiency of 10% to 25%; radiation therapy (of the testes or brain) seems to be more important than systemic chemotherapy for the development of androgen deficiency.[127,130,131] Although the scope and prevalence of secondary hypogonadism (and other pituitary dysfunction) in long-term survivors of childhood and early

---

Box 8
The potential lifetime prevalence of hypogonadism due to treatment of prostate cancer is high

Calculation: the lifetime prevalence or risk of hypogonadism due to androgen deprivation therapy in men aged 55 to 69 years who are undergoing prostate cancer screening at regular intervals is the ERSCP screening interval incidence rate of prostate cancer (13.3%) times the percentage of men with high risk prostate cancer in the ERSCP (21%) equals a lifetime prevalence of 2.8% for men between ages 55 and 70 years.[110] Age 70 years was chosen because a man diagnosed with prostate cancer at age 69 years might not receive androgen deprivation therapy until at least age 70 years.

> **Box 9**
> **Treatment of testicular cancer is a common cause of male hypogonadism**
>
> Calculation: the lifetime prevalence of androgen deficiency in men due to treatment of testicular cancer is the lifetime prevalence of testicular cancer (0.14%) times the incidence of therapeutic bilateral orchidectomy (1%) plus lifetime prevalence (0.14%) times incidence of chemotherapy- or radiation-induced hypogonadism (40%) equals 0.06% (6:10,000) lifetime prevalence.

adulthood cancers is unknown, it is likely that the prevalence will significantly increase as the treatments of these relatively rare childhood and early adult cancers (<1% of all new cancers annually) continue to improve, and survival and longevity increases.[131]

Androgen deficiency due to radiation therapy for benign and malignant tumors
Radiation therapy that directly or indirectly (by scatter) affects the testicles, pituitary, or hypothalamus may cause hypogonadism. The testes are generally shielded during pelvic radiation for treatment of nontesticular cancer. Although there are reports of androgen deficiency after pelvic radiation for rectal cancer, this adverse effect is rare.[132,133] However, brain tumors or head and neck cancers are commonly treated with external radiation that might cause damage to hypothalamic or pituitary dysfunction and lead to secondary hypogonadism. The frequency of radiation therapy for treatment of brain tumors is not known, but we shall attempt to estimate the range of secondary hypogonadism due to this treatment modality for intracranial neoplasms.

Androgen deficiency due to radiation therapy for benign brain tumors
The overall global lifetime prevalence of patients with primary benign brain tumors is unknown.[134] The prevalence of all benign tumors (pituitary plus nonpituitary tumors) is not known, but the prevalence of patients with benign pituitary tumors (eg, pituitary adenomas) is approximately 8 to 12:10,000 people.[69,73,134–136] About 50% of pituitary adenomas are macroadenomas.[66–69] Women are modestly more likely (~5:4) to be diagnosed with pituitary adenomas, but men are about modestly more likely to present with pituitary macroadenomas.[66] For the estimation, the authors use a male prevalence of pituitary adenomas 12:10,000 and macroadenomas 6:10,000, respectively. (Microadenomas are not typically radiated.) The incidence rate of benign pituitary tumors (eg, adenomas) is 0.4:10,000 patient-years, and the incidence rate for benign nonpituitary tumors is 1.3:10,000 patient-years.[66,134–136] Because patients with benign pituitary tumors have a generally excellent prognosis that is at least comparable to other benign brain tumors (eg, meningioma), it is conservative to assume a similar prevalence to incidence ratio (30–1) for all benign nonpituitary brain tumors. (The authors acknowledge the crudeness of this assumption and estimation.) Using this assumption, the prevalence of benign nonpituitary brain tumors would be ~39:10,000 men (assuming equal prevalence between men and women).

Many of the benign extrapituitary tumors and most of the benign pituitary tumors will not be treated with external beam radiation. For example, a 2021 study of a US national database indicated that external beam radiation therapy was used in only 3% of benign pituitary adenomas in 2014 (down from 8% in 2004).[137] The incidence of secondary hypogonadism is radiation dose–dependent and increases for years after sellar radiation of pituitary tumors. In studies that include at least 5-year follow-up data of patients with pituitary macroadenomas treated with cranial radiation, the percentage of men with androgen deficiency due to secondary hypogonadism ranged from ~5% -25% of men.[138–144] Assuming that 5% of patients with benign pituitary tumors are treated with cranial radiation and 25% of patients will have developed permanent gonadotrope dysfunction 5 years after sellar radiation, the lifetime prevalence of secondary hypogonadism due to radiation of benign pituitary tumors is less than or equal to 1:10,000 men (**Box 10**).

Similarly, a minority of benign nonpituitary primary brain tumors are treated with cranial radiation therapy. For example, meningiomas constitute greater than 70% of all benign nonpituitary brain tumors, and intracranial radiation is used as primary or adjunctive therapy in less than 10% of these tumors.[134,135,145] Up to 35% of patients with meningiomas (or other benign primary brain tumors) may develop hypogonadism after high dosages of radiation therapy (>30 cGy), but these high dosages are used primarily in the minority of tumors that are incompletely resected or recur after surgery.[146–149] Vestibular schwannomas, the second most common benign nonpituitary tumors, account for ∼10%-12% of the benign nonpituitary brain tumors.[134,135] Schwannomas are often treated with radiation therapy, but the dosage is typically less than 20 cGy, a dosage that is not likely to cause pituitary dysfunction.[150–152] Assuming that 10% of patients with benign nonpituitary tumors (mostly meningiomas) are treated with high dosages (>30 cGy) and that 35% of these patients develop secondary hypogonadism with long-term follow-up, the life-time prevalence of secondary male hypogonadism due to radiotherapy of benign nonpituitary tumors is up to 1.4:10,000 men (**Box 11**).

Androgen deficiency due to radiation of primary malignant brain tumors, brain metastases, or due to total body irradiation for bone marrow transplantation
The global prevalence of primary malignant brain tumors is estimated to be less than 2:10,000 because the survival time after diagnosis is generally low.[134,153] The prevalence in the United States is higher but still low (∼6:10,000).[135] For example, glioblastoma, the most common primary brain malignancy (∼50% of all primary brain malignancies), has an estimated prevalence of 0.5 to 1.0:10,000 and a median life expectancy of 8 to 14 months.[134,135,153] Although the incidence rate of brain metastases from solid tumors might be 10 to 30;100,000 patient-years, the prevalence of metastatic brain cancer is very low because the median time to death is just a few months.[154] However, hypopituitarism might occur within a few months of brain radiation for primary or metastatic brain cancer and might be clinically significant.[155] Similarly, total body irradiation for bone marrow transplantation is potentially associated with very high prevalence of androgen deficiency, but this procedure is too infrequently performed to affect the prevalence in androgen deficiency in the overall global male population.[129,131,156,157] Thus, although radiation therapy for primary or metastatic brain cancer and total body irradiation for bone marrow transplantation do not significantly contribute to the overall prevalence of male hypogonadism, further investigation about the epidemiology and the potential risks and benefits of testosterone therapy to these patients would be valuable.

Box 10
Radiation therapy of a pituitary adenoma is a rare cause of male hypogonadism

Calculation: the lifetime prevalence of male secondary hypogonadism due to radiation therapy of a benign pituitary tumor is the prevalence of macroadenomas in men (4–6:10,000) times the percentage of benign pituitary tumors treated with sellar radiation (5%) times the percentage of men with chronic gonadotrope dysfunction after radiation of a benign pituitary tumor (25%) equals 0.05-0.1:10,000 men. (Note that this range assumes that the androgen deficiency is due to radiation and not the macroadenoma. In addition, this calculation assumes that lifetime prevalence of men who develop secondary hypogonadism due to cranial radiation does not significantly increase 5–10 years after radiation therapy.)

Box 11
Radiation therapy of benign nonpituitary brain tumors is an uncommon cause of male hypogonadism

Calculation: the life-time prevalence of secondary hypogonadism due to radiation therapy of a benign nonpituitary brain tumor is the prevalence of benign nonpituitary brain tumors (39:10,000) times the percentage of benign nonpituitary tumors treated with cranial radiation (10%) times the percentage of patients with chronic gonadotrope dysfunction after radiation of a benign nonpituitary brain tumor (35%) equals 1.4:10,000. (Note that this calculation uses the same assumption as **Box 9**: the lifetime prevalence of secondary hypogonadism due to cranial radiation does not significantly increase 5–10 years after radiation therapy.)

Androgen deficiency due to radiation therapy for primary head and neck cancer
Head and neck cancer is common worldwide, and it is often treated with radiation therapy.[158,159] The incidence rate of secondary hypogonadism after head and neck irradiation ranges from 10% to 35% (depending on the radiation dosage, radiation field size and exposure to the sella turcica, and length of follow-up interval).[149,160] A recent, exhaustive systematic review cited at least a 35% incidence of secondary hypogonadism in childhood cancer survivors who have been treated with cranial radiation including for head and neck cancers that are not primary brain tumors.[129] However, the prevalence of androgen deficiency in survivors of head and neck cancers is unknown because we lack information on the global incidence of radiation therapy for head and neck cancer, and we need large, long-term follow-up studies of the gonadal function of these patients before and after head and neck irradiation.

Secondary hypogonadism due to medication-induced hyperprolactinemia, iatrogenic Cushing syndrome, (iatrogenic) opioids, and androgenic steroid abuse
There are few data on the dosage effects of exogenous corticosteroids, opioids, or drugs that induce hyperprolactinemia on the male gonadal axis, and there are not accurate data about the worldwide frequency, dosage, and duration of use of prescription corticosteroids, opioids, or medications that raise prolactin concentrations. Unlike the other 3 drug classes discussed earlier, chronic, current abuse of androgenic steroids does not cause hypogonadism during use, but cessation of chronic, long-term androgenic steroid abuse might cause persistent suppression of the gonadal axis and symptoms and signs of male hypogonadism in normal men, but recovery of normal gonadal function typically occurs (often within 1 year of discontinuation).[161] Because of the potential legal consequences and stigma attached to androgen abuse, there is even less known about the incidence, prevalence, and long-term effects and withdrawal from androgen abuse than the epidemiology of hypogonadism due to use of corticosteroids, opioids, or drugs that raise serum prolactin concentrations.[161]

There is no basis to estimate or determine the regional and global prevalence of these iatrogenic causes of hypogonadism, but these drugs could have a significant effect on the epidemiology of androgen deficiency in men.

SUMMARY OF IATROGENIC CAUSES OF MALE HYPOGONADISM

In general, iatrogenic causes are probably the most common causes of male hypogonadism.

Cancer therapies such as androgen deprivation therapy for the treatment of prostate cancer; surgical, medical, and radiation treatment of testicular cancer; radiation therapy of malignant benign nonpituitary brain tumors and head and neck cancers; and systemic chemotherapy for lymphoma and leukemia may commonly cause androgen deficiency. Chronic medication-induced hyperprolactinemia, supraphysiologic corticosteroid therapy, and opioid prescription are also likely common causes of secondary hypogonadism. High-quality studies of incidence rate and prevalence of permanent androgen deficiency in men with these conditions or exposures would be invaluable.

SUMMARY

The best available evidence indicates that the most common endogenous pathologic cause of hypogonadism is Klinefelter syndrome (affecting up to ~0.2% of the male population). Common iatrogenic causes include systemic androgen deprivation for prostate cancer, and surgical, medical, and radiation therapy for testicular cancer are common causes of hypogonadism. There are many important gaps in knowledge about the epidemiology of male hypogonadism including a lack of data about the longitudinal incidence and lifetime prevalence of androgen deficiency in men with Klinefelter and Down syndrome and men with a history of TBI or a history of chronic use of supraphysiological dosages of corticosteroids, drugs that raise serum prolactin concentrations, or opioids. In addition, we need better information about long-term follow-up of survivors who have been treated with radiation therapy (+/− chemotherapy) for cancers affecting the head, brain, neck, and pelvis. Finally, we need high-quality long-term studies of middle-aged to older men with "possible hypogonadism."

Overall, the prevalence of male hypogonadism due to known endogenous pathologic causes is low (likely <1%). Iatrogenic causes of male hypogonadism may significantly raise the prevalence of male hypogonadism, particularly in middle-aged and older men who are more likely to be affected by these iatrogenic causes. These iatrogenic causes are readily identified by taking a careful history. There is much to learn about the epidemiology of male hypogonadism (infertility and androgen deficiency), but the current evidence indicates that there is a discordance between the likely true (low) prevalence of endogenous male androgen deficiency and the widespread perception that it is a common malady in young and old men.

CLINICS CARE POINTS

- Klinefelter syndrome is by far the most common endogenous cause of male androgen deficiency that is underdiagnosed (with 25%–50% of affected men not being diagnosed during their lifetimes).

- Serum karyotyping (for Klinefelter syndrome) should be considered in all men with primary hypogonadism.

- Congenital causes of male hypogonadism (with androgen deficiency) are rare, and they generally have extragonadal symptoms or signs such as abnormalities affecting sight or the sense of smell; cerebellar abnormalities such as ataxia, dyskinesia, and synkinesis; and midline abnormalities such as coloboma or cleft palate.

- The prevalence of male androgen deficiency due to known pathologic causes is low, and the prevalence of low serum testosterone concentrations is high in men older than 40 years. Screening for male hypogonadism in adults is not warranted.

- Iatrogenic causes are the most common causes of persistent or permanent male hypogonadism.

- When evaluating a man with male hypogonadism (androgen deficiency) or suspected male hypogonadism, the clinician should query about any history of cancer and oncotherapy (particularly radiation therapy that might have affected the pelvis or brain), significant

- traumatic head injury (defined as loss of consciousness for at least several seconds), and a history of recent use of medications that increase serum prolactin, corticosteroids, or opioids.
- Classic causes of secondary hypogonadism including nonfunctional pituitary macroadenomas, prolactinomas, endogenous Cushing syndrome, and iron overload syndromes (eg, hereditary hemochromatosis or thalassemia) are rare.
- For older men with isolated secondary hypogonadism (ie, normal serum thyroxine and thyrotropin concentrations) and unsuppressed serum gonadotropins, sellar imaging is generally not necessary.
- For men with secondary hypogonadism, the evaluation should include serum prolactin.
- For men with secondary hypogonadism, the history and physical examination suffices to exclude Cushing syndrome as the cause.
- Assessment of iron studies to exclude hemochromatosis is most useful for men younger than 40 years and men who have secondary hypogonadism and other manifestations of hemochromatosis such as chondrocalcinosis of the hands or progressive hyperpigmentation of the skin.

REFERENCES

1. Anawalt BD. Approach to male infertility and induction of spermatogenesis. J Clin Endocrinol Metab 2013;98:3532–42.
2. Barratt CLR, Björndahl L, De Jonge CJ, et al. The diagnosis of male infertility: an analysis of the evidence to support the development of global WHO guidance-challenges and future research opportunities. Hum Reprod Update 2017;23: 660–80.
3. Bhasin S, Brito JP, Cunningham GR, et al. Testosterone therapy in men with hypogonadism: an Endocrine Society clinical practice guideline. J Clin Endocrinol Metab 2018;103:1715–44.
4. Mulhall JP, Trost LW, Brannigan RE, et al. Evaluation and management of testosterone deficiency: AUA guideline. J Urol 2018;200:423–32.
5. Kwong JCC, Krakowsky Y, Grober E. Testosterone deficiency: a review and comparison of current guidelines. J Sex Med 2019;16:812–20.
6. Travison TG, Vesper HW, Orwoll E, et al. Harmonized reference ranges for circulating testosterone levels in men of four cohort studies in the United States and Europe. J Clin Endocrinol Metab 2017;102:1161–73.
7. Martins PRJ, De Vito FB, Resende GAD, et al. Male sickle cell patients, compensated transpubertal hypogonadism and normal final growth. Clin Endocrinol (Oxf) 2019;91:676–82.
8. Ribeiro APMR, Silva CS, Zambrano JCC, et al. Compensated hypogonadism in men with sickle cell disease. Clin Endocrinol (Oxf) 2021;94:968–72.
9. Huang AW, Muneyyirci-Delale O. Reproductive endocrine issues in men with sickle cell anemia. Andrology 2017;5:679–90.
10. Pleasants S. Epidemiology: a moving target. Nature 2014;515:S2–3.
11. Harman SM, Metter EJ, Tobin JD, et al. Longitudinal effects of aging on serum total and free testosterone levels in healthy men. Baltimore Longitudinal Study of Aging. J Clin Endocrinol Metab 2001;86:724–31.
12. Bhasin S, Pencina M, Jasuja GK, et al. Reference ranges for testosterone in men generated using liquid chromatography tandem mass spectrometry in a community-based sample of healthy nonobese young men in the Framingham Heart Study and applied to three geographically distinct cohorts. J Clin Endocrinol Metab 2011;96:2430–9.

13. Wu FC, Tajar A, Beynon JM, et al. Identification of late-onset hypogonadism in middle-aged and elderly men. N Engl J Med 2010;363:123–35.
14. Tajar A, Huhtaniemi IT, O'Neill TW, al at. Characteristics of androgen deficiency in late-onset hypogonadism: results from the European Male Aging Study (EMAS). J Clin Endocrinol Metab 2012;97:1508–16.
15. Handelsman DJ, Yeap B, Flicker L, et al. Age-specific population centiles for androgen status in men. Eur J Endocrinol 2015;173:809–17.
16. Araujo AB, Esche GR, Kupelian V, et al. Prevalence of symptomatic androgen deficiency in men. J Clin Endocrinol Metab 2007;92:4241–7.
17. Araujo AB, O'Donnell AB, Brambilla DJ, et al. Prevalence and incidence of androgen deficiency in middle-aged and older men: estimates from the Massachusetts Male Aging Study. J Clin Endocrinol Metab 2004;89:5920–6.
18. Liu YJ, Shen XB, Yu N, et al. Prevalence of late-onset hypogonadism among middle-aged and elderly males in China: results from a national survey. Asian J Androl 2021;23:170–7.
19. Nguengang Wakap S, Lambert DM, Olry A, et al. Estimating cumulative point prevalence of rare diseases: analysis of the Orphanet database. Eur J Hum Genet 2020;28:165–73.
20. Herlihy AS, Halliday JL, Cock ML, et al. The prevalence and diagnosis rates of Klinefelter syndrome: an Australian comparison. Med J Aust 2011;194:24–8.
21. Bojesen A, Juul S, Gravholt CH. Prenatal and postnatal prevalence of Klinefelter syndrome: a national registry study. J Clin Endocrinol Metab 2003;88:622–6.
22. Berglund A, Viuff MH, Skakkebæk A, et al. Changes in the cohort composition of Turner syndrome and severe non-diagnosis of Klinefelter, 47,XXX and 47,XYY syndrome: a nationwide cohort study. Orphanet J Rare Dis 2019;14:16.
23. Gravholt CH, Chang S, Wallentin M, et al. Klinefelter syndrome: integrating genetics, neuropsychology, and endocrinology. Endocr Rev 2018;39:389–423.
24. Groth KA, Skakkebæk A, Høst C, et al. Clinical review: Klinefelter syndrome–a clinical update. J Clin Endocrinol Metab 2013;98:20–30.
25. Brauner R, Neve M, Allali S. Clinical, biological and genetic analysis of anorchia in 26 boys. PLoS One 2011;6:e23292.
26. Presson AP, Partyka G, Jensen KM, et al. Current estimate of down syndrome population prevalence in the United States. J Pediatr 2013;163:1163–8.
27. De Graaf G, Vis JC, Haveman M, et al. Assessment of prevalence of persons with down syndrome: a theory-based demographic model. J Appl Res Intellect Disabil 2011;24:247–62.
28. Sakadamis A, Angelopoulou N, Matziari C, et al. Bone mass, gonadal function and biochemical assessment in young men with trisomy 21. Eur J Obstet Gynecol Reprod Biol 2002;100:208–12.
29. Parizot E, Dard R, Janel N, et al. Down syndrome and infertility: what support should we provide? J Assist Reprod Genet 2019;36:1063–7.
30. McKelvey KD, Fowler TW, Akel NS, et al. Low bone turnover and low bone density in a cohort of adults with down syndrome. Osteoporos Int 2013;24:1333–8.
31. Hsiang YH, Berkovitz GD, Bland GL, et al. Gonadal function in patients with down syndrome. Am J Med Genet 1987;27:449–58.
32. Whooten R, Schmitt J, Schwartz A. Endocrine manifestations of down syndrome. Curr Opin Endocrinol Diabetes Obes 2018;25:61–6.
33. Roberts AE, Allanson JE, Tartaglia M, et al. Noonan syndrome. Lancet 2013;381:333–42.
34. Romano AA, Allanson JE, Dahlgren J, et al. Noonan syndrome: clinical features, diagnosis, and management guidelines. Pediatrics 2010;126:746–59.

35. Ankarberg-Lindgren C, Westphal O, Dahlgren J. Testicular size development and reproductive hormones in boys and adult males with Noonan syndrome: a longitudinal study. Eur J Endocrinol 2011;165:137–44.
36. Moniez S, Pienkowski C, Lepage B, et al. Noonan syndrome males display Sertoli cell-specific primary testicular insufficiency. Eur J Endocrinol 2018;179:409–18.
37. Thornton CA. Myotonic dystrophy. Neurol Clin 2014;32:705–19.
38. Al-Harbi TM, Bainbridge LJ, McQueen MJ, et al. Hypogonadism is common in men with myopathies. J Clin Neuromuscul Dis 2008;9:397–401.
39. Vazquez JA, Pinies JA, Martul P, et al. Hypothalamic-pituitary-testicular function in 70 patients with myotonic dystrophy. J Endocrinol Invest 1990;13:375–9.
40. Husebye ES, Anderson MS, Kämpe O. Autoimmune polyendocrine syndromes. N Engl J Med 2018;378:1132–41.
41. Kahaly GJ, Frommer L. Polyglandular autoimmune syndromes. J Endocrinol Invest 2018;41:91–8.
42. Dalla Costa M, Bonanni G, Masiero S, et al. Gonadal function in males with autoimmune Addison's disease and autoantibodies to steroidogenic enzymes. Clin Exp Immunol 2014;176:373–9.
43. Wisniewski AB, Batista RL, Costa EMF, et al. Management of 46,XY differences/disorders of sex development (DSD) throughout life. Endocr Rev 2019;40:1547–72.
44. Delvecchio M, Iacoviello M, Pantaleo A, et al. Clinical spectrum associated with Wolfram syndrome type 1 and type 2: a review on genotype-phenotype correlations. Int J Environ Res Public Health 2021;18:4796.
45. Rothblum-Oviatt C, Wright J, Lefton-Greif MA. Ataxia telangiectasia: a review. Orphanet J Rare Dis 2016;11:159–80.
46. Cassidy SB, Schwartz S, Miller JL, et al. Prader-Willi syndrome. Genet Med 2012;14:10–26.
47. Randhawa H, Blankstein U, Davies T. Scrotal trauma: a case report and review of the literature. Can Urol Assoc J 2019;13(6 Suppl4):S67–71.
48. Kitrey ND, Djakovic N, Gonsalves M, et al. EAU guidelines on urological trauma. European Association of Urology; 2016. Available at: https://uroweb.org/individual-guidelines/non-oncology-guidelines/. Accessed September 24, 2021.
49. Grigorian A, Livingston JK, Schubl SD, et al. National analysis of testicular and scrotal trauma in the USA. Res Rep Urol 2018;10:51–6.
50. Zhao LC, Lautz TB, Meeks JJ, et al. Pediatric testicular torsion epidemiology using a national database: incidence, risk of orchiectomy and possible measures toward improving the quality of care. J Urol 2011;186:2009–13.
51. Huang WY, Chen YF, Chang HC, et al. The incidence rate and characteristics in patients with testicular torsion: a nationwide, population-based study. Acta Paediatr 2013;102:e363–7.
52. Jacobsen FM, Rudlang TM, Fode M, et al, CopMich Collaborative. The impact of testicular torsion on testicular function. World J Mens Health 2020;38:298–307.
53. Davis NF, McGuire BB, Mahon JA, et al. The increasing incidence of mumps orchitis: a comprehensive review. BJU Int 2010;105:1060–5.
54. Ternavasio-de la Vega HG, Boronat M, Ojeda A, et al. Mumps orchitis in the post-vaccine era (1967–2009): a single-center series of 67 patients and review of clinical outcome and trends. Medicine 2010;89:96–116.
55. Gregory LC, Dattani MT. The molecular basis of congenital hypopituitarism and related disorders. J Clin Endocrinol Metab 2020;105:dgz184.

56. Vaaralahti K, Raivio T, Koivu R, et al. Genetic overlap between holoprosence-phaly and Kallmann syndrome. Mol Syndromol 2012;3:1–5.

57. Cangiano B, Swee DS, Quinton R, et al. Genetics of congenital hypogonado-tropic hypogonadism: peculiarities and phenotype of an oligogenic disease. Hum Genet 2021;140:77–111.

58. Laitinen EM, Vaaralahti K, Tommiska J, et al. Incidence, phenotypic features and molecular genetics of Kallmann syndrome in Finland. Orphanet J Rare Dis 2011; 6:41.

59. Brioude F, Bouligand J, Trabado S, et al. Non-syndromic congenital hypogona-dotropic hypogonadism: clinical presentation and genotype-phenotype relation-ships. Eur J Endocrinol 2010;162:835–51.

60. Fang Q, George AS, Brinkmeier ML, et al. Genetics of combined pituitary hor-mone deficiency: roadmap into the genome era. Endocr Rev 2016;37:636–75.

61. Kyritsi EM, Sertedaki A, Charmandari E, et al. Familial or sporadic adrenal hypo-plasia syndromes. In: Feingold KR, Anawalt B, Boyce A, et al, editors. Endotext [Internet]. South Dartmouth, MA: MDText.com, Inc; 2018.

62. de Geus CM, Free RH, Verbist BM, et al. Guidelines in CHARGE syndrome and the missing link: Cranial imaging. Am J Med Genet C Semin Med Genet 2017; 175:450–64.

63. Forsythe E, Beales PL. Bardet-Biedl syndrome. Eur J Hum Genet 2013;21:8–13.

64. Kim YJ, Osborn DP, Lee JY, et al. WDR11-mediated Hedgehog signalling de-fects underlie a new ciliopathy related to Kallmann syndrome. EMBO Rep 2018;19:269–89.

65. Lofrano-Porto A, Barra GB, Giacomini LA, et al. Luteinizing hormone beta muta-tion and hypogonadism in men and women. N Engl J Med 2007;357:897–904.

66. Daly AF, Beckers A. The epidemiology of pituitary adenomas. Endocrinol Metab Clin North Am 2020;49:347–55.

67. Fernandez A, Karavitaki N, Wass JA. Prevalence of pituitary adenomas: a community-based, cross-sectional study in Banbury (Oxfordshire, UK). Clin En-docrinol (Oxf) 2010;72:377–82.

68. Sigurdsson G, Thorsson AV, Carroll PV, et al. The epidemiology of pituitary ad-enomas in Iceland, 1955-2012: a nationwide population-based study. Eur J En-docrinol 2015;173:655–64.

69. Day PF, Loto MG, Glerean M, et al. Incidence and prevalence of clinically rele-vant pituitary adenomas: retrospective cohort study in a health management or-ganization in Buenos Aires, Argentina. Arch Endocrinol Metab 2016;60:554–61.

70. Freda PU, Bruce JN, Khandji AG, et al. Presenting features in 269 patients with clinically nonfunctioning pituitary adenomas enrolled in a prospective study. J Endocr Soc 2020;4:bvaa021.

71. Tresoldi AS, Carosi G, Betella N, et al. Clinically nonfunctioning pituitary inciden-talomas: characteristics and natural history. Neuroendocrinology 2020;110: 595–603.

72. Chen L, White WL, Spetzler RF, et al. A prospective study of nonfunctioning pi-tuitary adenomas: presentation, management, and clinical outcome. J Neurooncol 2011;102:129–38.

73. Vaninetti NM, Clarke DB, Zwicker DA, et al. A comparative, population-based analysis of pituitary incidentalomas vs clinically manifesting sellar masses. En-docr Connect 2018;7:768–76.

74. Trifanescu R, Ansorge O, Wass JA, et al. Rathke's cleft cysts. Clin Endocrinol (Oxf) 2012;76:151–60.

75. Nguyen R, Fiest KM, McChesney J, et al. The international incidence of traumatic brain injury: a systematic review and meta-analysis. Can J Neurol Sci 2016;43:774–85.

76. Lauzier F, Turgeon AF, Boutin A, et al. Clinical outcomes, predictors, and prevalence of anterior pituitary disorders following traumatic brain injury: a systematic review. Crit Care Med 2014;42:712–21.

77. Karaca Z, Tanrıverdi F, Unluhızarcı K, et al. GH and pituitary hormone alterations after traumatic brain injury. Prog Mol Biol Transl Sci 2016;138:167–91.

78. Park KD, Kim DY, Lee JK, et al. Anterior pituitary dysfunction in moderate- to-severe chronic traumatic brain injury patients and the influence on functional outcome. Brain Inj 2010;24:1330–5.

79. Caputo M, Mele C, Prodam F, et al. Clinical picture and the treatment of TBI-induced hypopituitarism. Pituitary 2019;22:261–9.

80. Klose M, Feldt-Rasmussen U. Chronic endocrine consequences of traumatic brain injury - what is the evidence? Nat Rev Endocrinol 2018;14:57–62.

81. Krewer C, Schneider M, Schneider HJ, et al. Neuroendocrine disturbances one to five or more years after traumatic brain injury and aneurysmal subarachnoid hemorrhage: data from the German database on hypopituitarism. J Neurotrauma 2016;33:1544–53.

82. Can A, Gross BA, Smith TR, et al. Pituitary dysfunction after aneurysmal subarachnoid hemorrhage: a systematic review and meta-analysis. Neurosurgery 2016;79:253–64.

83. Etminan N, Han-Sol C, Hackenberg K, et al. Subarachnoid hemorrhage according to region, time period, blood pressure, and smoking prevalence in the population: a systematic review and meta-analysis. JAMA Neurol 2019;76:588–97.

84. Rackauskaite D, Svanborg E, Andersson E, et al. Prospective study: long-term outcome at 12-15 years after aneurysmal subarachnoid hemorrhage. Acta Neurol Scand 2018;138:400–7.

85. Briet C, Salenave S, Bonneville JF, et al. Pituitary apoplexy. Endocr Rev 2015;36: 622–45.

86. Rajasekaran S, Vanderpump M, Baldeweg S, et al. UK guidelines for the management of pituitary apoplexy. Clin Endocrinol (Oxf) 2011;74:9–20.

87. Wildemberg LE, Glezer A, Bronstein MD, et al. Apoplexy in nonfunctioning pituitary adenomas. Pituitary 2018;21:138–44.

88. Chiloiro S, Giampietro A, Bianchi A, et al. DIAGNOSIS OF ENDOCRINE DISEASE: Primary empty sella: a comprehensive review. Eur J Endocrinol 2017; 177:R275–85.

89. Guitelman M, Garcia Basavilbaso N, Vitale M, et al. Primary empty sella (PES): a review of 175 cases. Pituitary 2013;16:270–4.

90. Auer MK, Stieg MR, Crispin A, et al. Primary empty sella syndrome and the prevalence of hormonal dysregulation. Dtsch Arztebl Int 2018;115:99–105.

91. McDermott JH, Walsh CH. Hypogonadism in hereditary hemochromatosis. J Clin Endocrinol Metab 2005;90:2451–5.

92. Kowdley KV, Brown KE, Ahn J, et al. ACG clinical guideline: hereditary hemochromatosis. Am J Gastroenterol 2019;114:1202–18.

93. Pelusi C, Gasparini DI, Bianchi N, et al. Endocrine dysfunction in hereditary hemochromatosis. J Endocrinol Invest 2016;39:837–47.

94. De Sanctis V, Soliman AT, Yassin MA, et al. Hypogonadism in male thalassemia major patients: pathophysiology, diagnosis and treatment. Acta Biomed 2018; 89(2-S):6–15.

95. Ho PJ, Tay L, Lindeman R, et al. Australian guidelines for the assessment of iron overload and iron chelation in transfusion-dependent thalassaemia major, sickle cell disease and other congenital anaemias. Intern Med J 2011;41:516–24.

96. Soto-Pedre E, Newey PJ, Bevan JS, et al. The epidemiology of hyperprolactinaemia over 20 years in the Tayside region of Scotland: the Prolactin Epidemiology, Audit and Research Study (PROLEARS). Clin Endocrinol (Oxf) 2017; 86:60–7.

97. Karavitaki N, Dobrescu R, Byrne JV, et al. Does hypopituitarism recover when macroprolactinomas are treated with cabergoline? Clin Endocrinol (Oxf) 2013; 79:217–23.

98. Tirosh A, Benbassat C, Lifshitz A, et al. Hypopituitarism patterns and prevalence among men with macroprolactinomas. Pituitary 2015;18:108–15.

99. Liu W, Zahr RS, McCartney S, et al. Clinical outcomes in male patients with lactotroph adenomas who required pituitary surgery: a retrospective single center study. Pituitary 2018;21:454–62.

100. Luton JP, Thieblot P, Valcke JC, et al. Reversible gonadotropin deficiency in male Cushing's disease. J Clin Endocrinol Metab 1977;45(3):488–95.

101. McKenna TJ, Lorber D, Lacroix A, et al. Testicular activity in Cushing's disease. Acta Endocrinol (Copenh) 1979;91:501–10.

102. Pivonello R, De Martino MC, De Leo M, et al. Cushing's syndrome. Endocrinol Metab Clin North Am 2008;37:135–49.

103. Shekhar S, McGlotten R, Auh S, et al. The hypothalamic-pituitary-thyroid axis in Cushing syndrome before and after curative surgery. J Clin Endocrinol Metab 2021;106:e1316–31.

104. Pivonello R, De Leo M, Cozzolino A, et al. The treatment of Cushing's disease. Endocr Rev 2015;36:385–486.

105. Lindholm J, Juul S, Jørgensen JO, et al. Incidence and late prognosis of Cushing's syndrome: a population-based study. J Clin Endocrinol Metab 2001;86: 117–23.

106. Etxabe J, Vasquez JA. Morbidity and mortality in Cushing's disease: an epidemiological approach. Clin Endocrinol (Oxf) 1994;40:479–84.

107. Pishgar F, Ebrahimi H, Saeedi Moghaddam S, et al. Global, regional and national burden of prostate cancer, 1990 to 2015: results from the Global Burden of Disease Study 2015. J Urol 2018;199:1224–32.

108. Sung H, Ferlay J, Siegel RL, et al. Global Cancer Statistics 2020: GLOBOCAN estimates of incidence and mortality worldwide for 36 cancers in 185 countries. CA Cancer J Clin 2021;71:209–49.

109. Shore ND, Antonarakis ES, Cookson MS, et al. Optimizing the role of androgen deprivation therapy in advanced prostate cancer: challenges beyond the guidelines. Prostate 2020;80:527–44.

110. Wang L, Paller CJ, Hong H, et al. Comparison of systemic treatments for metastatic castration-sensitive prostate cancer: a systematic review and network meta-analysis. JAMA Oncol 2021;7:412–20.

111. Lowrance WT, Breau RH, Chou R, et al. Advanced prostate cancer: AUA/ASTRO/SUO guideline PART I. J Urol 2021;205:14–21.

112. Lowrance WT, Breau RH, Chou R, et al. Advanced prostate cancer: AUA/ASTRO/SUO guideline PART II. J Urol 2021;205:22–9.

113. Wolters T, Roobol MJ, Steyerberg EW, et al. The effect of study arm on prostate cancer treatment in the large screening trial ERSPC. Int J Cancer 2010;126: 2387–93.

114. Schröder FH, Hugosson J, Roobol MJ, et al. Screening and prostate cancer mortality: results of the European Randomised Study of Screening for Prostate Cancer (ERSPC) at 13 years of follow-up. Lancet 2014;384:2027–35.

115. Hugosson J, Roobol MJ, Månsson M, et al. A 16-yr follow-up of the European randomized study of screening for prostate cancer. Eur Urol 2019;76:43–51.

116. US Preventive Services Task Force, Grossman DC, Curry SJ, Owens DK, et al. Screening for prostate cancer: US Preventive Services Task Force recommendation statement. JAMA 2018;319:1901–13.

117. Symeonidis EN, Tsifountoudis I, Anastasiadis A, et al. Synchronous bilateral testicular cancer with discordant histopathology occurring in a 20-year-old patient: a case report and review of the literature. Urologia 2021. https://doi.org/10.1177/03915603211028556.

118. Abu Zaid M, Dinh PC, Monahan PO, et al. Adverse health outcomes in relationship to hypogonadism after chemotherapy: a multicenter study of testicular cancer survivors. J Natl Compr Canc Netw 2019;17:459–68.

119. Rogol AD, Anawalt BD. Should survivors of childhood cancer or testicular cancer be screened for androgen deficiency? Clin Endocrinol (Oxf) 2018;89:397–8.

120. Masterson TA, Tagawa ST. A 25-year review of advances in testicular cancer: perspectives on evaluation, treatment, and future directions/challenges. Urol Oncol 2021;39:561–8.

121. Huddart RA, Norman A, Moynihan C, et al. Fertility, gonadal and sexual function in survivors of testicular cancer. Br J Cancer 2005;93:200–7.

122. Wiechno P, Demkow T, Kubiak K, et al. The quality of life and hormonal disturbances in testicular cancer survivors in cisplatin era. Eur Urol 2007;52:1448–54.

123. Gerl A, Muhlbayer D, Hansmann G, et al. The impact of chemotherapy on Leydig cell function in long term survivors of germ cell tumors. Cancer 2001;91:1297–303.

124. Kurobe M, Kawai K, Suetomi T, et al. High prevalence of hypogonadism determined by serum free testosterone level in Japanese testicular cancer survivors. Int J Urol 2018;25:457–62.

125. Bandak M, Jørgensen N, Juul A, et al. Testosterone deficiency in testicular cancer survivors - a systematic review and meta-analysis. Andrology 2016;4:382–8.

126. Sklar CA, Antal Z, Chemaitilly W, et al. Hypothalamic-pituitary and growth disorders in survivors of childhood cancer: an Endocrine Society clinical practice guideline. J Clin Endocrinol Metab 2018;103:2761–84.

127. Seejore K, Kyriakakis N, Murray RD. Is chemotherapy implicated in the development of hypopituitarism in childhood cancer survivors? J Clin Endocrinol Metab 2020;105:dgz132.

128. Isaksson S, Bogefors K, Ståhl O, et al. High risk of hypogonadism in young male cancer survivors. Clin Endocrinol (Oxf) 2018;88:432–41.

129. van Iersel L, Li Z, Srivastava DK, et al. Hypothalamic-pituitary disorders in childhood cancer survivors: prevalence, risk factors and long-term health outcomes. J Clin Endocrinol Metab 2019;104:6101–15.

130. Steffens M, Beauloye V, Brichard B, et al. Endocrine and metabolic disorders in young adult survivors of childhood acute lymphoblastic leukaemia (ALL) or non-Hodgkin lymphoma (NHL). Clin Endocrinol (Oxf) 2008;69:819–27.

131. Gebauer J, Higham C, Langer T, et al. Long-term endocrine and metabolic consequences of cancer treatment: a systematic review. Endocr Rev 2019;40:711–67.

132. Yau I, Vuong T, Garant A, et al. Risk of hypogonadism from scatter radiation during pelvic radiation in male patients with rectal cancer. Int J Radiat Oncol Biol Phys 2009;74:1481–6.

133. Hermann RM, Henkel K, Christiansen H, et al. Testicular dose and hormonal changes after radiotherapy of rectal cancer. Radiother Oncol 2005;75:83–8.

134. de Robles P, Fiest KM, Frolkis AD, et al. The worldwide incidence and prevalence of primary brain tumors: a systematic review and meta-analysis. Neuro Oncol 2015;17:776–83.

135. Ostrom QT, Patil N, Cioffi G, et al. CBTRUS statistical report: primary brain and other central nervous system tumors diagnosed in the United States in 2013-2017. Neuro Oncol 2020;22(12 Suppl 2):iv1–96.

136. Molitch ME. Diagnosis and treatment of pituitary adenomas: a review. JAMA 2017;317:516–24.

137. Fathy R, Kuan E, Lee JYK, et al. Factors associated with and temporal trends in the use of radiation therapy for the treatment of pituitary adenoma in the national cancer database. J Neurol Surg B Skull Base 2021;82:285–94.

138. Brada M, Rajan B, Traish D, et al. The long-term efficacy of conservative surgery and radiotherapy in the control of pituitary adenomas. Clin Endocrinol (Oxf) 1993;38:571–8.

139. Langsenlehner T, Stiegler C, Quehenberger F, et al. Long-term follow-up of patients with pituitary macroadenomas after postoperative radiation therapy: analysis of tumor control and functional outcome. Strahlenther Onkol 2007;183:241–7.

140. Bir SC, Murray RD, Ambekar S, et al. Clinical and radiologic outcome of gamma knife radiosurgery on nonfunctioning pituitary adenomas. J Neurol Surg B Skull Base 2015;76:351–7.

141. Minniti G, Flickinger J, Tolu B, et al. Management of nonfunctioning pituitary tumors: radiotherapy. Pituitary 2018;21:154–61.

142. Oh JW, Sung KS, Moon JH, et al. Hypopituitarism after gamma knife surgery for postoperative nonfunctioning pituitary adenoma. J Neurosurg 2018;129(Suppl1):47–54.

143. Castinetti F, Nagai M, Morange I, et al. Long-term results of stereotactic radiosurgery in secretory pituitary adenomas. J Clin Endocrinol Metab 2009;94:3400–7.

144. Cohen-Inbar O, Ramesh A, Xu Z, et al. Gamma knife radiosurgery in patients with persistent acromegaly or Cushing's disease: long-term risk of hypopituitarism. Clin Endocrinol (Oxf) 2016;84:524–31.

145. Agarwal V, McCutcheon BA, Hughes JD, et al. Trends in management of intracranial meningiomas: analysis of 49,921 cases from modern cohort. World Neurosurg 2017;106:145–51.

146. Lamba N, Bussiere MR, Niemierko A, et al. Hypopituitarism after cranial irradiation for meningiomas: a single-Institution experience. Pract Radiat Oncol 2019;9:e266–73.

147. Agha A, Sherlock M, Brennan S, et al. Hypothalamic-pituitary dysfunction after irradiation of nonpituitary brain tumors in adults. J Clin Endocrinol Metab 2005;90:6355–60.

148. Goldbrunner R, Stavrinou P, Jenkinson MD, et al. EANO guideline on the diagnosis and management of meningiomas. Neuro Oncol 2021;23:1821–34.

149. Kyriakakis N, Lynch J, Orme SM, et al. Pituitary dysfunction following cranial radiotherapy for adult-onset nonpituitary brain tumours. Clin Endocrinol (Oxf) 2016;84:372–9.

150. Goldbrunner R, Weller M, Regis J. EANO guideline on the diagnosis and treatment of vestibular schwannoma. Neuro Oncol 2020;22:31–45.

151. Jacob JT, Pollock BE, Carlson ML, et al. Stereotactic radiosurgery in the management of vestibular schwannoma and glomus jugulare: indications, techniques, and results. Otolaryngol Clin North Am 2015;48:515–26.

152. Kalogeridi MA, Kougioumtzopoulou A, Zygogianni A, et al. Stereotactic radiosurgery and radiotherapy for acoustic neuromas. Neurosurg Rev 2020;43: 941–9.

153. Zhang AS, Ostrom QT, Kruchko C, et al. Complete prevalence of malignant primary brain tumors registry data in the United States compared with other common cancers, 2010. Neuro Oncol 2017;19:726–35.

154. Habbous S, Forster K, Darling G, et al. Incidence and real-world burden of brain metastases from solid tumors and hematologic malignancies in Ontario: a population-based study. Neurooncol Adv 2021;3:1–14.

155. Mehta P, Fahlbusch FB, Rades D, et al. Are hypothalamic- pituitary (HP) axis deficiencies after whole brain radiotherapy (WBRT) of relevance for adult cancer patients? - a systematic review of the literature. BMC Cancer 2019;19:1213.

156. Shalitin S, Pertman L, Yackobovitch-Gavan M. Endocrine and metabolic disturbances in survivors of hematopoietic stem cell transplantation in childhood and adolescence. Horm Res Paediatr 2018;89:108–21.

157. Wei C, Albanese A. Endocrine disorders in childhood cancer survivors treated with haemopoietic stem cell transplantation. Children (Basel) 2014;1:48–62.

158. Colevas AD, Yom SS, Pfister DG, et al. NCCN guidelines insights: head and neck cancers, version 1.2018. J Natl Compr Canc Netw 2018;16:479–90.

159. Global Burden of Disease Cancer Collaboration, Fitzmaurice C, Abate D, Abbasi N, et al. Global, regional, and national cancer incidence, mortality, years of life lost, years lived with disability, and disability-adjusted life-years for 29 cancer groups, 1990 to 2017: a systematic analysis for the Global Burden of Disease Study. JAMA Oncol 2019;5:1749–68.

160. Appelman-Dijkstra NM, Malgo F, Neelis KJ, et al. Pituitary dysfunction in adult patients after cranial irradiation for head and nasopharyngeal tumours. Radiother Oncol 2014;113:102–7.

161. Anawalt BD. Diagnosis and management of anabolic androgenic steroid use. J Clin Endocrinol Metab 2019;104:2490–500.

Regulation of the Hypothalamic-Pituitary-Testicular Axis: Pathophysiology of Hypogonadism

Aditi Sharma, MBBCh, MRCP,
Channa N. Jayasena, MA, PhD, MRCP, FRCPath,
Waljit S. Dhillo, FRCP, FRCPath, PhD*

KEYWORDS

- Testosterone • Gonadotropins • Hypogonadism • Testes
- Hypothalamic-pituitary-testicular axis

KEY POINTS

- The hypothalamic-pituitary-testicular axis (HPT) is central to the normal testicular function of steroidogenesis and spermatogenesis.
- KNDy (kisspeptin/neurokinin B/dynorphin A) neurones in the infundibular nucleus/arcuate nucleus of the hypothalamus are important regulators of gonadotropin-releasing hormone (GnRH) secretion.
- Pulsatile GnRH stimulates gonadotropins (luteinizing hormone, LH and follicle-stimulating hormone, FSH) from the anterior pituitary which in turn stimulates the testis to secrete testosterone and spermatogenesis, respectively.
- Congenital and acquired conditions may lead to failure of hormone synthesis or action at any level of the HPT axis resulting in male hypogonadism.

INTRODUCTION

The hypothalamic-pituitary-testicular axis (HPT) regulates the testicular functions of steroidogenesis and spermatogenesis in both humans and animals.[1] The synchronized pulsatile secretion of gonadotropin-releasing hormone (GnRH) from neurones in the hypothalamus is mediated by the hypothalamic network of kisspeptin/neurokinin B/dynorphin A (KNDy) neurones.[2] GnRH is released into the hypophyseal portal system and stimulates luteinizing hormone (LH) and follicle-stimulating hormone (FSH) secretion from the anterior pituitary. LH acts via specific receptors on testicular Leydig cells, stimulating the enzymatic conversion of precursor cholesterol into testosterone. FSH stimulates spermatogenesis and production of Inhibin B from the

Section of Investigative Medicine, Imperial College London, Hammersmith Hospital, 6th Floor, Commonwealth Building, 150 Du Cane Road, London W12 0NN, UK
* Corresponding author.
E-mail address: w.dhillo@imperial.ac.uk

Endocrinol Metab Clin N Am 51 (2022) 29–45
https://doi.org/10.1016/j.ecl.2021.11.010
0889-8529/22/© 2021 Elsevier Inc. All rights reserved.

Sertoli cells of the testis. Testosterone exerts a negative feedback effect to decrease the production of LH and GnRH thereby decreasing endogenous testosterone levels. Similarly, inhibin B provides negative feedback at the pituitary for the action of FSH (**Fig. 1**).

Male hypogonadism is a clinical condition characterized by the diminished functional activity of the testes that results in diminished testosterone (+/− spermatozoa) production and secretion.[3] Recent studies observed that the prevalence of male hypogonadism has increased over the last 10 years, and this condition is underestimated and underdiagnosed.[4] Hypogonadism can be broadly subdivided into 2 categories: (1) primary (testicular) and (2) secondary (central or hypothalamic-pituitary) hypogonadism, according to whether the defect is inherent within the testes or lies outside of the testes (see **Fig. 1**). Primary hypogonadism (also called hypergonadotropic hypogonadism) is much less common and is typically due to hypofunction of the testes in the presence of normal function and anatomy of the hypothalamus and anterior pituitary. Hypothalamic-pituitary dysfunction leads to secondary hypogonadism (hypogonadotropic hypogonadism) which is much more common. Congenital and acquired conditions can disrupt the HPT axis at any level, resulting in male hypogonadism—age of onset, severity of androgen deficiency, and underlying cause of hypogonadism

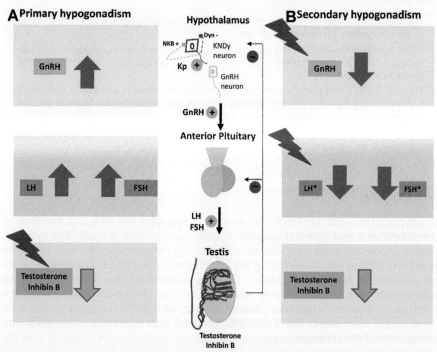

Fig. 1. Hypothalamic-pituitary-testicular axis and the pathophysiology of primary and secondary hypogonadism. (*A*) Primary hypogonadism is due to primary testicular pathology (red lightning sign at testis) with low testosterone, high gonadotropins (LH and FSH), and high GnRH. (*B*) Secondary hypogonadism is due to a defect at the hypothalamus or pituitary level (red lightning sign) with low testosterone, low or normal gonadotropins. LH luteinizing hormone, FSH follicle-stimulating hormone, GnRH gonadotropin-releasing hormone * LH and FSH can be low or normal. Level of defect depicted by the lightning sign. Broken line (—) depicts negative feedback.

determine the signs and symptoms of the condition.[5] In the setting of acquired hypogonadism, comorbidities such as obesity are often associated with hypogonadism.

GnRH PULSATILITY AND ITS REGULATION IN THE HYPOTHALAMIC-PITUITARY-TESTICULAR AXIS

GnRH is the principal neuropeptide in the HPT axis regulating sexual development, puberty, and maintenance of sex hormones in animals and humans. In humans, GnRH neurones extend from the preoptic area to the infundibular nucleus (homologous to the arcuate nucleus in other species) of the hypothalamus. Studies by Knobil and colleagues in the 1970s were the first to demonstrate that pulsatile GnRH secretion is a prerequisite for the maintenance of physiologic LH and FSH secretion from the anterior pituitary.[6] Conversely, continuous GnRH treatment paradoxically inhibited gonadotropin release. LH released from the anterior pituitary gland is used as a surrogate marker of GnRH pulse generator activity in humans based on its validation in several animal models as a reliable surrogate marker of GnRH secretion[7,8]

Kisspeptin/neurokinin B/dynorphin A neurones

Despite the central role of GnRH neurones in HPT axis (see **Fig. 1**), they do not express sex steroid receptors in particular oestradiol receptor alpha, ERα, required for feedback for gonadotropin secretion. Recent evidence suggests that a major hypothalamic regulatory network namely KNDy (co-expressing kisspeptin, neurokinin B (NKB), dynorphin A (Dyn)) neurons in the infundibular (humans)/arcuate (rodent and ruminant) nucleus are major regulators of GnRH neuron activity.[2] Increasing evidence suggests that these neurons are strongly conserved across a range of species from rodents to humans.[9] With direct projections onto GnRH neurones, KNDy neurones incorporate sex steroid, environmental and metabolic cues (e.g. from leptin) to regulate GnRH secretion.[10] KNDy neurones mediate a paracrine stimulatory role of NKB and inhibitory action of Dyn to coordinate the pulsatile release of kisspeptin, which in turn drives the pulsatile secretion of GnRH and LH.[11] Similarly, sex steroid negative feedback on KNDy neurones leads to the suppression of kisspeptin and NKB and stimulation of Dyn, which act synergistically to reduce the activity of GnRH neurones, and subsequent gonadotropin secretion (see **Fig. 1**).

Kisspeptin, neurokinin B and dynorphin A

Kisspeptin is a 54 amino acid peptide, encoded by the *Kiss-1* gene which acts as a ligand to the previously orphaned G-protein coupled receptor, GPR54, now termed KISS1R.[12] It is secreted by specialized kisspeptin neurones that are primarily located in the rostral preoptic area and infundibular nucleus of the hypothalamus in humans (arcuate nucleus in rodents).[12,13] Studies observed that kisspeptin administered to humans in different isoforms, routes and doses is a powerful stimulus for GnRH-induced LH secretion and LH pulse frequency in mammalian species.[14] These effects were blocked by GnRH antagonists suggestive of the action of kisspeptin on GnRH in the HPT axis. Interestingly, in males, the stimulatory effects of kisspeptin on FSH are much smaller compared with LH.[15] Mutations in the hypothalamic KISS1/KISS1R system can lead to multiple reproductive disorders; inactivating mutations cause lack of pubertal maturation and hypogonadotropic hypogonadism, conversely activating mutations cause precocious puberty.[16,17] Recent evidence suggests the role of kisspeptin in modulating limbic brain activity specifically in response to sexual and emotional stimuli using functional MRI.[18] There is also recent evidence of peripheral KISS1/KISS1R expression and peptide distribution in the cells of the testes of multiple animal species. However, variability is observed in the testicular cell types expressing KISS1/KISS1R, with direct testicular action on steroidogenesis or spermatogenesis yet to be determined in both animals and humans.[19]

NKB, encoded by the *Tac3* gene, is a tachykinin peptide that binds to the receptor NK3R. In humans, NKB is called TAC3 and binds to the receptor TAC3R.[20] Administration of TAC3R antagonist decreased LH and testosterone secretion in healthy men.[21] However, administration of NKB did not significantly change LH, FSH or testosterone secretion.[22] Inactivating mutations in TAC3/TAC3R leads to impaired GnRH secretion and subsequent congenital hypogonadotropic hypogonadism,[20] while pulsatile GnRH administration reverses the gonadotropin deficiency observed in patients with TAC3/TACR mutations.[23]

Dyn, encoded by the *Pdyn* gene, is an endogenous opioid peptide that binds to the kappa opioid receptor. Animal studies suggest that NKB is an excitatory stimulus, while Dyn is an inhibitory stimulus to kisspeptin release from kisspeptin neurones in the hypothalamus[24] (see **Fig. 1**).

Leptin

Leptin is a key metabolic signal regulating reproduction. Leptin is encoded by the *ob* gene in adipose tissue such that circulating serum leptin levels correlate positively with adiposity. The central role of leptin at the hypothalamus has been studied such that congenital leptin deficiency (for example by loss of mutations in *ob* or *ObR* genes) is associated with early-onset obesity, hyperphagia, and delayed onset of puberty due to hypogonadotropic hypogonadism.[25,26] There is evidence of leptin "cross-talk" with other central neuronal mediators involved in energy intake and reproductive function. In mice, OB-R has been co-localized with agouti-related peptide/neuropeptide Y (AgRP/NPY, orexigenic neuropeptides), proopiomelanocortin (POMC, anorexigenic neuropeptide), and Kiss1 neurones. This suggests an indirect action of leptin in regulating gonadotropin secretion by modulating KNDy neurones in the arcuate nucleus, with metabolic cues from the above orexigenic and anorexigenic neuropeptides.[27] Furthermore, animal studies have shown a local secretion of leptin at the pituitary with Ob-R also expressed in anterior pituitary suggestive of potential paracrine and autocrine actions of leptin in gonadotropin secretion.[28] However, the exact neuronal mechanisms of leptin action at the hypothalamus and pituitary and its implications are yet to be unequivocally confirmed.

In addition to the central actions of leptin, there is recent evidence of leptin expression in seminiferous tubules and spermatozoa in humans, and leptin receptor has been isolated from Sertoli, Leydig and testicular germ cells in rodents,[29] and Leydig cells and seminiferous tubules in humans,[30] suggesting that leptin may also directly modulate testicular functions. Furthermore, elevated leptin levels (leptin resistance) may have a direct inhibitory signal for testicular steroidogenesis.[31] This link is observed in men with obesity with low testosterone levels (hypogonadism) and hyper-leptinaemia (see section on Obesity). The underlying molecular pathways are yet to be fully understood but the reduction of several steroidogenic genes such as steroidogenic factor-1 (Nr5a1), steroidogenic acute regulatory protein (StAR), and cytochrome P450 cholesterol side-chain cleavage (CYP11A1) enzyme involved in testosterone synthesis may have a postulated role.[32]

ONTOGENY OF HYPOTHALAMIC-PITUITARY-TESTICULAR AXIS

In humans, the pattern of GnRH-induced gonadotropin secretion changes in different stages of life: (1) peak at mid-gestation leading to incomplete functional sexual development and maturation during intrauterine life, (2) peak after birth (mini-puberty) with functional quiescence during childhood, and (3) final reactivation during puberty.[33] As a result, the age of onset of hypogonadism leads to varying phenotype: testosterone deficiency or impaired action during fetal life may lead to a disorder of sexual differentiation; the occurrence of testosterone deficiency after birth but before pubertal development may lead to delayed puberty with delayed or absent secondary sexual characteristics; and adult-onset hypogonadism may present with symptoms of testosterone deficiency with normal secondary sexual characteristics. An understanding of the sequence of GnRH-induced activation during different developmental stages can help elucidate the pathophysiology of hypogonadism.

Fetal life: Masculinization of the fetus with appropriate development of male reproductive tissues depends on androgen exposure and action particularly during 'masculinization programming window' in late first to early second trimester.[34] *During 1st trimester,* early fetal testosterone production is stimulated by placental human chorionic gonadotropin, hCG (instead of GnRH), which stimulates the LH receptor in differentiating fetal testicular mesenchymal cells to Leydig cells for testosterone production essential for the development of male urogenital structures from the Wolffian duct.

GnRH neurones develop from the epithelium of the medial olfactory placode and migrate to the fetal hypothalamus reflecting the close association of reproductive and olfactory systems, hence why genetic mutations involved in embryonic migration of these GnRH neurones lead to both anosmia and hypogonadotropic hypogonadism (see section on congenital GnRH deficiency). The pituitary develops the ability to secrete LH and FSH at 9 weeks gestation approximately[35] with these peptide hormones detected in fetal blood at around 12 to 14 weeks gestation.[36] Contrary to 1st trimester that is dependent on hCG control (GnRH independent-LH release), GnRH peaks at mid-gestation with stimulation of GnRH-dependent gonadotropin secretion from mid to later fetal life, *(i.e. 2nd and 3rd trimester).*[37] The high testosterone levels at mid-gestation are essential for penile growth, testicular descent, and seminiferous tubule maturation. Fetal testis also produces insulin-like factor 3 (INSL3) and anti-Mullerian hormone (AMH); AMH secreted from fetal Sertoli cells results in regression of Mullerian ducts which prevents the formation of internal feminine genitalia, while INSL3 with testosterone controls the descent of the testis. There is also some evidence suggesting a shift from kisspeptin independent to KISS1/KISS1R-dependent GnRH-induced LH/FSH release from 30th week of gestation.[38] GnRH, thereafter, declines toward term coinciding with the development of functioning sex steroid negative feedback mechanisms from maternal placental oestrogens which lead to the suppression of the fetal HPG axis.[39]

Neonatal and childhood life: There is a postnatal surge in GnRH secretion or mini-puberty which stimulates testosterone production from the testis, peaking between 1 and 3 months of postnatal life. This transient activity of the HPT axis exhibits sexual dimorphism with higher LH in boys, while FSH predominates in girls. Clinically, a mild increase in testicular volume (TV) and penis is observed during mini-puberty. This period also provides a diagnostic window for early detection and treatment of congenital hypogonadotropic hypogonadism (CHH) (see section on congenital GnRH deficiency). Thereafter, GnRH, LH, and testosterone levels markedly decrease in amplitude by 6 months of age.[40] The HPT axis remains suppressed during childhood with low pulse frequency and low amplitude GnRH secretion (juvenile pause), low gonadotrophins, and sex steroids. During this period, diagnosis of hyper or hypogonadism is no longer possible until puberty. The precise mechanisms underlying this quiescent HPT axis are not elucidated. However, makorin ring finger protein 3, encoded by is the *MKRN3* gene, may be implicated in central inhibition of GnRH secretion such that the loss of function mutations of *MKRN3* result in the early activation of GnRH secretion and central precocious puberty.[41,42] Furthermore, androgen receptor expression remains low in the testis till about 4 years of age, hence why spermatogenesis does not occur in mini-puberty or infancy.

Puberty: Puberty is a complex process triggered by the sleep-entrained reactivation of the HPT axis with kisspeptin as the potential proximal stimulus[43] with marked increase in the amplitude of GnRH-induced LH pulses with more modest changes in frequency.[44] This nocturnal augmentation of LH secretion stimulates testicular testosterone with intratesticular testosterone levels up to 100 times those of systemic circulation boosting TV (to adult size, normal defined as >15mL on Prader orchidometer) and spermatogenesis. FSH stimulates Sertoli cells to secrete inhibin B which is an important biomarker of testicular function reflecting the pubertal maturation process and provides negative feedback of pituitary FSH secretion.[45] Leptin signaling is also postulated to be important for normal puberty, as reflected by identified gene mutations of leptin and its receptors causing CHH, presenting with delayed or absent puberty (and obesity).[26]

Adulthood: In the adult male, GnRH and gonadotropins are secreted in a high amplitude, regular pulsatile manner with parallel changes in testosterone levels. Testosterone has a diurnal rhythm with morning levels higher than at other times of the day; therefore, the diagnosis of adult-onset hypogonadism is recommended by checking early morning fasting testosterone levels.[46]

TESTOSTERONE AND ITS METABOLITES

In the postpubertal male, the testes contribute greater than 95% of circulating total testosterone (TT), with 5% of TT from adrenal glands. Free unbound form of testosterone (FT) represents 1% to 4% while the remainder is bound to carrier proteins: 65% to sex hormone-binding globulin (SHBG) with high affinity and 33% to albumin with low affinity. FT and albumin-bound testosterone is referred to as "bioavailable" testosterone to reflect the notion that albumin-bound testosterone can dissociate within tissue capillaries especially in organs with long transit times such as the liver and brain and become potentially available for tissue action.[1] These binding proteins play an important part in regulating the transport, distribution, metabolism, and biological activity of the sex steroid hormones. Changes in these carrier proteins particularly SHBG due to certain conditions such as obesity and aging can affect the level of TT and FT in men.[47] Testosterone is converted to 2 other active metabolites, oestradiol, and dihydrotestosterone from conversion by the aromatase or 5α reductase enzymes respectively, which can exert negative feedback and modulate gonadotropin release.

DISORDERS OF HYPOTHALAMIC-PITUITARY-TESTICULAR AXIS

The complex regulation of the HPT axis makes it susceptible to dysfunction by a variety of genetic or acquired insults resulting in different degrees of hypogonadism. We hereby discuss common congenital and acquired causes of hypothalamic-pituitary (secondary) and testicular (primary) hypogonadism (**Box 1**).

HYPOTHALAMIC-PITUITARY DYSFUNCTION/SECONDARY HYPOGONADISM
Congenital Gonadotropin-Releasing Hormone Deficiency

GnRH deficiency represents conditions with a failure of GnRH secretion, action, or impaired pituitary GnRH receptor function. Its phenotype varies with its age of onset (congenital vs acquired) and its severity. Biochemically, it is characterized by

---

Box 1
Congenital and acquired causes of primary and secondary hypogonadism

Secondary hypogonadism
  Congenital
    Genetic causes, for example, Kallmann syndrome, CHH
  Acquired
    Structural: hypothalamic-pituitary lesions, inflammatory diseases such as sarcoidosis, TB
    Functional: stress/excessive exercise, eating disorders
    Obesity
    Medications such as GnRH analogs, glucocorticoids, psychotropic agents
    Idiopathic

Primary hypogonadism
  Congenital
    Genetic causes, for example, Klinefelter syndrome and variants
    Congenital cryptorchidism
  Acquired
    Infections, for example, mumps orchitis
    Testicular trauma, torsion, or malignancy
    Chemotherapy, pelvic irradiation, or surgery
    Medications such as cimetidine, spironolactone, and flutamide
    Aging
    Idiopathic

Abbreviations: CHH, congenital hypogonadotropic hypogonadism; GnRH: gonadotropin releasing hormone; TB, tuberculosis.

---

inappropriately low gonadotropins in the context of low testosterone, in the absence of anatomic abnormalities in the hypothalamic and pituitary region, and otherwise normal anterior pituitary hormones.

- Isolated GnRH deficiency (IGD)

IGD is a multifaceted genetic disease with a global prevalence of 1 per 40,000 to 100,000 boys, with varying incidence in different populations.[48] Typically, patients with central hypogonadotropic hypogonadism and hyposmia or anosmia (hypoplasia or aplasia of olfactory bulbs) are given the diagnosis of Kallmann syndrome (KS) (50%–60% of all patients with IGD), and those with normal olfaction are diagnosed with normosmic CHH (40%–50% of all patients with IGD); albeit presence of both KS and CHH phenotypes can exist in the same family. CHH can be associated with a variety of developmental anomalies such as midline facial defects such as cleft lip/palate, renal agenesis, dental agenesis, or skeletal defects.[49]

- Prenatal/postnatal: Defective HPG axis activation during prenatal development is reflected by inappropriately low gonadotropins and testosterone in association with clinical signs at birth such as micro-penis, cryptorchidism, and/or micro-orchidism. These signs are related to the impairment of HPT axis ontogeny (see section above on the ontogeny of HPT axis) prenatally or at mini-puberty postnatally.
- Puberty: More typically, diagnosis of GnRH deficiency is made at adolescence with incomplete or failure of pubertal sexual development or delayed puberty which is defined as the absence of testicular development (TV < 4 mLs) by the age of 14 years in boys with subsequent initiation then arrest (partial puberty) or normal progression of sexual development[48]; the latter perhaps represents the mildest end of the phenotypic spectrum of IGD.

- Adulthood: Adult-onset CHH presents with symptoms of androgen deficiency and/or infertility. Interestingly, CHH reversal has been reported in 10% to 20% of patients, with normal activity of the HPT axis after the discontinuation of GnRH or gonadotropin treatment in adults, further reflecting its complex genotype–phenotype association.[50] However, prognostic characteristics to predict the reversal of CHH have not yet been identified with reported reversal even in the context of severe IGD.

Genetics: KS (IGD with anosmia) was originally thought to be a monogenic disorder secondary to mutation in the X-chromosome gene, KAL-1, that encodes anosmin-1, a protein involved in the embryonic migration of olfactory axons. However, IGD is now recognized to have a highly heterogeneous genetic component with an association with several genes expressed at multiple levels of the HPT axis (Table 1).[50] These include genes involved in correct embryonic development and migration of GnRH neurons such as KAL-1 and nasal embryonic LH releasing hormone factor (NELF), upstream genes involved in hypothalamic GnRH activation such as KISS1/KISS1R,[16]

Table 1
Gene mutations associated with congenital hypogonadotropic hypogonadism and Kallmann syndrome

Development and migration of GnRH Neurones (KS Phenotype: Anosmic HH)	Disruption of GnRH Secretion or its action on Pituitary* (Normosmic CHH) **CHH with Obesity	Both KS and CHH Phenotype
KAL1(ANOS1)	GNRH1	FGFR1
NELF	KISS1	FGF8
FGFR1	KISS1R (GPR54)	PROK2
FGF8	TAC3	PROK2R
PROK2	TAC3R	HS6ST1
PROK2R		CHD7
HS6ST1	GNRHR*	WDR11
CHD7		SEMA3A
WDR11	LEP**	SEMA3E
SEMA3A	LEPR**	CCDC141
SEMA3E		FEZF1
CCDC141		
FEZF1		

Abbreviations: ANOS1, anosmin1; CCDC141, coiled-coil domain containing 141; CHD7, CHARGE syndrome locus: eye coloboma, choanal atresia, growth and developmental retardation, genitourinary anomalies, ear anomalies; CHH, congenital hypogonadotropic hypogonadism; FEFF1, family zinc factor 1; FGF8, fibroblast growth factor 8; FGFR1, fibroblast growth factor receptor 1; GnRH1, gonadotropin-releasing hormone 1; GnRHR, GnRH receptor; HS6ST1, Heparin Sulfate 6-0-sulfotransferae 1; IGSF10, Immunoglobulin Superfamily Member10; KAL1, Kallmann syndrome interval-1; Kiss1, kisspeptin1; KISS1R, kisspeptin 1 receptor; KS: Kallmann syndrome; Lep, leptin; LEPR; leptin receptor; NELF, nasal embryonic luteinizing hormone-releasing hormone factor; PROK2, prokineticin 2; Prok2R, prokineticin 2 receptor; SEMA3A, semaphorin 3A; SEMA3E, semaphoring 3E; Tac3, tachykinin 3; Tac3R, tachykinin 3 receptor, WDR11, WD repeat-domain 11.
* is to identify gene mutation that causes disruption of GnRH action on pituitary.
** is to identify gene mutation that causes CHH with obesity.
Data from Refs.[3,33]

TAC3 and TAC3R,[51] or the action of GnRH itself on the pituitary, such as mutations in GnRH receptor, *GNRHR*.[52] Lastly, some genes have "overlapping" effects such as prokineticin 2 and its receptor (*PROK2/PROK2R*) and fibroblast growth factor receptor 1 and fibroblast growth factor 8 (*FGFR1/FGF8*) which may give overlapping KS and normosmic CHH phenotypes.[53] Lastly, leptin or leptin receptor mutations result in morbid obesity along with CHH[54] (see **Table 1**). The complex genetics and epigenetics contribute to the variable expressivity, penetrance, modes of inheritance (autosomal dominant, autosomal recessive or X linked), clinical phenotype, progression within and across IGD families. Despite recent acceleration in the discovery of mutations associated with congenital IGD, the genetic basis of around 50% of cases remains unknown.[49]

Acquired Gonadotropin-Releasing Hormone Deficiency

Acquired causes affect the HPT axis by either suppressing GnRH synthesis or secretion from hypothalamus or preventing GnRH from reaching the gonadotrophs by stalk injury or a pituitary defect. These are predominantly secondary to (1) structural or (2) functional abnormalities, albeit many causes remain idiopathic. Typically, these are patients who had age-appropriate puberty followed by postpubertal hypogonadism with near-normal testicular size (contrary to congenital GnRH deficiency). Biochemically, it is characterized by low or inappropriately normal gonadotropins in the context of low sex steroids (see **Fig. 1**). Hypogonadism may be transient or permanent. Obesity, chronic prescription opioid use, and anabolic-steroid withdrawal hypogonadism are commonly recognized causes of acquired HPT axis dysfunction.[55]

Structural

Structural lesions of the hypothalamus and/or pituitary can interfere with the normal pattern of GnRH synthesis, secretion, or stimulation of gonadotrophs. These include space-occupying lesions such as benign/malignant tumors, infiltrative/inflammatory disorders such as sarcoidosis, lymphocytic hypophysitis, or pituitary apoplexy. These patients can be distinguished from those with CHH or KS by the presence of multiple pituitary hormone deficiencies and/or by the identification of an anatomic lesion on MRI of the hypothalamic-pituitary region.[56] Men may present with either symptoms of hypogonadism such as low libido or erectile dysfunction, symptoms from other pituitary hormone excess or deficiency, or mass effect such as visual field defect or headache from the hypothalamic-pituitary lesion itself. One of the most common causes of acquired GnRH deficiency is hyperprolactinaemia, either from a functioning pituitary micro- or macro-adenoma or a hypothalamic/pituitary lesion with "stalk effect" that interrupts hypothalamic dopaminergic inhibition of prolactin secretion or iatrogenic from the use of dopamine antagonist medications. Prolactin inhibits hypothalamic *Kiss1* gene expression resulting in the suppression of downstream GnRH and gonadotropin secretion, whereas kisspeptin administration restored GnRH and gonadotropin secretion.[57]

Functional

HPT axis is sensitive to alterations in energy/nutritional balance, emotional stress, and illness.[58] These functional causes including eating disorders or chronic illnesses which may suppress the testosterone by suppressing central GnRH/LH pulses. Although it is primarily a disease recognized in women, nearly 5%–15% of all patients with anorexia nervosa are men.[59] Furthermore, moderate to severe dietary restriction in otherwise healthy men have been observed to decrease testosterone levels due to suppressed GnRH secretion;[60] albeit the suppression is reversible analogous to hypothalamic amenorrhoea in women. Similarly, longitudinal studies in men, especially in those engaging in ultraendurance exercise such as marathons have reported reductions in serum testosterone by up to 70%.[61] Proposed mechanisms include (1) central suppression of the HPT axis by the dysregulation of regulators of GnRH pulsatility, for example, KNDy neurones, leptin signaling, or proinflammatory cytokines[62] and (2) testosterone production disrupted by inhibitory hormones in a stress response cascade, for example, cortisol or prolactin.[63] Moreover, increased susceptibility to GnRH dysregulation in these energy deficit states may be governed by concomitant unidentified genetic factors.

- Obesity

Epidemiologic studies have concluded that obesity is an important factor associated with symptomatic low testosterone, overriding the effects of aging and other comorbidities.[64] In the large European Male Aging Study (EMAS), 73% of men with reduced testosterone were overweight or obese, and TT and FT of men with a body mass index (BMI) > 30 kg/m^2 was 5.1 nmol/L (30%) and 53.7 pmol/L (18%) lower, respectively, with decreased or unchanged LH compared with normal weight (BMI < 25 kg/m^2) men, suggestive of hypothalamic-pituitary dysfunction.[65] Similarly, among 1822 men from the Boston Area Community Health survey, central obesity was the most important contributor to symptomatic testosterone deficiency, more than age or overall health status.[4]

Several studies have reported a negative correlation between BMI and weight with TT, FT, testosterone:oestradiol ratio, and SHBG.[66,67] Some authors concluded that decreased SHBG allowed for normalization of FT in the context of low TT,[68] while others have observed a decrease in both FT and TT independent of the simultaneous decrease in SHBG.[65] Recent evidence has further highlighted the "bidirectional" relationship between obesity and hypogonadism, whereby low testosterone may further contribute to the accumulation of fat tissue because of reduced lipolysis.[55] In contrast, bariatric surgery is associated with an increase in TT, FT, and gonadotropins with reduction in oestradiol levels reflecting the reactivation of the HPT axis with weight loss.[69] Similarly, combined diet and exercise-induced weight loss were associated with increases in TT and FT when compared with baseline.[70]

Several key mechanisms have been implicated from animal and/or human studies to explain the obesity-associated HPT axis suppression[68,71,72]:

- Increased peripheral conversion of testosterone to oestradiol by aromatase enzyme in adipose tissue contributes to oestradiol-mediated negative HPT feedback
- Proinflammatory cytokines such as interleukin 2 (IL-2) have been shown to suppress the HPT axis both at the level of hypothalamus and Leydig cells
- Hyper-leptinaemia and hyper-insulinaemia secondary to leptin and insulin resistance of obesity leads to negative feedback at the hypothalamic (KNDy neurones) and pituitary (gonadotrophs) level suppressing the HPT axis.
- Decrease in SHBG production by the liver due to insulin resistance associated with obesity reduces the "travel capacity" of testosterone.
- Lastly, obesity is associated with other comorbidities that may independently contribute to HPT axis suppression such as sleep apnoea or hyperlipidemia.

- Medications

Numerous prescribed and nonprescribed medications have been reported to be associated with acquired GnRH deficiency. These include prolonged administration of GnRH analogs (eg, used in prostate cancer), glucocorticoids, and psychotropic agents which may suppress the intrinsic hypothalamic GnRH pulsatility.

Long-term glucocorticoids act at glucocorticoid receptors at the KNDy and GnRH neurones to suppress GnRH pulsatility; however, the exact mechanism in humans is not confirmed. One study of 16 men with chronic lung disease who received high dose glucocorticoid therapy for at least 1 month had mean TT reduction of nearly half of that of age and disease-matched controls.[73] Psychotropic drugs including antipsychotics, antidepressants and mood stabilizers modulate dopamine, serotonin, and GABA impairing hypothalamic-pituitary regulation of GnRH secretion.[74] Similarly, secondary hypogonadism is the most common endocrine side effect from chronic prescription opioid use and anabolic androgenic steroid (AAS) withdrawal. These 2 conditions have emerged as the 2 most prevalent antecedents of testosterone prescriptions in the United States. Androgens may cause hypothalamic hypogonadism due to negative feedback on the HPT axis. Furthermore, discontinuation of AAS may lead to the development of withdrawal symptoms. A recent study reported that these negative effects of androgen abuse on the HPT axis are slowly reversible (apart from SHBG and TV) in most men in 6 to 18 months after stopping androgen use.[75] Opioid use may inhibit KNDy neuronal activity and downregulate GnRH secretion. Antagonizing the opioid receptors with naloxone or naltrexone was found to increase GnRH and LH secretion.[76] A recent systematic review with 3250 patients using opioids for chronic pain or maintenance treatment of opioid addiction (with methadone being the most frequently used opioid) reported that factors including the type of opioid, higher doses, and longer durations of action were the strongest factors associated with the onset of secondary hypogonadism.[77]

In summary, many of these adverse effects of medication use or misuse are usually dose- and time-dependent, with increased accumulative risk with higher repeated doses, and improvements in hypogonadism with the cessation of therapy.

TESTICULAR FAILURE/PRIMARY HYPOGONADISM

Primary hypogonadism or hypergonadotropic hypogonadism occurs due to the failure of the testis to produce sufficient amounts of testosterone with compensatory "positive feedback" increase in pituitary gonadotropins. Klinefelter syndrome is the most common congenital cause of primary hypogonadism, while acquired forms of hypergonadotropic hypogonadism include mumps orchitis and male aging.

Congenital Primary Hypogonadism

Klinefelter syndrome and uncorrected cryptorchidism, the 2 main causes of primary hypogonadism are discussed below.

- Klinefelter syndrome

Klinefelter syndrome (Ks) is the most common genetic aneuploidy resulting in primary hypogonadism. It has a global prevalence of 1 in 500 to 1000 male live births.[78] The 47XXY karyotype is the most prevalent in 80% to 90% of patients with Ks; however, mosaicism with 47XXY/46XY (10%–20% of patients with Ks) leads to significant phenotypic variation and milder disease. Testicular germ cell degeneration begins in fetal and early postnatal life and accelerates during prepuberty. The classical phenotype is that of a small firm testis, gynaecomastia, and/or infertility (azoospermia). The endocrine profile reveals low-normal testosterone levels, raised LH and FSH, and undetectable inhibin B reflecting both seminiferous tubular degeneration and impaired Leydig cell function. Typical testicular histology may include extensive fibrosis, hyalinization of seminiferous tubules, loss of germ cells, Sertoli cell degeneration, and Leydig cell hyperplasia.[78] Patients with Ks have increased overall mortality and risk of cardiovascular disease, venous thromboembolism, breast and lung cancer, non-Hodgkin's lymphoma, and autoimmune diseases.

- Congenital cryptorchidism

Undescended testis (UDT) or cryptorchidism is the most common congenital urogenital malformation in boys. It is associated with impaired spermatogenesis due to Sertoli cell dysfunction; however, steroidogenesis may also be impaired due to Leydig cell dysfunction. Furthermore, germ cell loss in the UDT is proportional to the duration of the condition; therefore, it is recommended to correct with orchidopexy between 6 and 18 months of age to reduce the risk of infertility, androgen deficiency, and testicular cancer. INSL-3 together with testosterone during fetal development is suggested to be the main regulator of testicular descent, with novel mutations in INSL3 associated with cryptorchidism. Biochemically boys with UDT may have normal (or low) testosterone levels but slightly elevated LH levels compared with healthy boys; this high gonadotrophin drive may compensate for mild Leydig cell dysfunction in cryptorchidism.[79] Increasing recent evidence suggests that cryptorchidism, hypospadias, impaired spermatogenesis, and testicular cancer are components of "testicular dysgenesis syndrome" and maybe related to common genetic and environmental perturbations including the effects of endocrine-disrupting factors (EDC).[80] These EDCs may exert antiandrogenic effects or directly induce testicular toxicity. Several animal and in vitro studies have suggested that exposure to EDCs during different stages of life has dose-dependent antiandrogenic or direct toxic effects on steroidogenesis and spermatogenesis by impairing Leydig and Sertoli cell function, respectively.[81] However, clinical evidence is currently limited due to the inability to use interventional clinical trials (RCTs).

Acquired Primary Hypogonadism

Testes are vulnerable to injury from infections, trauma, malignancy, or medications. Other cases remain idiopathic.

- Epididymo-orchitis may be caused by mumps virus or other viruses such as echovirus or group B arbovirus, with 10% to 30% of cases being bilateral. Testicular function may recover completely in many men after orchitis; however, 30% to 50% of cases may develop testicular atrophy.[82] Pathogenesis involves lymphocyte infiltration of the testicular interstitial space with interstitial edema; however, the exact mechanism of Leydig cell dysfunction resulting in symptomatic hypogonadism is unknown. An observational study reported significantly increased mean basal LH and FSH even 10 to 12 months after the acute phase of mumps, despite normalizing of testosterone levels suggesting that mumps orchitis may impair Leydig cell function on a medium to long-term basis.[83]
- Testicular germ cell tumors are the most frequent type of cancer in postpubertal young men. Risk factors include uncorrected UDT, gonadal dysgenesis, and contralateral germ cell tumor. Nearly 25% of men with testicular malignancy develop symptomatic testosterone deficiency after treatment of the cancer.[84] Testicular surgery, radiotherapy, and chemotherapeutic agents can all cause Leydig and germ cell impairment resulting in hypogonadism.[85]
- Multiple medications have been reported to be associated with direct testicular dysfunction. These include cimetidine, spironolactone, and flutamide that have peripheral antiandrogenic effects by androgen receptor antagonism and/or inhibition of steroidogenic enzymes (17α-hydroxylase/17,20-lyase) involved in testosterone biosynthesis.[86]

CLINICS CARE POINTS

- Hypogonadism can be broadly subdivided into 2 categories: (1) primary (testicular) and (2) secondary (central or hypothalamic-pituitary) hypogonadism, according to whether the defect is inherent within the testes or lies outside of the testes.

- Age of onset, severity of androgen deficiency, and underlying cause of hypogonadism (congenital vs acquired) determine the signs and symptoms of the condition.

- Mini-puberty (1–2 months postnatal) provides a diagnostic window for early detection and treatment of congenital hypogonadotropic hypogonadism.

- Obesity is a risk factor for male hypogonadism and predominantly impairs central hypothalamic-pituitary function.

DISCLOSURE

The Section of Endocrinology and Investigative Medicine is funded by grants from the MRC, NIHR and is supported by the NIHR Imperial Biomedical Research Centre (BRC) Funding Scheme. The following authors have grant funding as follows: AS, Imperial College Healthcare Charity Fellowship; CNJ, NIHR Post-Doctoral Fellowship & Imperial BRC; WSD, NIHR Senior Investigator Award. The views expressed are those of the authors and not necessarily those of the above-mentioned funders, the NHS, the NIHR, or the Department of Health.

REFERENCES

1. Corradi PF, Corradi RB, et al. Physiology of the hypothalamic pituitary gonadal axis in the male. Urol Clin North Am 2016;43(2):151–62.
2. Lehman MN, Coolen LM, Goodman RL. Minireview: Kisspeptin/Neurokinin B/ Dynorphin (KNDy) cells of the arcuate nucleus: a central node in the control of gonadotropin-releasing hormone secretion. Endocrinology 2010;151(8): 3479–89.
3. Ross A, Bhasin S. Hypogonadism: its prevalence and diagnosis. Urol Clin North Am 2016;43(2):163–76.
4. Hall SA, Esche GR, Araujo AB, et al. Correlates of Low testosterone and symptomatic androgen deficiency in a population-based sample. J Clin Endocrinol Metab 2008;93(10):3870–7.
5. Salonia A, Rastrelli G, Hackett G, et al. Paediatric and adult-onset male hypogonadism. Nat Rev Dis Primers 2019;5(1):38.
6. Belchetz PE, Plant TM, Nakai Y, et al. Hypophysial responses to continuous and intermittent delivery of hypothalamic gonadotropin-releasing hormone. Science 1978;202(4368):631–3.
7. Clarke IJ, Cummins JT. The temporal relationship between gonadotropin releasing hormone (GnRH) and luteinizing hormone (LH) secretion in ovariectomized ewes. Endocrinology (Philadelphia) 1982;111(5):1737–9.
8. Levine JE, Pau KY, Ramirez VD, et al. Simultaneous measurement of luteinizing hormone-releasing hormone and luteinizing hormone release in unanesthetized, ovariectomized sheep. Endocrinology 1982;111(5):1449–55.
9. Ohkura S, Takase K, Matsuyama S, et al. Gonadotrophin-Releasing Hormone Pulse Generator Activity in the Hypothalamus of the Goat. J Neuroendocrinol 2009;21(10):813–21.
10. Pinilla L, Aguilar E, Dieguez C, et al. Kisspeptins and reproduction: physiological roles and regulatory mechanisms. Physiol Rev 2012;92(3):1235–316.

11. Nagae M, Uenoyama Y, Okamoto S, et al. Direct evidence that KNDy neurons maintain gonadotropin pulses and folliculogenesis as the GnRH pulse generator. Proc Natl Acad Sci U S A 2021;118(5). https://doi.org/10.1073/pnas.2009156118.

12. Kotani M, Detheux M, Vandenbogaerde A, et al. The Metastasis Suppressor Gene KiSS-1 Encodes Kisspeptins, the natural ligands of the orphan G protein-coupled Receptor GPR54. J Biol Chem 2001;276(37):34631–6.

13. Hrabovszky E, Ciofi P, Vida B, et al. The kisspeptin system of the human hypothalamus: sexual dimorphism and relationship with gonadotropin-releasing hormone and neurokinin B neurons. Eur J Neurosci 2010;31(11):1984–98.

14. Dhillo WS, Chaudhri OB, Patterson M, et al. Kisspeptin-54 stimulates the hypothalamic-pituitary gonadal axis in human males. J Clin Endocrinol Metab 2005;90(12):6609–15.

15. Jayasena CN, Nijher GMK, Comninos AN, et al. The effects of Kisspeptin-10 on reproductive hormone release show sexual dimorphism in humans. J Clin Endocrinol Metab 2011;96(12):E1963–72.

16. Seminara SB, Messager S, Chatzidaki EE, et al. The GPR54 Gene as a Regulator of Puberty. N Engl J Med 2003;349(17):1614–27.

17. de Roux N, Genin E, Carel J, et al. Hypogonadotropic hypogonadism due to loss of function of the KiSS1-Derived Peptide Receptor GPR54. Proc Natl Acad Sci U S A 2003;100(19):10972–6.

18. Comninos AN, Wall MB, Demetriou L, et al. Kisspeptin modulates sexual and emotional brain processing in humans. J Clin Invest 2017;127(2):709–19.

19. Sharma A, Thaventhiran T, Minhas S, et al. Kisspeptin and testicular function-is it necessary? Int J Mol Sci 2020;21(8):2958.

20. Topaloglu AK, Reimann F, Guclu M, et al. TAC3 and TACR3 mutations in familial hypogonadotropic hypogonadism reveal a key role for Neurokinin B in the central control of reproduction. Nat Genet 2009;41(3):354–8.

21. Skorupskaite K, George JT, Veldhuis JD, et al. Neurokinin 3 receptor antagonism decreases gonadotropin and testosterone secretion in healthy men. Clin Endocrinol (Oxf) 2017;87(6):748–56.

22. Jayasena CN, Comninos AN, De Silva A, et al. Effects of Neurokinin B Administration on reproductive hormone secretion in healthy men and women. J Clin Endocrinol Metab 2014;99(1):E19–27.

23. Young J, Bouligand J, Francou B, et al. TAC3 and TACR3 Defects Cause Hypothalamic Congenital Hypogonadotropic Hypogonadism in Humans. J Clin Endocrinol Metab 2010;95(5):2287–95.

24. Yen SS, Quigley ME, Reid RL, et al. Neuroendocrinology of opioid peptides and their role in the control of gonadotropin and prolactin secretion. Am J Obstet Gynecol 1985;152(4):485–93.

25. Guy-Grand B, Cassuto D, Dina C, et al. A mutation in the human leptin receptor gene causes obesity and pituitary dysfunction. Nature 1998;392(6674):398–401.

26. Farooqi IS, Wangensteen T, Collins S, et al. Clinical and molecular genetic spectrum of congenital deficiency of the leptin receptor. N Engl J Med 2007;356(3):237–47.

27. Wahab F, Atika B, Ullah F, et al. Metabolic Impact on the Hypothalamic Kisspeptin-Kiss1r Signaling Pathway. Front Endocrinol (Lausanne) 2018;9:123.

28. Jin L, Zhang S, Burguera BG, et al. Leptin and leptin receptor expression in rat and mouse pituitary cells. Endocrinology 2000;141(1):333–9.

29. El-Hefnawy T, Ioffe S, Dym M. Expression of leptin receptor during germ cell development in the mouse testis. Endocrinology 2000;141(7):2624–30.

30. Ishikawa T, Fujioka H, Ishimura T, et al. Expression of leptin and leptin receptor in the testis of fertile and infertile patients. Andrologia 2007;39(1):22–7.
31. Tena-Sempere M, Pinilla L, Gonzalez L, et al. Leptin inhibits testosterone secretion from adult rat testis in vitro. J Endocrinol 1999;161(2):211–8.
32. Landry D, Sormany F, Haché J, et al. Steroidogenic genes expressions are repressed by high levels of leptin and the JAK/STAT signaling pathway in MA-10 Leydig cells. Mol Cell Biochem 2017;433(1):79–95.
33. Abreu AP, Kaiser UB. Pubertal development and regulation. Lancet Diabetes Endocrinol 2016;4(3):254–64.
34. O'Shaughnessy PJ, Antignac JP, Le Bizec B, et al. Alternative (backdoor) androgen production and masculinization in the human fetus. PLoS Biol 2019; 17(2):e3000002.
35. Hagen C, McNeilly AS. The gonadotrophins and their subunits in foetal pituitary glands and circulation. J Steroid Biochem 1977;8(5):537–44.
36. Clements JA, Reyes FI, Winter JS, et al. Studies on human sexual development. III. Fetal Pituitary and Serum, and Amniotic Fluid Concentrations of LH, CG, and FSH. J Clin Endocrinol Metab 1976;42(1):9–19.
37. Castillo RH, Matteri RL, Dumesic DA. Luteinizing hormone synthesis in cultured fetal human pituitary cells exposed to gonadotropin-releasing hormone. J Clin Endocrinol Metab 1992;75(1):318–22.
38. Guimiot F, Chevrier L, Dreux S, et al. Negative Fetal FSH/LH Regulation in Late Pregnancy Is Associated with Declined Kisspeptin/KISS1R Expression in the Tuberal Hypothalamus. J Clin Endocrinol Metab 2012;97(12):E2221–9.
39. Massa G, de Zegher F, Vanderschueren-Lodeweyckx M. Serum levels of immunoreactive inhibin, FSH, and LH in human infants at preterm and term birth. Bio Neonate 1992;61(3):150–5.
40. Winter JS, Faiman C, Hobson WC, et al. Pituitary-gonadal relations in infancy. I. Patterns of serum gonadotropin concentrations from birth to four years of age in man and chimpanzee. J Clin Endocrinol Metab 1975;40(4):545–51.
41. Abreu AP, Dauber A, Macedo DB, et al. Central precocious puberty caused by mutations in the imprinted gene MKRN3. N Engl J Med 2013;368(26):2467–75.
42. Macedo DB, Abreu AP, Reis ACS, et al. Central precocious puberty that appears to be sporadic caused by paternally inherited mutations in the imprinted gene Makorin Ring Finger 3. J Clin Endocrinol Metab 2014;99(6):E1097–103.
43. Terasawa E, Guerriero KA, Plant TM. Kisspeptin and puberty in mammals. Kisspeptin Signaling in reproductive biology. New York: Springer New York; 2013. p. 253–73.
44. Boyar RM, Rosenfeld RS, Kapen S, et al. Human puberty. Simultaneous augmented secretion of luteinizing hormone and testosterone during sleep. J Clin Invest 1974;54(3):609–18.
45. Andersson A, Skakkebæk NE. Serum inhibin B levels during male childhood and puberty. Mol Cell Endocrinol 2001;180(1):103–7.
46. Dohle GR, Arver S, Bettocchi C, et al. Guidelines on male hypogonadism. Available at: https://uroweb.org/wp-content/uploads/EAU-Guidelines-Male-Hypogonadism-2015.pdf. Accessed 20 May, 2021.
47. Rastrelli G, Corona G, Cipriani S, et al. Sex hormone-binding globulin is associated with androgen deficiency features independently of total testosterone. Clin Endocrinol (Oxf) 2018;88(4):556–64.
48. Bonomi M, Vezzoli V, Krausz C, et al. Characteristics of a nationwide cohort of patients presenting with isolated hypogonadotropic hypogonadism (IHH). Eur J Endocrinol 2018;178(1):23–32.

49. Boehm U, Bouloux P, Dattani MT, et al. Expert consensus document: European Consensus Statement on congenital hypogonadotropic hypogonadism–pathogenesis, diagnosis and treatment. Nat Rev Endocrinol 2015;11(9):547–64.

50. Pitteloud N, Durrani S, Raivio T, et al. Complex genetics in idiopathic hypogonadotropic hypogonadism. Kallmann syndrome and hypogonadotropic hypogonadism. Basel (Switzerland): S. Karger AG; 2010. p. 142–53.

51. Ramaswamy S, Seminara SB, Ali B, et al. Neurokinin B Stimulates GnRH Release in the Male Monkey (Macaca mulatta) and Is Colocalized with Kisspeptin in the Arcuate Nucleus. Endocrinology (Philadelphia) 2010;151(9):4494–503.

52. Themmen APN, Huhtaniemi IT. Mutations of gonadotropins and gonadotropin receptors: elucidating the physiology and pathophysiology of pituitary-gonadal function. Endocr Rev 2000;21(5):551–83.

53. Pitteloud N, Acierno J, James S, et al. Mutations in fibroblast growth factor receptor 1 cause both kallmann syndrome and normosmic idiopathic hypogonadotropic hypogonadism. Proc Natl Acad Sci U S A 2006;103(16):6281–6.

54. Strosberg AD, Ozata M, Issad T, et al. A leptin missense mutation associated with hypogonadism and morbid obesity. Nat Genet 1998;18(3):213–5.

55. Carrageta DF, Oliveira PF, Alves MG, et al. Obesity and male hypogonadism: Tales of a vicious cycle. Obes Rev 2019;20(8):1148–58.

56. Kim SY. Diagnosis and treatment of hypopituitarism. Endocrinol Metab (Seoul) 2015;30(4):443–55.

57. Sonigo C, Bouilly J, Carré N, et al. Hyperprolactinemia-induced ovarian acyclicity is reversed by kisspeptin administration. J Clin Invest 2012;122(10):3791–5.

58. Rolih CA, Ober KP. The endocrine response to critical illness. Med Clin North Am 1995;79(1):211–24.

59. Robergeau K, Joseph J, Silber TJ. Hospitalization of children and adolescents for eating disorders in the State of New York. J Adolesc Health 2006;39(6):806–10.

60. Veldhuis JD, Iranmanesh A, Evans WS, et al. Amplitude suppression of the pulsatile mode of immunoradiometric luteinizing hormone release in fasting-induced hypoandrogenemia in normal men. J Clin Endocrinol Metab 1993;76(3):587–93.

61. Geesmann B, Gibbs JC, Mester J, et al. Association between energy balance and metabolic hormone suppression during ultraendurance exercise. Int J Sports Physiol Perform 2017;12(7):984–9.

62. Wong HK, Hoermann R, Grossmann M. Reversible male hypogonadotropic hypogonadism due to energy deficit. Clin Endocrinol (Oxf) 2019;91(1):3–9.

63. Brownlee KK, Moore AW, Hackney AC. Relationship between circulating cortisol and testosterone: influence of physical exercise. J Sports Sci Med 2005;4(1):76–83.

64. Tajar A, Forti G, O'Neill TW, et al. Characteristics of secondary, primary, and compensated hypogonadism in aging men: evidence from the european male ageing study. J Clin Endocrinol Metab 2010;95(4):1810–8.

65. Wu FC, Tajar A, Beynon JM, et al. Identification of late-onset hypogonadism in middle-aged and elderly men. N Engl J Med 2010;363(2):123–35.

66. Osuna CJA, Gomez-Perez R, Arata-Bellabarba G, et al. Relationship between BMI, total testosterone, sex hormone binding-globulin, leptin, insulin and insulin resistance in obese men. Arch Androl 2006;52(5):355–61.

67. Tsai EC, Matsumoto AM, Fujimoto WY, et al. Association of bioavailable, free, and total testosterone with insulin resistance: influence of sex hormone-binding globulin and body fat. Diabetes Care 2004;27(4):861–8.

68. Schneider G, Kirschner MA, Berkowitz R, et al. Increased estrogen production in obese men. J Clin Endocrinol Metab 1979;48(4):633–8.
69. Corona G, Rastrelli G, Monami M, et al. Body weight loss reverts obesity-associated hypogonadotropic hypogonadism: a systematic review and meta-analysis. Eur J Endocrinol 2013;168(6):829–43.
70. Håkonsen LB, Thulstrup AM, Aggerholm AS, et al. Does weight loss improve semen quality and reproductive hormones? results from a cohort of severely obese men. Reprod Health 2011;8(1):24.
71. Tsatsanis C, Dermitzaki E, Avgoustinaki P, et al. The impact of adipose tissue-derived factors on the hypothalamic-pituitary-gonadal (HPG) axis. Hormones (Athens) 2015;14(4):549–62.
72. Tena-Sempere M. Interaction between energy homeostasis and reproduction: central effects of leptin and ghrelin on the reproductive axis. Horm Metab Res 2013;45(13):919–27.
73. Macadams MR, White RH, Chipps BE. Reduction of serum testosterone levels during chronic glucocorticoid therapy. Ann Intern Med 1986;104(5):648–50.
74. Ilgin S. The adverse effects of psychotropic drugs as an endocrine disrupting chemicals on the hypothalamic-pituitary regulation in male. Life Sci 2020;253: 117704.
75. Shankara-Narayana N, Yu C, Savkovic S, et al. Rate and extent of recovery from reproductive and cardiac dysfunction due to androgen abuse in men. J Clin Endocrinol Metab 2020;105(6):1827–39.
76. Veldhuis JD, Rogol AD, Samojlik E, et al. Role of endogenous opiates in the expression of negative feedback actions of androgen and estrogen on pulsatile properties of luteinizing hormone secretion in man. J Clin Invest 1984;74(1): 47–55.
77. Wehbeh L, Dobs AS. Opioids and the hypothalamic-pituitary-gonadal (HPG) Axis. J Clin Endocrinol Metab 2020;105(9):e3105–13.
78. Aksglaede L, Link K, Giwercman A, et al. 47,XXY Klinefelter syndrome: Clinical characteristics and age-specific recommendations for medical management. Am J Med Genet C Semin Med Genet 2013;163C(1):55–63.
79. Toppari J, Kaleva M, Virtanen HE, et al. Luteinizing hormone in testicular descent. Mol Cell Endocrinol 2007;269(1):34–7.
80. Sharpe RM, Skakkebaek NE. Testicular dysgenesis syndrome: mechanistic insights and potential new downstream effects. Fertil Steril 2008;89(2):e33–8.
81. Sharma A, Mollier J, Brocklesby RWK, et al. Endocrine-disrupting chemicals and male reproductive health. Reprod Med Biol 2020. https://doi.org/10.1002/rmb2. 12326.
82. Senanayake SN. Mumps: a resurgent disease with protean manifestations. Med J Aust 2008;189(8):456–9.
83. Adamopoulos DA, Lawrence DM, Vassilopoulos P, et al. Pituitary-testicular inter-relationships in mumps orchitis and other viral infections. Br Med J 1978;1(6121): 1177–80.
84. Eberhard J, Ståhl O, Cwikiel M, et al. Risk factors for post-treatment hypogonad-ism in testicular cancer patients. Eur J Endocrinol 2008;158(4):561–70.
85. Nord C, Bjøro T, Ellingsen D, et al. Gonadal hormones in long-term survivors 10 years after treatment for unilateral testicular cancer. Eur Urol 2003;44(3):322–8.
86. Wang C, Lai C, Lam K, et al. Effect of cimetidine on gonadal function in man. Br J Clin Pharmacol 1982;13(6):791–4.

Diagnosis and Evaluation of Hypogonadism

Alvin M. Matsumoto, MD[a,b,]*

KEYWORDS

- Hypogonadism • Testosterone • Gonadotropins • Testes • Pituitary

KEY POINTS

- Symptoms and signs of testosterone deficiency should be established before testosterone testing and other causes of manifestations that could be managed without testosterone should be considered.
- In the presence of conditions that transiently suppress serum testosterone concentrations (eg, acute illness; certain medications, such as opioids; and states of energy deficit), laboratory testing for testosterone should be delayed until these conditions are completely resolved.
- The diagnosis of hypogonadism should be confirmed by measuring serum testosterone in the morning after an overnight fast on at least 2 separate days, using an accurate and reliable standardized total testosterone assay.
- In presence of conditions that alter sex hormone–binding globulin (SHBG) or of serum total testosterone concentrations near the lower limit of the normal adult male reference range (eg, 200–400 ng/dL [6.9–13.9 nmol/L]), free testosterone should be measured by an accurate method (ie, free testosterone by equilibrium dialysis or calculated free testosterone).
- Serum LH and FSH concentrations should be measured to distinguish primary from secondary hypogonadism and a specific etiology and whether the cause is reversible (functional) or irreversible (organic) to guide management.

INTRODUCTION

Over the last 20 years, large database surveys of several countries reported consistent two- to four-fold increases in the rates of testosterone testing and prescriptions from 2000 to 2014.[1] Increases in prescription rates were temporally associated with the availability of transdermal testosterone formulations and direct-to-consumer advertising of testosterone treatment of age-related symptoms associated with low serum

a Division of Gerontology & Geriatric Medicine, Department of Medicine, University of Washington School of Medicine, Seattle, WA, USA; b Geriatric Research, Education and Clinical Center, V.A. Puget Sound Health Care System, 1660 South Columbian Way (S-182-GRECC), Seattle, WA 98108, USA
* Geriatric Research, Education and Clinical Center, V.A. Puget Sound Health Care System, 1660 South Columbian Way (S-182-GRECC), Seattle, WA 98108.
E-mail address: alvin.matsumoto@va.gov

Endocrinol Metab Clin N Am 51 (2022) 47–62
https://doi.org/10.1016/j.ecl.2021.11.001
0889-8529/22/© 2021 Elsevier Inc. All rights reserved.

testosterone concentrations ("low T"). Following initial observational studies that reported possible increased cardiovascular events associated with testosterone treatment (although not confirmed in subsequent studies) and Food and Drug Administration warnings, testosterone prescription rates declined in 2014, but remained higher than in 2000.[1,2] These findings suggested considerable overtesting for testosterone that likely resulted in increased finding of low testosterone concentrations and subsequent overtreatment with testosterone.

The primary indication for testosterone treatment is a diagnosis of hypogonadism. According to evidence-based Endocrine Society clinical practice guidelines (published initially in 2006 and updated most recently in 2018), hypogonadism is defined as symptoms or signs of testosterone deficiency and consistently low serum testosterone concentrations on at least two occasions.[3] However, numerous studies found that testosterone therapy was often initiated in the absence of a diagnosis of hypogonadism as specified by guideline recommendations.[1] In these studies, a minority (10%–40%) of men had at least two testosterone measurements and 12% to 46% had no testosterone levels measured in the year before initiating testosterone therapy.

To avoid an inappropriate testosterone treatment, an accurate diagnosis of hypogonadism is imperative. However, for many practitioners, the nonspecific clinical manifestations of testosterone deficiency and complexities associated with serum testosterone measurements present challenges in making a proper diagnosis of hypogonadism. This review highlights these challenges and provides a systematic and practical approach to making a rigorous guideline-based diagnosis and evaluation of hypogonadism.

APPROACH TO THE DIAGNOSIS AND EVALUATION OF HYPOGONADISM

A structured approach is necessary to make a reliable diagnosis of hypogonadism and identify men who are the most appropriate candidates for testosterone replacement and the most likely to respond. The following is a summary of the orderly diagnostic strategy that is recommended to diagnose hypogonadism (**Fig. 1**):

- Establish the presence of symptoms and signs of testosterone deficiency.
- Consider other causes of largely nonspecific symptoms and signs that might be managed without testosterone treatment.
- Delay laboratory testing for testosterone until conditions that transiently suppress serum testosterone concentrations are completely resolved.
- Confirm the diagnosis of hypogonadism by measuring serum total testosterone in the morning after an overnight fast on at least 2 separate days, using an accurate and reliable standardized assay.
- Measure serum free testosterone using an accurate and reliable method in patients who have conditions that alter sex hormone–binding globulin (SHBG) or if serum total testosterone concentrations are near the lower limit of the normal adult male reference range.
- In men found to have hypogonadism, measure serum luteinizing hormone (LH) and follicle-stimulating hormone (FSH) concentrations to distinguish primary versus secondary hypogonadism.
- Establish the specific cause of hypogonadism and determine whether the cause of hypogonadism is a potentially reversible or treatable (functional hypogonadism) or an irreversible congenital or destructive disorder (organic hypogonadism) to guide management.

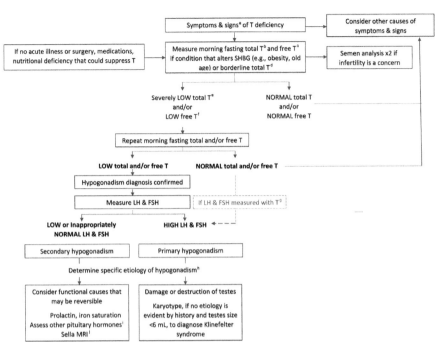

Fig. 1. Approach to the diagnosis and evaluation of hypogonadism. [a]Symptoms and signs of testosterone deficiency are summarized in **Table 1**. [b]Total testosterone should be measured in morning (7:00–10:00 AM) after an overnight fast, using an accurate and reliable standardized CDC-certified assay, or an assay that is certified by an accuracy-based quality control program. A harmonized reference interval for CDC-certified total testosterone assays in healthy, young nonobese men is 264 to 916 ng/dL (9.2–31.8 nmol/L).[19] If nonstandardized assays are used, total testosterone concentrations and reference ranges vary greatly depending on the specific assay and may not accurately identify men with hypogonadism. [c]Free testosterone should be measured by an accurate and reliable method, that is, free testosterone by equilibrium dialysis or calculated free testosterone (using total testosterone, SHBG, albumin concentrations, and published algorithms that yield values comparable with free testosterone by equilibrium dialysis). Direct free testosterone using tracer analogue immunoassays is inaccurate and should not be used. The reference range for free testosterone varies with the specific assay method used. [d]The indications for measurement of free testosterone by equilibrium dialysis or calculated free testosterone are summarized in **Table 2**. [e]If serum total testosterone concentration is severely low (eg, <150 ng/dL [5.2 nmol/L]), a free testosterone measurement is not needed. [f]If serum total and free testosterone are measured on initial laboratory evaluation, findings of a low total testosterone with free testosterone and normal to high-normal total testosterone with low free testosterone, that is, low free testosterone irrespective of total testosterone, concentrations are consistent with biochemical hypogonadism. [g]If serum LH and FSH are measured initially in conjunction with testosterone, a normal serum total and/or free testosterone associated with high LH and FSH concentrations suggests mild or subclinical hypogonadism (also known as compensated hypogonadism). [h]Specific causes of potentially reversible functional and irreversible organic etiologies of primary and secondary hypogonadism are summarized in **Table 4**. [i]If there is clinical evidence of hypopituitarism, sella abnormality on imaging, or polyuria, evaluation of other pituitary or hypothalamic hormones should be performed (eg, free thyroxine, morning cortisol or corticotropin stimulation test if clinical adrenal insufficiency is suspected, water deprivation test to exclude diabetes insipidus). [j]Sella MRI to exclude hypothalamic and/or pituitary tumor or infiltrative disease should be performed

PRESENCE OF CLINICAL MANIFESTATIONS OF TESTOSTERONE DEFICIENCY

Hypogonadism should be suspected in a man who has symptoms and signs of testosterone deficiency.[3] Therefore, before measuring serum testosterone and pursuing a diagnosis of hypogonadism, it is important to assess whether a man has clinical manifestations of testosterone deficiency. However, the symptoms and signs of testosterone are mostly nonspecific and occur commonly, especially in older men with multiple comorbidities. The symptoms and signs of testosterone deficiency are broadly classified as sexual, physical, and psychological manifestations (**Table 1**).

Clinical manifestations depend on the severity and duration of testosterone deficiency. Although uncommon, many individuals with congenital or structural disorders of the testes (eg, Klinefelter syndrome), or hypothalamus or pituitary gland (eg, congenital hypogonadotropic hypogonadism, androgen deprivation therapy in older men with prostate cancer) who have severe testosterone deficiency demonstrate most of the symptoms and signs summarized in **Table 1**.

Although most symptoms and signs of testosterone deficiency are nonspecific, eunuchoidism (inadequate sexual development), decreased androgen-dependent hair, and very small testes are specific signs that are characteristic of severe testosterone deficiency.[4] A clinical finding that is pathognomonic of severe prepubertal testosterone deficiency is eunuchoidism, which is characterized by extremely small penis and testes (prepubertal testis volume <2–4 mL), poorly developed scrotum, lack of androgen-dependent hair pattern (facial, axillary, chest, and pubic hair), a high-pitched voice, and a eunuchoidal body habitus (poor upper body muscle mass; prepubertal fat distribution in hips, chest, and face; and arms and legs >5 cm longer than height). Although usually detected in boys who present with delayed puberty, eunuchoidism may also be found in adult males who are not diagnosed at an earlier age. In men, decreased or loss of androgen-dependent hair is a specific sign of long-standing, severe testosterone deficiency. Decreased testes size is an indicator of impaired spermatogenesis because seminiferous tubules comprise 80% to 90% of the testes volume. However, very small testes (eg, <6 mL) are characteristic of Klinefelter syndrome, which is associated with impairments of testosterone and sperm production.

In contrast to these manifestations, other sexual, physical, and psychological symptoms and signs of testosterone deficiency are nonspecific and may be caused by coexisting comorbidities, illnesses, or medications. In addition to the severity and duration of testosterone deficiency, clinical manifestations of hypogonadism may be modified by previous testosterone therapy, age, comorbid conditions, medications, and variations in target-organ androgen sensitivity, all of which contribute to variability in clinical presentation.

Sexual symptoms, especially reduced libido (sexual interest or desire), loss of spontaneous (nighttime and morning) erections, erectile dysfunction, and reduced sexual

---

in men with severely low serum testosterone (eg, <150 ng/dL [5.2 nmol/L]), LH, and FSH concentrations; persistent hyperprolactinemia after discontinuation of medications that elevate prolactin; panhypopituitarism; or space-occupying tumor mass symptoms or signs (eg, new-onset headache, visual impairment, visual field defects, cerebrospinal fluid rhinorrhea). Computed tomography scan is sufficient to detect a pituitary macroadenoma and is useful to evaluate parasellar bone involvement. CDC, Centers for Disease Control and Prevention; FSH, follicle-stimulating hormone; LH, luteinizing hormone; SHBG, sex hormone–binding globulin; T, testosterone.

Table 1
Symptoms and signs of testosterone deficiency

Sexual	Physical	Psychological
Eunuchoidism	**Decreased androgen-dependent hair**	Decreased energy and vitality
Decreased libido	**Very small testes (eg, <6 mL)**	Decreased motivation and self-confidence
Decreased sexual activity	Gynecomastia	Depressed mood, irritability
Loss of spontaneous erections	Decreased muscle mass and strength	Hot flashes, sweats
Erectile dysfunction	Low bone density, osteoporosis	Sleep disturbance
Infertility	Normochromic, normocytic anemia	Poor concentration and memory

Signs in bold print are specific for prepubertal (eunuchoidism) or long-standing severe testosterone deficiency.

activity, are common symptoms of testosterone deficiency that are responsive to testosterone treatment. In the middle-aged and older male participants of the European Male Aging Study (EMAS), sexual symptoms (decreased frequency of sexual thoughts, erectile dysfunction, and decreased frequency of morning erections) demonstrated a stronger syndromic association with low serum testosterone concentrations (total testosterone <230–320 ng/dL [8–11 nmol/L] and free testosterone <64 pg/mL [220 pmol/L]) than physical or behavioral symptoms.[5] In healthy older men (aged 60–80 years) with experimental hypogonadism (induced by gonadotropin-releasing hormone [GnRH] agonist administration) who were treated with various doses of testosterone, sexual desire and erectile dysfunction were progressively decreased at serum testosterone concentrations less than 300 ng/dL (10.4 nmol/L), but significantly only at testosterone level less than 100 ng/dL (3.5 nmol/L), compared with placebo-treated men.[6] A meta-analysis of randomized, placebo-controlled clinical trials of testosterone treatment in men who had a morning total testosterone less than or equal to 300 ng/dL (10.4 nmol/L) and at least one symptom or sign of testosterone deficiency (a more rigorous diagnosis of hypogonadism than used in previous meta-analyses) found that testosterone treatment for 3 months or longer increased sexual desire, erectile function, and sexual satisfaction, but had no consistent significant effect on energy or mood.[7]

CONSIDER OTHER CAUSES OF SYMPTOMS AND SIGNS

Because the clinical manifestations of hypogonadism are nonspecific, it is important to consider the differential diagnosis or contribution of other causes of symptoms and signs to identify those that could be managed and treated independently of testosterone therapy.[4,8] Comorbid illnesses and conditions (eg, depression), and medications may contribute significantly to symptoms and signs consistent with testosterone deficiency. Consideration of other causes of symptoms and signs is particularly relevant for a patient who has an isolated or predominant symptom or sign consistent with testosterone deficiency. For example, in an older man who presents with low bone mineral density, potential contributing causes in addition to hypogonadism might include immobility or reduced activity, smoking, excessive alcohol intake, low calcium intake, vitamin D deficiency, medications (eg, glucocorticoids, anticonvulsants), and chronic kidney disease. Of note, in healthy older men with experimental hypogonadism induced by GnRH agonist treated with various doses of testosterone, L4 trabecular bone mineral density by computed tomography was only decreased in men who had serum testosterone levels less than 200 ng/dL (6.9 nmol/L), compared with placebo-treated men.[9]

DELAY LABORATORY TESTING UNTIL CONDITIONS THAT TRANSIENTLY SUPPRESS TESTOSTERONE ARE RESOLVED

Acute illness or surgery, use of certain medications (eg, opioids or glucocorticoids), and nutritional deficiency that causes an energy deficit (eg, eating disorders, malnutrition, or excessive exercise associated with inadequate energy intake) can transiently suppress gonadotropin and testosterone production.[3,4] Therefore, measurements should be delayed until these conditions are completely resolved to avoid an incorrect diagnosis of testosterone deficiency and hypogonadism and subsequent inappropriate testosterone therapy.

REPEATED FASTING MORNING TESTOSTERONE MEASUREMENTS USING AN ACCURATE ASSAY TO CONFIRM HYPOGONADISM

To confirm a diagnosis of hypogonadism in men with symptoms and signs of testosterone deficiency, serum total testosterone concentrations should be measured in morning (eg, 7:00–10:00 AM) samples after overnight fasting and measurements should be repeated on at least 2 separate days.[3] For the most rigorous and accurate diagnosis of hypogonadism, an accurate and reliable total testosterone assay should be used, preferably an assay that is standardized and certified by an accuracy-based quality control program (eg, Centers for Disease Control and Prevention [CDC] Hormone Standardization Program).

Serum testosterone levels exhibit a circadian variation with higher values in the morning that is blunted but still present in older compared with young men.[10] More than half of men older than 65 years of age who had low testosterone in the afternoon were found to have normal levels measured in the morning. Testosterone concentrations also demonstrate substantial day-to-day variability. Approximately 30% to 35% of men who had a single low testosterone level on initial sampling were subsequently found to have a normal testosterone level on repeat sampling.[11] In community-dwelling middle-aged to older men who had a single initial serum testosterone less than 250 ng/dL (8.7 nmol/L), 20% had an average testosterone greater than 300 ng/dL (10.4 nmol/L) on repeated sampling over the subsequent 6 months; a single testosterone measurement was inadequate to define an individual's serum concentrations.[12] In contrast, no men who had an initial average testosterone less than 250 ng/dL on two or more samples drawn on separate days had an average testosterone greater than 300 ng/dL on repeated sampling over the subsequent 6 months. Finally, testosterone levels are suppressed by glucose administration and food intake.[13,14] These finding provide a strong scientific rationale for using a standardized approach of repeated blood sampling in the morning after an overnight fast to reduce the influence of biologic variability of serum testosterone measurements that contributes to inaccurate diagnosis of hypogonadism.

Currently, most testosterone measurements are not standardized and performed by automated platform-based immunoassays and few are performed by mass spectrometry–based assays, which are more accurate but may not be standardized. As a result, testosterone assays exhibit considerable assay-to-assay variation in the values measured. A College of American Pathologists peer-based quality control sample from a hypogonadal man measured in 1133 laboratories using 14 different assays reported testosterone values that ranged from 45 to 365 ng/dL (1.6–12.7 nmol/L), that is, values that ranged from clearly hypogonadal to eugonadal concentrations.[15] In contrast, the same sample measured in five different mass spectrometry–based assays ranged from 60 to 72 ng/dL (2.1–2.5 nmol/L).[15] This extreme interassay and interlaboratory variability is caused by the lack of standardization of most total testosterone assays. As a result, measured values and reference ranges for total testosterone differ from assay-to-assay and laboratory-to-laboratory. The extreme variability in reference ranges is highlighted in two recent surveys of laboratories in the United States and United Kingdom. In 120 laboratories in the United States, the lower limit of the reference range ranged from 160 to 300 ng/dL (5.5–10.4 nmol/L) with the lower limit in 50% of laboratories less than or equal to 241 ng/dL (8.4 nmol/L).[16] In 60 laboratories in the United Kingdom, the lower limit of the reference ranges ranged 141 to 317 ng/dL (4.9–11 nmol/L) with the lower limit in 50% of laboratories less than 231 ng/dL (8.0 nmol/L).[17]

Clearly, the use of a uniform lower limit of normal, such as total testosterone less than 300 ng/dL (10.4 nmol/L) as used by some clinical practice guidelines,[18] is inappropriate for all total testosterone assays and results in an increasing likelihood of overdiagnosis or underdiagnosis of hypogonadism. The Endocrine Society clinical practice guideline recommends the use of a standardized testosterone assay, such as a CDC-certified assay or similar accuracy-based assay standardization program.[3] CDC-certified total testosterone assays (mostly mass spectrometry and some immunoassays) are listed and regularly updated at https://www.cdc.gov/labstandards/hs_certified_participants.html. Most major commercial reference laboratories offer CDC-certified total testosterone assays. However, clinicians should be careful when ordering because some reference laboratories offer CDC-certified and non-CDC-certified total testosterone assays.

A harmonized reference range that cross-calibrated testosterone values to CDC reference standards was established in 9054 community-dwelling men.[19] The harmonized reference range for young (18–39 year old), healthy, nonobese men was 264 to 916 ng/dL (9.2–31.8 nmol/L). This range is used as a uniform reference range for all CDC-certified total testosterone assays. If nonstandardized assays are used, total testosterone concentrations and reference ranges vary greatly depending on the specific assay and may not accurately identify men with hypogonadism.

Consistent use of accurate and reliable CDC-certified standardized assays in clinical trials of hypogonadism (eg, The Testosterone Trials[20]), clinical practice guidelines (eg, Endocrine Society guidelines[3]), and endocrine practice will facilitate translation of research findings to clinical practice. Standardized testosterone assays will also prevent an inaccurate diagnosis of hypogonadism with subsequent inappropriate testosterone treatment and potential adverse events and increased health care costs associated with treatment.

INDICATIONS FOR ACCURATE AND RELIABLE FREE TESTOSTERONE MEASUREMENTS

Serum total testosterone is affected by alterations in SHBG concentrations (**Table 2**) and the high level of assay imprecision in the total testosterone immunoassays in the low range increases the risk of misdiagnosis when the measured total testosterone concentrations are at or slightly higher or lower than the lower limit of the normal adult male reference range. Therefore, in men being evaluated for hypogonadism who have conditions that alter SHBG or serum total testosterone concentrations that are moderately higher or lower than the lower limit of the normal adult male reference range (eg, 200–400 ng/dL [6.9–13.9 nmol/L]), an accurate measurement of free testosterone (free

Table 2
Indications for free testosterone by equilibrium dialysis or calculated free testosterone

Conditions that Alter Sex Hormone-Binding Globulin	
Decreased SHBG Concentration	**Increased SHBG Concentration**
Obesity, type 2 diabetes mellitus	Advanced age
Androgens, progestins, glucocorticoids	Estrogens, anticonvulsants
Nephrotic syndrome	Hepatitis, hepatic cirrhosis
Untreated clinical hypothyroidism	Untreated clinical hyperthyroidism
Acromegaly	HIV disease
SHBG gene mutations or polymorphisms	SHBG gene polymorphisms
Borderline Total Testosterone Concentration: total testosterone around lower limit of normal range (200–400 ng/dL [6.9–13.9 nmol/L])	

Adapted from Bhasin S, Brito JP, Cunningham GR, et al. Testosterone Therapy in Men With Hypogonadism: An Endocrine Society Clinical Practice Guideline. *J Clin Endocrinol Metab.* 2018;103(5):1715-1744.

testosterone by equilibrium dialysis or calculated free testosterone estimate) should be used to confirm testosterone deficiency.[3]

In circulation, testosterone is mostly bound to serum proteins, primarily tightly bound to SHBG with high affinity and loosely bound to albumin with low affinity, and only 2% to 4% circulating testosterone is unbound to proteins, that is, free testosterone.[21] Free testosterone and loosely albumin-bound testosterone is referred to as bioavailable testosterone. According to the free hormone hypothesis, free testosterone is the biologically active circulating fraction and testosterone loosely bound to albumin can dissociate in capillaries and become potentially biologically available in some tissues with long capillary transit times (eg, liver and brain).

Serum total testosterone assays measure protein-bound and free testosterone. Therefore, conditions associated with alterations in SHBG concentrations (not necessarily outside the normal reference range) affect total testosterone levels in the same direction; conditions associated with low SHBG levels (eg, obesity) result in low total testosterone and conditions associated with high SHBG levels (eg, advanced old age) result in high total testosterone concentrations. Because free testosterone is the biologically active fraction that is regulated by negative feedback control of gonadotropin secretion, abnormalities in total testosterone caused solely by alterations of SHBG levels are typically not associated with abnormalities of free testosterone levels.

The importance of free testosterone levels on symptoms of testosterone deficiency is supported by findings in middle-aged to older men in EMAS.[22] Compared with eugonadal men who had normal total and free testosterone (≥303 ng/dL [10.5 nmol/L] and ≥65 pg/mL [226 pmol/L], respectively), men who had low total testosterone but normal free testosterone levels were more obese, had lower SHBG, and lacked sexual or physical symptoms of testosterone deficiency; in contrast, men with normal total testosterone but low free testosterone concentrations were older and in poorer health, and reported sexual and physical symptoms of testosterone deficiency. In a subsequent prospective study, eugonadal men in EMAS who had normal total (≥303 ng/dL [10.5 nmol/L]) and free testosterone (≥49 pg/mL [170 nmol/L]) and normal LH (>9.4 IU/L) were followed for a median of 4.3 years.[23] At follow-up, most (93.2%) remained persistently eugonadal, but based on total testosterone concentrations, 6.8% developed apparent secondary hypogonadism with low total testosterone and normal LH levels. However, of the men who had low total testosterone concentrations, only those who also had low free testosterone levels developed or had worsening of sexual symptoms of testosterone deficiency (decreased sexual thoughts, erectile dysfunction, and decreased morning erections), compared with those with low total testosterone but normal free testosterone concentrations and eugonadal men who remained persistently free of sexual symptoms. Finally, a man who demonstrated undetectable SHBG because of a homozygous missense mutation of SHBG and very low serum total, but normal free testosterone was found to have normal serum gonadotropins, semen analysis, and sexual development, supporting the importance of free rather than total testosterone on these sensitive objective indicators of testosterone action.[24]

In a large cohort of men (3672 male Veterans; mean age, 59.7 years) who had laboratory evaluation with a panel comprised of total testosterone, SHBG, and albumin measurements and calculated free testosterone, 61.7% of men with low total testosterone had normal calculated free testosterone (<34 pg/mL [118 pmol/L]), whereas only 38.3% of those with low total testosterone had low calculated free testosterone; 2.1% of men with normal total testosterone had low calculated free testosterone.[25] These results suggest that reliance only on total testosterone concentrations could result in considerable overdiagnosis of testosterone deficiency and hypogonadism. In these men, low free testosterone could be excluded reliably only when total testosterone exceeded 350 to 400 ng/dL (12.1–13.9 nmol/L) and low free testosterone could only be reliably predicted when total testosterone was less than 150 to 200 ng/dL (5.2–6.9 nmol/L). Therefore, measurement of free testosterone in men with total testosterone concentrations 200 to 400 ng/dL (6.9–13.9 nmol/L) should improve the accuracy of biochemical evaluation of hypogonadism. In men with very low total testosterone levels (eg, <150 ng/dL [5.2 nmol/L]), free testosterone measurements are not needed because the likelihood of finding a normal free testosterone is extremely low.

Accurate and reliable methods that are available to measure serum free testosterone concentrations include equilibrium dialysis and calculated free testosterone.[3,21] Preferably, free testosterone should be measured by an equilibrium dialysis method, the gold standard method. If equilibrium dialysis is not accessible, clinically useful accurate estimates of free testosterone relative to equilibrium dialysis is calculated using measurements of total testosterone, SHBG, and albumin concentrations and various published formulae that use algorithms based on the binding affinity of testosterone to SHBG and albumin. However, it is important to recognize that the accuracy of calculated free testosterone values depends on the accuracy of total testosterone, SHBG, and albumin assays. Therefore, calculated free testosterone values should be cross-calibrated against those measured using equilibrium dialysis. Recent studies suggest that SHBG circulates as a dimer with allosterically coupled binding sites on each of the two monomers; the binding of testosterone to SHBG is a multistep process that involves an allosteric interaction between the two binding sites.[21,26] Calculated free testosterone estimates using an ensemble allosteric model yielded free testosterone concentrations that closely approximated those measured by equilibrium dialysis.

Accurate and reliable free testosterone assays are not available in most local laboratories. Therefore, free testosterone by equilibrium dialysis and calculated free testosterone should be measured in a dependable reference laboratory. Limitations of using free testosterone by equilibrium dialysis and calculated free testosterone concentrations in practice are the lack of assay standardization, an accuracy-based quality control program, and a harmonized reference range. Until these limitations are addressed, free testosterone by equilibrium dialysis and calculated free testosterone should use reference ranges established by individual laboratories or their specific assay method.

Many local laboratories and some reference laboratories still measure direct free testosterone levels by a testosterone tracer analogue immunoassay on an automated assay platform. Free testosterone immunoassays are inaccurate, resulting in values that are an order of magnitude lower than free testosterone by equilibrium dialysis and calculated free testosterone and they should not be used to evaluate men for hypogonadism.[21] Bioavailable testosterone is measured by an ammonium sulfate precipitation method, which is technically demanding or calculated from total testosterone, SHBG, and albumin measurements using the same algorithms that are used for calculating free testosterone. The major limitation of using bioavailable testosterone concentrations for clinical evaluation is the relative lack of clinical studies of testosterone deficiency and hypogonadism using bioavailable compared with those using free testosterone levels.

MEASURE GONADOTROPIN CONCENTRATIONS TO DISTINGUISH PRIMARY VERSUS SECONDARY HYPOGONADISM

If a diagnosis of hypogonadism is confirmed, serum gonadotropin, LH, and FSH concentrations should be measured to determine whether the origin of hypogonadism is a disorder of the testes (primary hypogonadism), or pituitary or hypothalamus (secondary hypogonadism).[3,4] Serum LH and FSH should be measured in the same sample as testosterone, usually together with a repeat testosterone measurement after an initial low testosterone level or less commonly with an initial testosterone measurement.

Men with primary hypogonadism exhibit repeatedly low testosterone with simultaneously high LH and FSH concentrations (FSH typically being higher than LH). High LH levels indicate reduced testosterone negative feedback and production by Leydig cells of the testes. High FSH levels indicate seminiferous tubule dysfunction (reflecting reduced inhibin B negative feedback) and impaired sperm production but is a more sensitive indicator of primary testicular dysfunction than high LH levels. If high LH and FSH are measured in the same sample as an initial testosterone measurement, men with normal serum testosterone with high LH and/or FSH concentrations might be identified. These men have mild or subclinical primary hypogonadism (also called compensated hypogonadism), analogous to subclinical hypothyroidism.

Men with secondary hypogonadism demonstrate repeatedly low testosterone with simultaneously low or inappropriately normal LH and FSH levels. Some causes of hypogonadism are associated with defects in the testes and pituitary or hypothalamus, which is combined primary and secondary hypogonadism. However, in most cases, a hormone profile of either primary or secondary hypogonadism predominates. For example, in men with hemochromatosis, iron overload results in defects in the testes and pituitary but the latter is the dominant defect that results in gonadotropin deficiency and a hormone profile of low serum testosterone and low gonadotropin concentrations consistent with secondary hypogonadism.[27]

Serum LH and FSH measurements are usually performed by automated platform-based immunoassays. Most LH and FSH assays have sufficient sensitivity to distinguish low-normal from low values but are susceptible to immunoassay interference (eg, by high-dose biotin use). Although gonadotropin assays are not standardized, differences in values and reference ranges are small. The reference ranges for serum LH and FSH concentrations in well-characterized, healthy fertile young men are 1.6 to 8.0 IU/L and 1.3 to 8.4 IU/L, respectively.[28] Assays with upper limits of reference range higher LH and FSH levels probably included older men or men with unrecognized impairment of spermatogenesis.

Distinguishing whether a patient has primary from secondary hypogonadism is clinically important.[3,4] Secondary hypogonadism is caused by a pituitary or hypothalamic tumor that might result in deficiency of or be associated with hypersecretion of other pituitary hormones and space-occupying tumor mass effects (eg, headaches, visual field defects, hydrocephalus, or cerebrospinal fluid rhinorrhea) that may require further management. Also, secondary hypogonadism is commonly caused by potentially reversible gonadotropin suppression in the presence a functionally intact hypothalamic-pituitary-testicular axis (ie, functional hypogonadism), whereas causes of primary hypogonadism are usually caused by irreversible pathologic disease (ie, organic hypogonadism). Finally, infertility caused by impaired spermatogenesis caused by gonadotropin deficiency in secondary hypogonadism is treatable with gonadotropin (or GnRH)-replacement therapy. In contrast, infertility caused by primary hypogonadism is usually not treatable with hormone therapy and requires other fertility options (eg, assisted reproductive technologies).

It is essential that LH and FSH are measured before initiating testosterone therapy. However, it is not uncommon that testosterone therapy is started without measurement of gonadotropin levels. In this situation, testosterone should be discontinued for at least 2 to 4 weeks for short-acting (transdermal, oral, transbuccal), 2 to 3 months for intermediate-acting (intramuscular testosterone cypionate or enanthate), and 6 to 12 months for long-acting (intramuscular testosterone undecanoate and testosterone pellets) before measuring testosterone and gonadotropins. However, even with more prolonged discontinuation of testosterone therapy, some men may experience persistent gonadotropin and testosterone suppression, especially older men and those receiving high dosages of exogenous testosterone for long periods of time.

FURTHER EVALUATION OF SPECIFIC CAUSE OF FUNCTIONAL VERSUS ORGANIC HYPOGONADISM

After determining whether a patient has primary or secondary hypogonadism, further evaluation should be performed to establish the specific cause of hypogonadism to guide further management, including the need for testosterone therapy.[3,4]

It is important to determine whether a man with hypogonadism has organic hypogonadism or functional hypogonadism to guide management (**Table 3**).[3,4,8] Organic (also known as "classical") hypogonadism is caused by irreversible structural, destructive, infiltrative, developmental, or congenital disorders of reproductive axis. Generally, it results in severe symptoms and signs of testosterone deficiency and consistently and severely low serum testosterone and high (primary organic hypogonadism) or distinctly low (secondary organic hypogonadism) serum LH and FSH concentrations for which testosterone treatment is indicated. In contrast, functional hypogonadism is caused by potentially reversible or treatable testosterone or gonadotropin suppression. Functional hypogonadism is more common than organic hypogonadism and it usually results in mild symptoms and signs of testosterone deficiency and slightly low serum testosterone and slightly high (functional primary hypogonadism) or normal to low-normal (functional secondary hypogonadism) LH and FSH levels. Some causes of functional secondary hypogonadism, such as long-acting opioid use, result in severe clinical manifestations of testosterone deficiency and severely low serum testosterone, LH, and FSH concentrations. Management of functional hypogonadism should initially focus on treatment of the underlying causative condition (eg, weight loss for obesity) or discontinuation of the offending medication (eg, glucocorticoids) rather than testosterone treatment. However, in men who have severe functional hypogonadism that is not readily reversible or treatable (eg, men taking methadone for opioid

Table 3
Comparison of organic versus functional hypogonadism

	Organic Hypogonadism	Functional Hypogonadism
Etiology	Irreversible pathologic HPT axis disease Structural, destructive, or congenital disorder	Potentially reversible, intact HPT axis Comorbidities or medications
Symptoms	Low libido, loss of spontaneous erections Severe	Erectile dysfunction, low energy, depressed mood Mild, occasionally severe
Signs	Eunuchoidism, loss of male hair, small testes	None
Serum T level	Consistently and severely low	Fluctuating, slightly low, occasionally severely low
Serum LH and FSH	Unequivocally high (primary) or low (secondary)	Slightly high (primary) or normal (secondary), occasionally low
Relationship of symptoms/ signs to low T	Causal	Ambiguous, confounded by comorbidities or medications
Treatment	T treatment indicated	Treatment of underlying condition or discontinuation of offending medication; T treatment, if irreversible or incompletely treated

Abbreviations: HPT, hypothalamic-pituitary-testicular; T, testosterone.

use disorder), testosterone treatment could be considered after acknowledgment and discussion of the inadequacy of high-quality evidence for potential benefits and risks of testosterone treatment.

Age-related hypogonadism in middle-aged to older men is mostly related to functional secondary hypogonadism and gonadotropin suppression caused by age-associated comorbidities (eg, obesity, illness, and use of medications). However, advanced age men (eg, >75 years of age) develop organic primary hypogonadism and testicular failure with elevated gonadotropin levels and reduced testicular responsiveness to LH and human chorionic gonadotropin.[29]

Evaluation to identify the specific cause of primary or secondary hypogonadism should begin with a careful history and physical examination.[4] In men with primary hypogonadism, evaluation should include inquiry about a history of undescended testes; mumps with testicular involvement; testes damage, torsion, or surgery; medications that reduce testosterone production (eg, alkylating agents); and end-stage kidney disease. In men with secondary hypogonadism, assessment should include questioning regarding a history of delayed puberty; anosmia or hyposmia; tumor mass symptoms (eg, headache, peripheral vison loss); hypothalamic/pituitary disease or surgery; trauma brain injury; medications that suppress gonadotropin secretion (eg, long-acting opioids, anabolic steroids, glucocorticoids); morbid obesity; reduced energy intake; excessive exercise; wasting syndromes; alcohol use disorder; type 2 diabetes mellitus; and chronic liver, heart, or lung failure.

If no cause is apparent in a man with primary hypogonadism and very small testes less than 6 mL (normal testis volume is 15–30 mL), a karyotype should be ordered to

Table 4
Causes of hypogonadism

Primary Hypogonadism		Secondary Hypogonadism	
Organic	**Functional**	**Organic**	**Functional**
Klinefelter syndrome and variants	End-stage renal disease*	Iron overload (eg, hemochromatosis, transfusion-associated)*	Opioid, anabolic steroid, progestin use, estrogen excess, glucocorticoid excess (Cushing syndrome)*, GnRH agonist/antagonist (for treatment of prostate cancer)
Testis damage, trauma, torsion, irradiation, orchidectomy	Malignancy (testicular cancer, lymphoma)	Hypothalamic or pituitary tumor	Severe obesity, obstructive sleep apnea
Bilateral cryptorchidism (uncorrected)	Androgen synthesis inhibitors (for treatment of prostate cancer)	Hypothalamic or pituitary infiltrative or destructive disease, irradiation, hypophysectomy	Relative energy deficit (energy expenditure/ exercise > energy/ food intake), malnutrition
Orchitis		Severe traumatic brain injury	Hyperprolactinemia
Cancer chemotherapy drugs (eg, alkylating agents)		Pituitary stalk section	Alcohol abuse*
Myotonic dystrophy, congenital disorders (eg, anorchia)		Congenital hypogonadotropic hypogonadism (isolated or associated with complex syndromes)	Chronic systemic disease (eg, type 2 diabetes, HIV disease), organ failure (liver, heart, respiratory failure)*
Advanced older age (eg, >75 y)			Comorbid illness– associated with aging

* denotes combined primary and secondary hypogonadism.
Adapted from Bhasin S, Brito JP, Cunningham GR, et al. Testosterone Therapy in Men With Hypogonadism: An Endocrine Society Clinical Practice Guideline. J Clin Endocrinol Metab. 2018;103(5):1715-1744.

diagnose Klinefelter syndrome.[3] In men with secondary hypogonadism, initial laboratory evaluation should include serum prolactin (to exclude hyperprolactinemia) and iron saturation (to screen for iron overload syndromes, such as hemochromatosis). If there is clinical evidence of hypopituitarism or unprovoked polyuria, assessment of other pituitary or hypothalamic hormones (eg, free T4, morning cortisol or corticotropin stimulation test if clinical suspicion of adrenal insufficiency, water deprivation test to exclude diabetes insipidus) should be performed. Sella MRI to exclude pituitary and/or hypothalamic tumors or infiltrative disease should be performed in men with severely low serum testosterone (eg, <150 ng/dL [5.2 nmol/L]), LH, and FSH concentrations; persistent hyperprolactinemia after discontinuation of medications that elevate prolactin; panhypopituitarism; or tumor mass symptoms or signs (eg, new-onset headache, visual impairment, visual field defects, cerebrospinal fluid rhinorrhea).

If fertility is an important concern and a man presents with infertility (inability of a sexually active couple to conceive after a year of unprotected intercourse) with or without co-occurring testosterone deficiency, seminal fluid analysis should be performed on an ejaculated semen sample obtained by masturbation after a 2- to 7-day period of abstinence from ejaculation.[3,4] Given the extreme variability in sperm concentrations, seminal fluid analysis should be performed on at least two occasions (separated by at least 1–2 weeks). World Health Organization criteria (based on men whose partners became pregnant in 1 year or less) for normal semen parameters include: sperm concentration greater than or equal to 15 million/mL; volume greater than or equal to 1.5 mL; count greater than or equal to 39 million/ejaculate; sperm motility greater than or equal to 40%; and morphology greater than or equal to 4% strict normal forms.[30]

In older men (especially, men >70 years old) who are at risk for falls and bone fractures, assessment of bone mineral density to exclude the presence of osteoporosis is advisable.[3,4]

CLINICS CARE POINTS

- When considering a diagnosis of hypogonadism, look for clinical manifestations of hypogonadism, especially poor sexual development, decreased male hair, and very small testes (eg, <6 mL).
- Before laboratory testing, consider causes of nonspecific symptoms and signs other than hypogonadism and rule out conditions that could transiently suppress serum testosterone levels.
- To confirm the diagnosis of hypogonadism, measure serum total testosterone in the morning after an overnight fast on at least 2 separate days, using an accurate and reliable standardized assay, or free testosterone (by equilibrium dialysis or calculated) in men who have conditions that alter sex hormone–binding globulin or if serum total testosterone concentrations are moderately lower or higher than the lower normal range.
- To determine whether the origin of testosterone deficiency is primary (testes) or secondary (hypothalamus or pituitary) hypogonadism, measure serum luteinizing hormone and follicle-stimulating hormone together with testosterone.
- To guide subsequent management, determine the specific cause of hypogonadism and whether it is potentially reversible or treatable (functional hypogonadism) or an irreversible congenital or destructive (organic hypogonadism) disorder.

ACKNOWLEDGMENTS

Dr. Matsumoto was supported by the Department of Veterans Affairs Geriatric Research, Education and Clinical Center and Puget Sound Health Care System.

DISCLOSURE

No disclosures.

REFERENCES

1. Jasuja GK, Bhasin S, Rose AJ. Patterns of testosterone prescription overuse. Curr Opin Endocrinol Diabetes Obes 2017;24(3):240–5.

2. Baillargeon J, Kuo YF, Westra JR, et al. Testosterone prescribing in the United States, 2002-2016. Jama 2018;320(2):200–2.

3. Bhasin S, Brito JP, Cunningham GR, et al. Testosterone therapy in men with hypogonadism: an Endocrine Society Clinical Practice Guideline. J Clin Endocrinol Metab 2018;103(5):1715–44.

4. Matsumoto AM, Anawalt BD. Testicular disorders. In: Melmed S, Auchus RJ, Goldfine AB, et al, editors. Williams textbook of endocrinology. 14th edition. Philadelphia (PA): Elsevier, Inc.; 2020. p. 668–755.

5. Wu FC, Tajar A, Beynon JM, et al. Identification of late-onset hypogonadism in middle-aged and elderly men. N Engl J Med 2010;363(2):123–35.

6. Finkelstein JS, Lee H, Burnett-Bowie SM, et al. Dose-response relationships between gonadal steroids and bone, body composition, and sexual function in aging men. J Clin Endocrinol Metab 2020;105(8):2779–88.

7. Ponce OJ, Spencer-Bonilla G, Alvarez-Villalobos N, et al. The efficacy and adverse events of testosterone replacement therapy in hypogonadal men: a systematic review and meta-analysis of randomized, placebo-controlled trials. J Clin Endocrinol Metab 2018;103(5):1745–54.

8. Matsumoto AM. Testosterone administration in older men. Endocrinol Metab Clin North Am 2013;42(2):271–86.

9. Finkelstein JS, Lee H, Leder BZ, et al. Gonadal steroid-dependent effects on bone turnover and bone mineral density in men. J Clin Invest 2016;126(3):1114–25.

10. Brambilla DJ, Matsumoto AM, Araujo AB, et al. The effect of diurnal variation on clinical measurement of serum testosterone and other sex hormone levels in men. J Clin Endocrinol Metab 2009;94(3):907–13.

11. Swerdloff RS, Wang C, Cunningham G, et al. Long-term pharmacokinetics of transdermal testosterone gel in hypogonadal men. J Clin Endocrinol Metab 2000;85(12):4500–10.

12. Brambilla DJ, O'Donnell AB, Matsumoto AM, et al. Intraindividual variation in levels of serum testosterone and other reproductive and adrenal hormones in men. Clin Endocrinol (Oxf) 2007;67(6):853–62.

13. Caronia LM, Dwyer AA, Hayden D, et al. Abrupt decrease in serum testosterone levels after an oral glucose load in men: implications for screening for hypogonadism. Clin Endocrinol (Oxf) 2013;78(2):291–6.

14. Plumelle D, Lombard E, Nicolay A, et al. Influence of diet and sample collection time on 77 laboratory tests on healthy adults. Clin Biochem 2014;47(1–2):31–7.

15. Rosner W, Auchus RJ, Azziz R, et al. Position statement: utility, limitations, and pitfalls in measuring testosterone: an Endocrine Society position statement. J Clin Endocrinol Metab 2007;92(2):405–13.

16. Le M, Flores D, May D, et al. Current practices of measuring and reference range reporting of free and total testosterone in the United States. J Urol 2016;195(5):1556–61.

17. Livingston M, Downie P, Hackett G, et al. An audit of the measurement and reporting of male testosterone levels in UK clinical biochemistry laboratories. Int J Clin Pract 2020;74(11):e13607.

18. Mulhall JP, Trost LW, Brannigan RE, et al. Evaluation and management of testosterone deficiency: AUA Guideline. J Urol 2018;200(2):423–32.

19. Travison TG, Vesper HW, Orwoll E, et al. Harmonized reference ranges for circulating testosterone levels in men of four cohort studies in the United States and Europe. J Clin Endocrinol Metab 2017;102(4):1161–73.

20. Snyder PJ, Bhasin S, Cunningham GR, et al. Effects of testosterone treatment in older men. N Engl J Med 2016;374(7):611–24.
21. Goldman AL, Bhasin S, Wu FCW, et al. A reappraisal of testosterone's binding in circulation: physiological and clinical implications. Endocr Rev 2017;38(4): 302–24.
22. Antonio L, Wu FC, O'Neill TW, et al. Low free testosterone is associated with hypogonadal signs and symptoms in men with normal total testosterone. J Clin Endocrinol Metab 2016;101(7):2647–57.
23. Rastrelli G, O'Neill TW, Ahern T, et al. Symptomatic androgen deficiency develops only when both total and free testosterone decline in obese men who may have incident biochemical secondary hypogonadism: prospective results from the EMAS. Clin Endocrinol (Oxf) 2018;89(4):459–69.
24. Vos MJ, Mijnhout GS, Rondeel JM, et al. Sex hormone binding globulin deficiency due to a homozygous missense mutation. J Clin Endocrinol Metab 2014;99(9): E1798–802.
25. Anawalt BD, Hotaling JM, Walsh TJ, et al. Performance of total testosterone measurement to predict free testosterone for the biochemical evaluation of male hypogonadism. J Urol 2012;187(4):1369–73.
26. Zakharov MN, Bhasin S, Travison TG, et al. A multi-step, dynamic allosteric model of testosterone's binding to sex hormone binding globulin. Mol Cell Endocrinol 2015;399:190–200.
27. McDermott JH, Walsh CH. Hypogonadism in hereditary hemochromatosis. J Clin Endocrinol Metab 2005;90(4):2451–5.
28. Sikaris K, McLachlan RI, Kazlauskas R, et al. Reproductive hormone reference intervals for healthy fertile young men: evaluation of automated platform assays. J Clin Endocrinol Metab 2005;90(11):5928–36.
29. Kaufman JM, Lapauw B, Mahmoud A, et al. Aging and the male reproductive system. Endocr Rev 2019;40(4):906–72.
30. Cooper TG, Noonan E, von Eckardstein S, et al. World Health Organization reference values for human semen characteristics. Hum Reprod Update 2010;16(3): 231–45.

Accurate Measurement and Harmonized Reference Ranges for Total and Free Testosterone Levels

Ravi Jasuja, PhD[1], Karol M. Pencina, PhD[1], Liming Peng, MSc,
Shalender Bhasin, MB, BS*

KEYWORDS

- Testosterone assays • Free testosterone • Total testosterone • Equilibrium dialysis
- Ensemble ALlstery Model • Harmonized reference ranges for testosterone
- Hypogonadism • Testosterone deficiency

KEY POINTS

- Accurate measurement of total testosterone concentrations and, if indicated, free testosterone concentrations is essential for establishing a diagnosis of testosterone deficiency in men.
- Total testosterone concentrations should be measured in the morning in a fasting state using an accurate assay, such as liquid chromatography–tandem mass spectrometry, preferably in a laboratory that is certified by the Centers for Disease Control and Prevention (CDC) Hormone Standardization (HoST) Program for testosterone.
- Free testosterone concentration should be measured in men who are being evaluated for testosterone deficiency when alterations in binding protein concentrations are suspected or when total testosterone concentrations are close to or only slightly below the lower limit of the normal male range.
- Free testosterone concentration preferably should be measured using an equilibrium dialysis method in a reliable laboratory. If an equilibrium dialysis method is not available, free testosterone concentration should be estimated using an equation that has been validated against the equilibrium dialysis method.
- Harmonized reference ranges for testosterone concentrations in community-dwelling men have been published and they can be used for assays that have been certified by the CDC's HoST Program.

Research Program in Men's Health: Aging and Metabolism, Boston Claude D. Pepper Older Americans Independence Center, Brigham and Women's Hospital, Harvard Medical School, 221 Longwood Avenue, Boston, MA 02115, USA
[1] These authors contributed equally.
* Corresponding author.
E-mail address: sbhasin@bwh.harvard.edu

Endocrinol Metab Clin N Am 51 (2022) 63–75
https://doi.org/10.1016/j.ecl.2021.11.002
0889-8529/22/© 2021 Elsevier Inc. All rights reserved.

endo.theclinics.com

INTRODUCTION

A central tenet of endocrinology is that the hormones secreted by the endocrine glands circulate and regulate the function of distant organs. The circulating concentration of the hormone often is used as a marker of the functional state of that endocrine gland; there is an optimum or healthy range of hormone concentration, and deviations from this range are associated with disease. Thus, a diagnosis of clinical disorders associated with hormonal deficiency (eg, hypothyroidism) and hormonal excess (hyperthyroidism) is predicated crucially on accurate measurement of the circulating hormone concentration. Because hypogonadism in men is a syndrome characterized by symptoms and signs associated with consistently low testosterone levels, accurate and precise measurement of circulating testosterone concentration is an essential component of the diagnostic evaluation of patients suspected of testosterone deficiency.[1] The ability to diagnose and treat testosterone deficiency correctly requires accurate and precise measurement of total testosterone levels and free testosterone levels, reliable reference ranges derived in relevant populations, and an understanding of the relation between circulating testosterone concentrations and disease outcomes. The assay accuracy and rigorously derived reference ranges have an impact on diagnosis and treatment of individual patients. The thresholds of hormone concentrations that distinguish healthy from diseased people in the general population influence the estimates of the disease prevalence and thereby health policy.

Circulating testosterone is bound mostly to human serum albumin (33% to 54%) and sex hormone–binding globulin (SHBG); the fraction of circulating testosterone bound to SHBG varies in men and women, with approximately 44% of testosterone bound to SHBG in men and 66% in women. A small fraction is bound to orosomucoid and cortisol-binding globulin; only 2% to 4% of circulating testosterone is unbound or free[2] (**Fig. 1**). Conditions associated with elevated SHBG concentrations include old age, hyperthyroidism, polymorphisms in the SHBG gene, liver disease, human immunodeficiency virus infection, inflammatory conditions, and some medications, such as estrogens and some antiepileptics. SHBG concentrations are decreased with obesity, type 2 diabetes mellitus, polymorphisms in the SHBG gene, hypothyroidism, acromegaly, nephrotic syndrome, advanced liver disease, and treatment with androgens, progestins, and glucocorticoids.

Total testosterone refers to the sum of bound and unbound testosterone concentrations in the circulation. Only the unbound or free fraction can enter the cell and exert its biological effects. The term, *bioavailable testosterone*, refers to the fraction of circulating testosterone that is not bound to SHBG and connotes the view that testosterone binds to human serum albumin with low affinity and can dissociate readily in the tissue capillaries, especially in organs with long transit times, such as the liver and brain[3,4] (see **Fig. 1**).

This article reviews the extant methods for the measurements of total testosterone concentrations and free testosterone concentrations, their relative merits and limitations, and the application of reference ranges to interpret the circulating concentrations of total testosterone and of free testosterone and offers an approach to increase diagnostic accuracy in the evaluation of men suspected of testosterone deficiency.

METHODS FOR THE MEASUREMENT OF TOTAL TESTOSTERONE IN HUMAN SERUM OR PLASMA

Serum total testosterone concentrations can be measured using antibody-based immunoassays, such as radioimmunoassays, enzyme-linked immunosorbent assays,

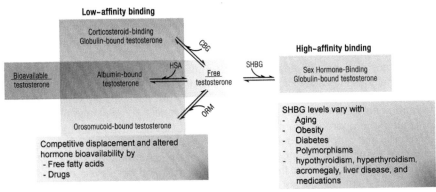

Fig. 1. Dynamic regulation of testosterone bioavailability in systemic circulation. Circulating testosterone binds with high affinity to SHBG and with a lower affinity weakly to other human serum albumin (HSA), orosomucoid (ORM), and corticosteroid-binding globulin (CBG). The bioavailability of testosterone is influenced by competitive displacement by other biomolecules and altered SHBG levels in many clinical conditions. Free testosterone refers to the fraction of circulating testosterone that is, not bound to any plasma protein and is able to cross the cell membrane. The term, *bioavailable testosterone*, refers to the fraction of circulating testosterone that is not bound to SHBG; this term reflects the view that testosterone bound to HSA, being bound with low affinity, can dissociate at the capillary level and become bioavailable in some tissues. Testosterone binds to multiple binding sites on HSA that are shared by free fatty acids and many commonly used drugs. In many physiologic and disease conditions, free fatty acids and some commonly used drugs can displace testosterone from these binding sites and influence its bioavailability. (*Adapted from* Goldman AL, Bhasin S, Wu FCW, Krishna M, Matsumoto AM, Jasuja R. A Reappraisal of Testosterone's Binding in Circulation: Physiological and Clinical Implications. Endocr Rev. 2017 Aug 1;38(4):302-324.)

and immunofluorometric or immunochemiluminescent assays; aptamer-based assays; or mass spectrometry-based assays. The immunoassays utilize a high-affinity antibody to recognize and bind the analyte with a high degree of specificity in the human serum or plasma (**Fig. 2**). For detection of the antigen-antibody complexes, the immunoassays use a variety of labels that are linked to the antibody and sometimes to the antigen. Some of the earliest immunoassays used radioactive tracers as labels and were referred to as radioimmunoassays. Enzyme-linked immunosorbent assays (ELISAs) and enzyme-multiplied immunoassays use an enzyme, such as horseradish peroxidase, alkaline phosphatase, or glucose oxidase, linked to the primary or secondary antibody to produce a color change in the presence of the analyte that can be detected quantitatively. Chemiluminescence immunoassays use chemical probes that generate light emission during the analytical reaction.

The first-generation radioimmunoassays for testosterone had limited sensitivity and significant cross-reactivity of dihydrotestosterone and some other steroids. To overcome the dual problems of limited sensitivity and cross-reactivity of these early assays, a large volume of serum or plasma was extracted using organic solvents, such as methanol or hexane, and the steroidal extract of serum or plasma was subjected to chromatography on activated silica gel, high-pressure liquid chromatography, or another chromatographic procedure to separate testosterone from potentially cross-reacting steroids prior to radioimmunoassay. The assays that used extraction and chromatography had better sensitivity and avoided nonspecificity due to cross-reacting steroids and interference from plasma proteins. Because these extraction immunoassays were labor intensive, platform-based assays were developed that eliminated the extraction and chromatographic steps to achieve high throughput and to reduce cost. Today, these platform-based direct immunoassays are widely used in clinical chemistry laboratories around the world because of their efficiency and relatively low cost but, as demonstrated by multiple studies,[5,6] these direct immunoassays suffer from problems of nonspecificity, limited sensitivity, and high imprecision in the low range; therefore, they are not suitable for testosterone measurements in women, prepubertal children, and hypogonadal men.[7,8] Wang and colleagues[6] compared serum total testosterone levels measured using several commonly used automated and manual immunoassay methods with measurements performed by liquid chromatography–tandem mass spectrometry (LC-MS/MS) and found that, in the low range, the immunoassays exhibited high levels of imprecision and inaccuracy and significant bias relative to an LC-MS/MS method.[6]

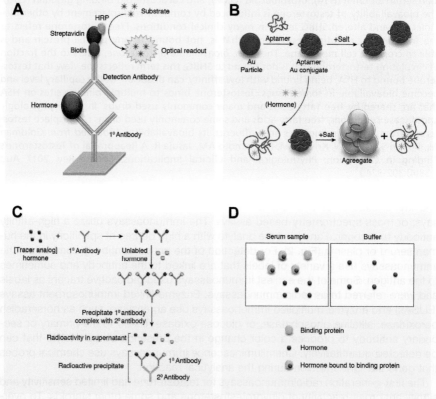

Fig. 2. Schematic depiction of the principles of common analytical assays used for the measurement of testosterone concentrations: (A) competitive binding immunoassay, (B) aptamer (synthetic ligand-binding oligonucleotides)-based assay, (C) tracer analog assay for free testosterone, and (D) equilibrium dialysis method for free testosterone. In the equilibrium dialysis method, human serum or plasma is dialyzed against a buffer with the ionic composition of human serum or plasma across a semipermeable membrane. At equilibrium, the dialyzed testosterone fraction can be measured directly by LC-MS/MS or a radiotracer-labeled testosterone is added to the sample and the dialyzed fraction can be counted to obtain an estimate of free testosterone.

Aptamers are single-stranded nucleic acids that can bind the targeted analyte with high affinity and specificity. Aptamers can be synthesized in vitro, characterized for their target specificity and binding affinity using high throughput in selection methods, and immobilized to a matrix, if needed.[9–12] The aptamers offer several advantages over antibodies including their greater stability, longer shelf-life, their amenability to in vitro synthesis, modification, and immobilization.[9–12] Few aptamer-based testosterone assays, however, are in clinical use at present.

LC-MS/MS has emerged as the method of choice with the highest specificity and sensitivity for the measurement of total testosterone in human serum or in plasma.[8,13,14] LC-MS/MS assays typically involve initial extraction of the serum or plasma using either solid phase extraction or liquid extraction using an organic solvent, followed by separation of compounds based on their polarity by high-pressure liquid chromatography.[15,16] The eluted compounds are transferred to the mass spectrometer, where the analytes are ionized and separated based on their mass and charge. In tandem mass spectrometry, the precursor ions are transferred to a chamber where they are bombarded with a collision gas, such as nitrogen or xenon, and fragmented into product ions, and the mass of the product ions is quantified in the detector. Deuterated testosterone is added to each sample as an internal standard to correct for recovery. Gas chromatography–mass spectrometry provides even greater specificity than LC-MS/MS, but LC-MS/MS offers higher throughput. Consequently, LC-MS/MS assays have become widely available from many large commercial and some research laboratories; however, they require greater initial investment in expensive equipment and a higher level of technical skill and remain more expensive than immunoassays. Unfortunately, despite their nonspecificity and imprecision in the low range, platform-based ELISAs and chemiluminescent immunoassays for testosterone continue to be used far more commonly than LC-MS/MS assays in hospital laboratories.

METHODS FOR THE DETERMINATION OF FREE TESTOSTERONE CONCENTRATIONS

Free testosterone concentrations can be measured either directly using one of several available methods or estimated from total testosterone, SHBG, and albumin concentrations. The methods for the direct measurement of free testosterone include equilibrium dialysis,[17,18] centrifugal ultrafiltration,[19,20] steady-state gel filtration,[21] flow dialysis,[22] and direct tracer analog immunoassays.[23] The equilibrium dialysis method employs dialysis of serum or plasma sample across a semipermeable membrane; the unbound testosterone crosses the dialysis membrane and equilibrates across the dialysis chambers whereas the protein-bound testosterone is retained on the sample side. The dialyzed fraction can be measured directly by LC-MS/MS; alternately, a tracer amount of radiolabeled testosterone can be added to the serum or plasma sample, and free testosterone concentration can be estimated by multiplying the percent of tracer in the dialyzed fraction with total testosterone concentration in the sample. The other methods, such as centrifugal centrifugation and gel filtration, use different techniques for separating unbound from bound testosterone. The equilibrium dialysis and centrifugal ultrafiltration methods have been shown to provide comparable results.[18,19] Several laboratories offer the measurement of salivary testosterone[24] as a marker of serum free testosterone concentrations; however, salivary testosterone assays have not been shown to be an accurate measure of serum free testosterone concentrations.[24] Additionally, uneven sample desiccation, potential from contamination of oral contents and bacteria, and the paucity of rigorously derived reference ranges have prevented wide adaption of salivary testosterone assays in clinical practice.

Equilibrium dialysis is considered the reference method against which all other methods are compared. Equilibrium dialysis methods are available from many large commercial laboratories but usually are not available in most local hospital laboratories. Furthermore, because of interlaboratory differences in assay procedures and lack of harmonized reference ranges, free testosterone should be measured in a reliable laboratory. Direct tracer analog methods are widely used in hospital laboratories; however, these assays are inaccurate and their use is not recommended.[1,25,26]

Algorithms for Estimating Free Testosterone Concentrations

Because of the complexities in the current methods of measuring free testosterone, several equations have been published for the calculation of free testosterone concentrations from total testosterone, SHBG, and albumin concentrations.[27–31] These equations can be broadly categorized into those that use the law of mass action equations[27,29,31] and those that are deriving empirically using regression methods.[30] The law of mass action equations, such as those published by Sodergard and colleagues,[27] Vermeulen and colleagues,[29] and Mazer,[31] are based on the assumptions of linear binding of testosterone to SHBG with a fixed association constant. Furthermore, these equations assume that testosterone binds to a single binding site on human serum albumin with low affinity. Recent studies using modern biophysical techniques have shown that the binding of testosterone and estradiol to SHBG is a dynamic nonlinear process that involves an allosteric interaction between the 2 SHBG monomers, such that the Kd varies dynamically across the range of sex hormone and SHBG concentrations[28,32] (**Fig. 3**). The estimates of free testosterone concentration using the novel Ensemble ALlstery Model match closely the concentrations measured derived by the equilibrium dialysis method.[28] All algorithms are highly dependent on the accuracy and sensitivity of the total testosterone and SHBG assays. Furthermore, recent studies of testosterone's binding to human serum albumin using

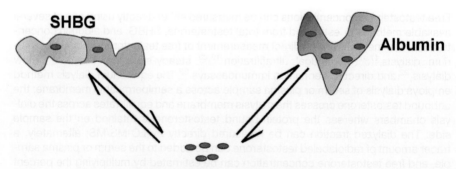

SHBG

Albumin

Testosterone or estradiol

Fig. 3. Nonlinear association and allosteric interactions between hormone binding sites on human serum albumin (HAS) and SHBG allow dynamic regulation of hormone bioavailability. SHBG is a dimeric glycoprotein; each monomer of SHBG dimer has a single binding site for testosterone and estradiol. HSA has multiple binding sites (at least 6, likely more) for testosterone that also can bind free fatty acids and some commonly used drugs. Binding of testosterone to 1 binding site on SHBG and HAS induces allosteric coupling with other binding sites. The allosteric coupling between the multiple sites on binding proteins alters the apparent binding affinity as relative and absolute concentrations change several orders of magnitude during reproductive and nonreproductive phases of a person's life.

2-dimensional nuclear magnetic resonance and fluorescence spectroscopy have revealed the presence of multiple, allosterically coupled binding sites for testosterone on albumin[33] (see **Fig. 3**). Testosterone shares these binding sites on human serum albumin with free fatty acids and many commonly used drugs, such as ibuprofen and warfarin, that could displace testosterone from human serum albumin under various physiologic states or disease conditions.[33]

Bioavailable Testosterone

Bioavailable testosterone can be measured directly using the ammonium sulfate precipitation method that precipitates SHBG-bound testosterone or can be calculated from total testosterone, SHBG, and albumin. The high level of imprecision of ammonium sulfate precipitation method and the lack of rigorously derived reference range, however, limit its utility in clinical practice.

OPTIMIZING THE MEASUREMENTS OF TOTAL TESTOSTERONE AND FREE TESTOSTERONE TO REDUCE DIAGNOSTIC INACCURACY

The circulating concentrations of total testosterone and free testosterone vary substantially among men and in the same individual over time due to biologic factors as well as measurement variation. A substantial fraction of the population-level variation in total testosterone levels among men is due to genetic factors, including genetic variants in the SHBG locus and on the X chromosome and some autosomes.[34–36] Testosterone levels vary over time due to its pulsatile secretion and its circadian and circannual secretory rhythms. Testosterone is secreted in bursts approximately once every 90 minutes. Testosterone levels are higher in the morning than in the late afternoon; this diurnal rhythm is dampened in older men. The seasonal variation has been reported more clearly in geographic areas exposed to wide seasonal variation in temperature and daylight (eg, Northern Norway)[37]; in these regions, serum testosterone levels are the lowest in summer and the highest in early winter months. Testosterone levels decline after a meal, especially after a glucose load.[38] Testosterone levels may be transiently suppressed during an acute illness; therefore, the evaluation of hypogonadism should be avoided during an acute illness.

Therefore, testosterone levels should be measured on 2 or more separate occasions within 4 hours to 5 hours of waking after an overnight fast.[1] Total testosterone level should be measured using an accurate assay, preferably an LC-MS/MS assay, that is certified by an accuracy-based standardization or quality control program (eg, Centers for Disease Control and Prevention's [CDC] Hormone Standardization Program for Testosterone [HoST]).[1]

Due to complexities of free testosterone measurements and lack of rigorously derived reference ranges, an expert panel of the Endocrine Society recommended the use of total testosterone as the initial test for screening men suspected of testosterone deficiency.[1] Free testosterone level should be measured in men with conditions associated with alterations in binding protein concentrations or in men in whom total testosterone concentrations are at or near the lower limit of the normal male range.[1] Free testosterone concentration should be measured directly, preferably using an equilibrium dialysis assay in a reliable laboratory; if equilibrium dialysis assay is not available, free testosterone concentration should be estimated using an equation that provides close approximation of values derived using the equilibrium dialysis method.[1] The direct tracer analog assays for free testosterone assays should be avoided.[8]

REFERENCE RANGES FOR TOTAL TESTOSTERONE LEVELS AND FREE TESTOSTERONE LEVELS
Reference Range for Total Testosterone in Men

The reference range refers to the distribution of the circulating concentration of a hormone or analyte in the general population and provides the foundational basis for distinguishing normal from low or high values.[26] Therefore, rigorously derived reference ranges are essential for establishing a diagnosis of hypogonadism. The authors and others have published reference ranges for circulating testosterone levels in the Framingham Heart Study (FHS) and in other populations.[39–42] Because of differences in the study populations, assay methodology, and calibrators, however, reference ranges derived in 1 population may not be applicable to other populations or assays. Accordingly, under the auspices of the Endocrine Society, the authors compared the distribution of total testosterone concentrations in epidemiologic studies that included men from different geographic regions of the United States and Europe and generated consensus reference ranges for total testosterone levels in men.[43] Serum testosterone levels were measured in 9054 community-dwelling men who were participants in 1 of 4 cohort studies in the United States and Europe: FHS, European Male Ageing Study (EMAS), Osteoporotic Fractures in Men Study, and Male Sibling Study of Osteoporosis.[43]

The assays used to measure testosterone concentrations in the 4 cohorts were cross-calibrated by measuring testosterone levels in serum samples from approximately 100 men in each cohort in the CDC Clinical Reference Laboratory using an assay calibrated to a higher-order reference materials and using serum-based reference materials as additional accuracy controls. Normalizing equations were generated using Passing-Bablok regression and used to generate harmonized values, from which standardized, age-specific reference ranges were derived. In healthy non-obese men, ages 19 years to 39 years; harmonized 2.5th, 5th, 95th, and 97.5th percentile values were 264 ng/dL, 303 ng/dL, 852 ng/dL, and 916 ng/dL (9.2 nmol/L, 10.3 nmol/L, 29.5 nmol/L, and 31.8 nmol/L, respectively) (**Table 1**). The median value was 531 ng/dL (18.4 nmol/L).[43] Age-specific harmonized testosterone

	Healthy, Nonobese Young Men (ng/dL)	All Young Men (ng/dL)
Table 1 The 2.5th and 5th percentile values for harmonized circulating total testosterone concentrations among nonobese and obese men, ages 19 years to 39 years		
Percentiles		
2.5	264	228
5	303	273

To generate harmonized reference ranges, the assays used to measure testosterone concentrations in the participating cohort studies were cross-calibrated by measuring testosterone levels in serum samples from approximately 100 men in each cohort in the CDC Clinical Reference Laboratory.[42] Normalizing equations were generated using Passing-Bablok regression and used to generate harmonized values, from which standardized, reference ranges were derived. The 2.5th and 5th percentile values of the harmonized values in healthy, nonobese men as well as in all men are shown in the table.

To convert total testosterone from nanograms per deciliter to nanomoles per liter (SI units), multiply the value nanograms per deciliter by 0.0347.

Data from Travison TG, Vesper HW, Orwoll E, Wu F, Kaufman JM, Wang Y, Lapauw B, Fiers T, Matsumoto AM, Bhasin S. Harmonized Reference Ranges for Circulating Testosterone Levels in Men of Four Cohort Studies in the United States and Europe. J Clin Endocrinol Metab. 2017;102(4):1161-73.

concentrations in nonobese men as well as in the entire study population also were derived, by decades of age, and were similar across cohorts.[43] These harmonized reference ranges can be applied to all assays and laboratories that are certified by the CDC HoST Program.[1]

The assay imprecision and substantial biologic variation in testosterone levels over time should be considered in interpreting the reference ranges, especially when the measured testosterone concentrations are at or within 2 SDs of the threshold that distinguishes normal and low values. A true value of 274 ng/dL (9.50 nmol/L) in an assay whose lower limit is reported as 275 ng/dL (9.53 nmol/L) has 95% probability of being reported within 2 SDs on either side of the true value if the measurements were to be repeated. Therefore, the lower limit of the normal range should not be viewed as an absolute cutpoint. The risk of misclassification is high when the measured concentrations are at, just below, or just above the cutpoint.

Reference Range for Free Testosterone

Harmonized reference ranges for free testosterone levels using equilibrium dialysis currently are not available, and clinicians have to rely on reference ranges provided by a laboratory. The populations included and the statistical methods used for generating these reference ranges are not published. Reference ranges for free testosterone concentrations estimated using the Ensemble ALlstery Model in male participants of the FHS have been published.[28] The distribution of free testosterone concentrations was studied in a reference sample of healthy young male participants (ages 19–40 years; N = 434) of the FHS: Generation 3, who were nonobese and nonsmokers and who did not have a diagnosis of cancer, cardiovascular disease, diabetes mellitus, hypertension, or hypercholesterolemia.[28,39] Only men with the wild-type SHBG (CC for rs6258 single nucleotide polymorphism) genotype, who constitute nearly 98% of the population, were included.[34] The 2.5th percentile value for free testosterone in nonobese men, ages 19 years to 40 years (mean age 32.6 years), in the FHS Generation 3, was 114.6 pg/mL[28]; the corresponding 2.5th percentile values for free testosterone level in FHS broad sample (ages 19–90 years; mean age 49.3 years) and the EMAS (ages 40–79 years; mean age 60 years)[44] were 69.7 pg/mL and 58 pg/mL, respectively. In the EMAS, the men with free testosterone levels more than 2 SDs below the mean of the reference sample (T score < −2) were at increased risk for having sexual symptoms and elevated LH associated. Several caveats should be considered when applying these reference ranges. The estimates of free testosterone concentrations are affected greatly by the method used to measure total testosterone and SHBG. The FHS population is predominantly white. The distribution of normative ranges generated in community-dwelling, healthy young men needs further validation in clinical populations and randomized trials. Efforts currently are under way to generate reference ranges for free testosterone concentrations using a standardized equilibrium dialysis method.

SYNOPSIS

Because hypogonadism is a syndrome characterized by a syndromic constellation of symptoms and signs in association with consistently low testosterone concentrations, accurate and precise measurement of total, and, if indicated, free testosterone concentration is necessary to establish its diagnosis. Variations in testosterone levels over time due to genetic factors, secretory rhythms, and effects of food, medications, age, obesity, and disease; imprecision and inaccuracy in the measurement of total testosterone concentrations and free testosterone concentrations; variations in binding protein concentrations; and suboptimal reference ranges contribute to diagnostic inaccuracies. The use of accurate assays, such as the LC-MS/MS for the measurement of total testosterone concentration in a laboratory certified by an accuracy-based program (eg, CDC HoST Program), multiple measurements of testosterone over time to confirm the diagnosis in fasting early morning samples, and measurement of free testosterone levels using the equilibrium dialysis method, when indicated, and the application of rigorously derived reference ranges can reduce the risk of disease misclassification and enhance diagnostic accuracy.

CLINICS CARE POINTS

- Measure testosterone levels on 2 or more days in early morning hours in a fasting state.
- Measure total testosterone concentration using an LC-MS/MS assay, if available, in a laboratory that is certified by an accuracy-based benchmark, such as the CDC HoST Program.
- Avoid making a diagnosis of testosterone deficiency based on 1 low value or only on the basis of testosterone levels.
- Avoid measuring testosterone levels during an acute illness.
- Measure free testosterone level when binding protein abnormality is suspected or when the total testosterone levels are at or near the lower limit of the normal range for men.
- Use an equilibrium dialysis method for the measurement of free testosterone level in a reliable laboratory.
- Avoid the use of tracer analog methods for free testosterone measurement.
- For total testosterone assays that are certified by the CDC HoST Program, the published harmonized references can be applied. The 2.5th, 5th, 95th, and 97.5th percentile values of the harmonized reference range for healthy young, nonobese men, ages 19 years to 40 years, are 264 ng/dL, 303 ng/dL, 852 ng/dL, and 916 ng/dL, respectively.
- Lack of standardization of the equilibrium dialysis method has retarded efforts to generate harmonized reference ranges for free testosterone levels. Clinicians have to rely on reference ranges provided by a laboratory. Reference ranges for free testosterone estimated using the ensemble allostery model have been published.

DISCLOSURES

Dr S. Bhasin reports receiving research grants from the National Institute on Aging, the National Institute of Child Health and Human Development, the National Institute of Nursing Research, the Patient-Centered Outcomes Research Institute (PCORI), Abb-Vie, Transition Therapeutics, Metro International Biotechnology, and Alivegen. These grants are managed by the Brigham and Women's Hospital. These conflicts are overseen and managed in accordance with the policies of the Office of Industry Interactions, Massachusetts General Brigham Healthcare System, Boston.

REFERENCES

1. Bhasin S, Brito JP, Cunningham GR, et al. Testosterone therapy in men with hypogonadism: an endocrine society clinical practice guideline. J Clin Endocrinol Metab 2018;103(5):1715–44.
2. Goldman AL, Bhasin S, Wu FCW, et al. A reappraisal of testosterone's binding in circulation: physiological and clinical implications. Endocr Rev 2017;38(4):302–24.

3. Manni A, Pardridge WM, Cefalu W, et al. Bioavailability of albumin-bound testosterone. J Clin Endocrinol Metab 1985;61(4):705–10.

4. Pardridge WM. Serum bioavailability of sex steroid hormones. Clin Endocrinol Metab 1986;15(2):259–78.

5. Taieb J, Mathian B, Millot F, et al. Testosterone measured by 10 immunoassays and by isotope-dilution gas chromatography-mass spectrometry in sera from 116 men, women, and children. Clin Chem 2003;49(8):1381–95.

6. Wang C, Catlin DH, Demers LM, et al. Measurement of total serum testosterone in adult men: comparison of current laboratory methods versus liquid chromatography-tandem mass spectrometry. J Clin Endocrinol Metab 2004; 89(2):534–43.

7. Herold DA, Fitzgerald RL. Immunoassays for testosterone in women: better than a guess? Clin Chem 2003;49(8):1250–1.

8. Rosner W, Auchus RJ, Azziz R, et al. Position statement: Utility, limitations, and pitfalls in measuring testosterone: an Endocrine Society position statement. J Clin Endocrinol Metab 2007;92(2):405–13.

9. Aquino-Jarquin G, Toscano-Garibay JD. RNA aptamer evolution: two decades of SELEction. Int J Mol Sci 2011;12(12):9155–71.

10. Gold L, Janjic N, Jarvis T, et al. Aptamers and the RNA world, past and present. Cold Spring Harb Perspect Biol 2012;4(3). https://doi.org/10.1101/cshperspect.a003582.

11. Sanghavi BJ, Moore JA, Chavez JL, et al. Aptamer-functionalized nanoparticles for surface immobilization-free electrochemical detection of cortisol in a microfluidic device. Biosens Bioelectron 2016;78:244–52.

12. Song KM, Lee S, Ban C. Aptamers and their biological applications. Sensors (Basel) 2012;12(1):612–31.

13. Vesper HW, Bhasin S, Wang C, et al. Interlaboratory comparison study of serum total testosterone [corrected] measurements performed by mass spectrometry methods. Steroids 2009;74(6):498–503.

14. Ketha H, Kaur S, Grebe SK, et al. Clinical applications of LC-MS sex steroid assays: evolution of methodologies in the 21st century. Curr Opin Endocrinol Diabetes Obes 2014;21(3):217–26.

15. Bui HN, Struys EA, Martens F, et al. Serum testosterone levels measured by isotope dilution-liquid chromatography-tandem mass spectrometry in postmenopausal women versus those in women who underwent bilateral oophorectomy. Ann Clin Biochem 2010;47(Pt 3):248–52.

16. Cawood ML, Field HP, Ford CG, et al. Testosterone measurement by isotope-dilution liquid chromatography-tandem mass spectrometry: validation of a method for routine clinical practice. Clin Chem 2005;51(8):1472–9.

17. Umstot ES, Baxter JE, Andersen RN. A theoretically sound and practicable equilibrium dialysis method for measuring percentage of free testosterone. J Steroid Biochem 1985;22(5):639–48.

18. Barini A, Liberale I, Menini E. Simultaneous determination of free testosterone and testosterone bound to non-sex-hormone-binding globulin by equilibrium dialysis. Clin Chem 1993;39(6):938–41.

19. Hammond GL, Nisker JA, Jones LA, et al. Estimation of the percentage of free steroid in undiluted serum by centrifugal ultrafiltration-dialysis. J Biol Chem 1980;255(11):5023–6.

20. Vlahos I, MacMahon W, Sgoutas D, et al. An improved ultrafiltration method for determining free testosterone in serum. Clin Chem 1982;28(11):2286–91.

21. Fisher RA, Anderson DC, Burke CW. Simultaneous measurement of unbound testosterone and estradiol fractions in undiluted plasma at 37 degrees C by steady-state gel filtration. Steroids 1974;24(6):809–24.

22. Moll GW Jr, Rosenfield RL. Testosterone binding and free plasma androgen concentrations under physiological conditons: chararacterization by flow dialysis technique. J Clin Endocrinol Metab 1979;49(5):730–6.

23. Wilke TJ, Utley DJ. Total testosterone, free-androgen index, calculated free testosterone, and free testosterone by analog RIA compared in hirsute women and in otherwise-normal women with altered binding of sex-hormone-binding globulin. Clin Chem 1987;33(8):1372–5.

24. Pearce S, Dowsett M, Jeffcoate SL. Three methods compared for estimating the fraction of testosterone and estradiol not bound to sex-hormone-binding globulin. Clin Chem 1989;35(4):632–5.

25. Rosner W. Errors in the measurement of plasma free testosterone. J Clin Endocrinol Metab 1997;82(6):2014–5.

26. Bhasin S, Zhang A, Coviello A, et al. The impact of assay quality and reference ranges on clinical decision making in the diagnosis of androgen disorders. Steroids 2008;73(13):1311–7.

27. Sodergard R, Backstrom T, Shanbhag V, et al. Calculation of free and bound fractions of testosterone and estradiol-17 beta to human plasma proteins at body temperature. J Steroid Biochem 1982;16(6):801–10.

28. Zakharov MN, Bhasin S, Travison TG, et al. A multi-step, dynamic allosteric model of testosterone's binding to sex hormone binding globulin. Mol Cell Endocrinol 2015;399:190–200.

29. Vermeulen A, Verdonck L, Kaufman JM. A critical evaluation of simple methods for the estimation of free testosterone in serum. J Clin Endocrinol Metab 1999; 84(10):3666–72.

30. Ly LP, Handelsman DJ. Empirical estimation of free testosterone from testosterone and sex hormone-binding globulin immunoassays. Eur J Endocrinol 2005;152(3):471–8.

31. Mazer NA. A novel spreadsheet method for calculating the free serum concentrations of testosterone, dihydrotestosterone, estradiol, estrone and cortisol: with illustrative examples from male and female populations. Steroids 2009;74(6): 512–9.

32. Jasuja R, Spencer D, Jayaraj A, et al. Estradiol induces allosteric coupling and partitioning of sex-hormone-binding globulin monomers among conformational states. iScience 2021;24(6):102414.

33. Jayaraj A, Schwanz HA, Spencer DJ, et al. Allosterically coupled multisite binding of testosterone to human serum albumin. Endocrinology 2021;162(2). https://doi.org/10.1210/endocr/bqaa199.

34. Ohlsson C, Wallaschofski H, Lunetta KL, et al. Genetic determinants of serum testosterone concentrations in men. PLoS Genet 2011;7(10):e1002313.

35. Mohammadi-Shemirani P, Chong M, Pigeyre M, et al. Effects of lifelong testosterone exposure on health and disease using Mendelian randomization. Elife 2020;9. https://doi.org/10.7554/eLife.58914.

36. Ruth KS, Day FR, Tyrrell J, et al. Using human genetics to understand the disease impacts of testosterone in men and women. Nat Med 2020;26(2):252–8.

37. Svartberg J, Jorde R, Sundsfjord J, et al. Seasonal variation of testosterone and waist to hip ratio in men: the Tromso study. J Clin Endocrinol Metab 2003;88(7): 3099–104.

38. Caronia LM, Dwyer AA, Hayden D, et al. Abrupt decrease in serum testosterone levels after an oral glucose load in men: implications for screening for hypogonadism. Clin Endocrinol (Oxf) 2013;78(2):291–6.

39. Bhasin S, Pencina M, Jasuja GK, et al. Reference ranges for testosterone in men generated using liquid chromatography tandem mass spectrometry in a community-based sample of healthy nonobese young men in the Framingham Heart Study and applied to three geographically distinct cohorts. J Clin Endocrinol Metab 2011;96(8):2430–9.

40. Sikaris K, McLachlan RI, Kazlauskas R, et al. Reproductive hormone reference intervals for healthy fertile young men: evaluation of automated platform assays. J Clin Endocrinol Metab 2005;90(11):5928–36.

41. Haring R, Hannemann A, John U, et al. Age-specific reference ranges for serum testosterone and androstenedione concentrations in women measured by liquid chromatography-tandem mass spectrometry. J Clin Endocrinol Metab 2012; 97(2):408–15.

42. Yeap BB, Alfonso H, Chubb SA, et al. Reference ranges and determinants of testosterone, dihydrotestosterone, and estradiol levels measured using liquid chromatography-tandem mass spectrometry in a population-based cohort of older men. J Clin Endocrinol Metab 2012;97(11):4030–9.

43. Travison TG, Vesper HW, Orwoll E, et al. Harmonized reference ranges for circulating testosterone levels in men of four cohort studies in the United States and Europe. J Clin Endocrinol Metab 2017;102(4):1161–73.

44. Wu FC, Tajar A, Beynon JM, et al. Identification of late-onset hypogonadism in middle-aged and elderly men. N Engl J Med 2010;363(2):123–35.

Testosterone Replacement Therapy in Hypogonadal Men

Christina Wang, MD[a],*, Ronald S. Swerdloff, MD[b]

KEYWORDS

- Transdermal gels • Oral capsules • Intramuscular injections • Implants
- Modified androgens • Selective androgen receptor modulators
- Endogenous testosterone stimulators

KEY POINTS

- Testosterone replacement is efficacious in elevating serum testosterone into the adult male range and improves symptoms in hypogonadal men.
- Many testosterone methods of delivery are available and are safe when used according to recommendations.
- The method of testosterone replacement is decided by the patient in consultation with the physician.
- Dose adjustment requires monitoring testosterone concentrations to achieve the desired testosterone concentration usually in the midadult male range.
- Modified androgens that are potentially hepatotoxic should not be used; those androgens that do not aromatize to estrogens should be used with caution because of bone loss.

INTRODUCTION

Testosterone replacement is indicated in men with symptoms or signs of testosterone insufficiency and persistently low circulating testosterone concentrations.[1] The diagnosis, indication, benefits versus risks, and monitoring of testosterone replacement for hypogonadal men are described in other chapters. This article focuses on the different formulations and routes of administration of testosterone used to achieve physiologic testosterone concentration and alleviate symptoms of testosterone insufficiency. We also discuss how to adjust the dose of testosterone replacement depending on the method used for testosterone replacement, goals of testosterone replacement, and patient preferences.

[a] Division of Endocrinology, Clinical and Translational Science Institute, The Lundquist Institute at Harbor-UCLA Medical Center, Harbor-UCLA Medical Center, 1124 West Carson Street, Torrance, CA 90502, USA; [b] Division of Endocrinology, The Lundquist Institute and Harbor-UCLA Medical Center, 1124 West Carson Street, Torrance, CA 90502, USA
* Corresponding author.
E-mail address: wang@lundquist.org

Endocrinol Metab Clin N Am 51 (2022) 77–98
https://doi.org/10.1016/j.ecl.2021.11.005
0889-8529/22/© 2021 Elsevier Inc. All rights reserved.

The decision on which formulation and route to replace testosterone depends on the patient's choice, his acceptance of different modalities, the pharmacokinetics of testosterone that best suit the patient, and the goals of treatment. This decision is made by the patient with information provided by the physician. Because long-acting androgens remain in the body for a longer time and there is a lack of a placebo-controlled long-term safety study to ascertain possible cardiovascular and prostate adverse events, long-acting testosterone replacement is usually reserved for younger men with hypogonadism. This recommendation may be revised when additional safety data are available. Shorter acting injections, gels, and oral testosterone are frequently used in the initiation of therapy in hypogonadal older men and those whereby a therapeutic trial of testosterone may be indicated. Testosterone gels and creams may be available from compounding pharmacies and from many Internet sites, but these compounded preparations are not recommended for testosterone replacement because their composition and the pharmacokinetics have not been verified.

- The decision on which testosterone preparation for replacement therapy resides with the patient after information on the differences between different modalities is provided by the health professional.

TRENDS IN TESTOSTERONE PRESCRIPTIONS

There was an increase in testosterone prescriptions reported from 2000 to 2011 throughout the world but the increase was most marked (more than threefold) in the United States.[2-4] Topical gel is the most used method of testosterone replacement in the United States; globally injections are the most prescribed testosterone formulation. Interestingly, long-term adherence to the prescribed testosterone treatment is relatively low; in one study, about 18% of the men only filled one prescription. The increase in testosterone prescriptions was the highest in men more than 60 years.[2] The striking increase in prescribed testosterone usage in the first decade of the 21st century may be related to the introduction of new testosterone gels in 2003; continued medical education for general physicians on recognition of testosterone deficiency; rising prevalence of blood testosterone testing, and direct marketing of testosterone products to the public. In the United States, there was substantial use of testosterone without testing of testosterone levels and for the treatment of men with symptoms despite normal testosterone levels.[3] The increase in prescribed testosterone has been viewed as the effects of direct-to-consumer marketing of testosterone products to the public. Many men, who were prescribed testosterone may not have hypogonadism with persistently low serum testosterone.[5] More recent data indicate that testosterone use in the United States declined by 48% from 2013 to 2016[6]; similar trends were observed in Canada.[7] This decline in testosterone prescription and use may be related to reports of possible adverse effects of testosterone therapy on cardiovascular disease and the change in the labeling of testosterone products to include possible but debatable increased risk of myocardial infarction and stroke.[8-12] In addition, the Food and Drug Administration (FDA) in the United States provided guidance that testosterone therapy should be used only in men with low testosterone concentration due to defined causes (testicular or hypothalamic–pituitary dysfunction) of hypogonadism.[8] Low testosterone in aging men is not regarded by the FDA as an indication for testosterone replacement. Physicians should discuss all the benefits and risks of testosterone replacement including the possible increased risk of cardiovascular events before starting testosterone replacement therapy. Each patient needs to be aware of the possible risks to himself and balance that against the proven beneficial effects of testosterone treatment.

- Testosterone prescriptions soared from 2000 to 2011 with the introduction of transdermal testosterone gels.
- About 18% of the men only filled testosterone prescription once.
- From 2013 to 2016, the prescriptions for testosterone replacement decreased following FDA and professional society recommendations to use testosterone therapy only for symptomatic men with consistently low testosterone.

TESTOSTERONE REPLACEMENT THERAPY

Table 1 shows the available testosterone replacement options in the United States (US) which includes topical patch and gels; nasal gel and buccal tablets; oral pills and capsules; injections and implants. The goal of testosterone replacement therapy is to relieve the symptoms and signs of testosterone insufficiency and maintain serum testosterone concentrations in the physiologic range. While reference ranges differ according to assay methodology,[13] the population used to determine the reference range, the lower reference range from published data is commonly between 250 and 300 ng/dL (8.7–10.4 nmol/L) and the upper reference levels between 950 to 1000 ng/dL (33.0–34.7 nmol/L).[14] In most hypogonadal patients receiving testosterone, the optimal average concentrations are in the midreference range (approximately 400–800 ng/dL; 13.9–27.8 nmol/L) although the exact ideal levels within the normal range are not known and may differ based on symptom relief and adverse effects in an individual.

Testosterone binds and activates the androgen receptors to exert its actions on the target tissues. It is converted by the 5 alpha-reductase enzymes to 5 alpha-dihydrotestosterone (**Fig. 1**) which also exerts its effect through the androgen receptor predominantly in the skin, hair follicles, and the male reproductive tract including the external genitalia, Wolffian duct-derived structures including the epididymis, vas deference, ejaculatory ducts, and seminal vesicle as well as the prostate.[15] Mutations of the 5 alpha-reductase gene cause underdevelopment of the external genitalia.[16,17] Testosterone is also aromatized to estradiol (see **Fig. 1**) and the absence of the aromatase enzyme results in low bone mass.[18] Placebo controlled clinical investigations in adult healthy men with induced hypogonadism demonstrate that after testosterone replacement the increase in concentrations of testosterone is related to increased hematocrit/hemoglobin, lean body mass, bone mineral density, and decreased fat mass in both young and older men.[19–23] In experimental studies, when an aromatase inhibitor was coadministered with testosterone to men with suppressed testosterone concentrations, the increase in bone mass and decrease in fat mass were lessened than testosterone treatment alone; these studies suggest that the aromatization of testosterone to estradiol may be required for greatest testosterone effects on bone density and reduction of fat mass.[22] Sexual desire and activity but not erectile function have been more recently shown to be related to increases in serum total and free testosterone as well as estradiol concentrations achieved after testosterone replacement in older hypogonadal men.[24] Taken together, these studies suggest that aromatizable androgens such as testosterone may be preferred over nonaromatizable modified androgens for androgen replacement in hypogonadal men.[25]

Some modified androgens are available in the US, such as methyltestosterone, mesterolone, oxandrolone oral tablets, and stanozolol injections, but are not recommended for testosterone replacement in hypogonadal men (see **Fig.1**). One reason for this reservation for their use in treating hypogonadal adult men is that they are

Table 1
Testosterone products approved by the Food and Drug Administration in Unites States (2021)

Delivery System/ Drug	Brand Name	Recommended Dose Regimen	Available Format
Topical/Transdermal			
Testosterone patch	Androderm	2 or 4 mg patch/day	4 mg starting dose Do not apply the patch to the same area within 7 days Apply to back, abdomen, upper arms
Testosterone gel	AndroGel	1% gel – 50 to 100 mg of testosterone per day	25 or 50 mg testosterone packets Apply to shoulders and upper arms
		1.62% gel – 40.5 to 81 mg of testosterone per day	20.25 mg testosterone, one pump actuation or a 20.25 mg packet 40.5 mg testosterone, two pump actuation or a 40.5 packet Apply to shoulders and upper arms
Testosterone gel	Testim	1% gel – 50 mg of testosterone/tube	50 mg/day starting dose Apply to shoulder and upper arms
Testosterone gel	Fortesta	2% gel 10 mg/0.5 g per pump actuation	40 mg (4 pump actuations)/day starting dose Apply to inner thighs
Testosterone gel	Vogelxo	1% gel 50 or 100 mg per tube or packet, 12.5 mg per actuation for pump	Generic testosterone gel
	Testosterone Gel	1.62% gel similar to AndroGel (1.62%)	Generic, same as AndroGel 1.62%
Testosterone lotion	Axiron	2% lotion 30 mg/pump actuation	Start with 60 mg Apply to axilla Discontinued
Buccal/Nasal			
Buccal tablets	Striant	30 mg twice/day	Apply to gum Dislodging of tablets Discontinued
Nasal gel	Natesto	11 mg gel intranasal three times per day	Start with one actuation (5.5 mg) into each nostril total 11 mg Apply to nose three times per day

(continued on next page)

Table 1
(continued)

Delivery System/ Drug	Brand Name	Recommended Dose Regimen	Available Format
Oral Capsule			
Testosterone undecanoate	Andriol	40 mg capsules two or three times a day	80 to 120 mg per day Not available in US
Testosterone undecanoate	Jatanzo	158 to 396 mg twice per day	Start with 237 mg twice a day with food
Testosterone undecanoate	Tlando	225 mg twice per day	Tentative approval by FDA
Injection			
Testosterone enanthate	Xyosted	50, 75 and 100 mg in 0.5 mL sesame oil	Autoinjector Start with 75 mg once per week subcutaneously injection to abdomen
	Delatestryl	200 mg/mL sesame oil	Intramuscular injection once in 2 weeks Not available in US
Testosterone cypionate	Depo-Testosterone	100 mg/mL or 200 mg/mL in cottonseed oil	Deep intramuscular injection to gluteal muscle once in 2 week or Inject subcutaneously to abdominal adipose tissue every week
Testosterone undecanoate	Aveed	750 mg/3 mL (250 mg/mL) in castor oil	Start with 750 mg deep intramuscular injection Deep into gluteal muscle Repeat 750 mg injection after 4 weeks and then every 10 weeks 30 minutes observation for pulmonary oil embolism
Implants			
Testosterone		Testopel pellets 75 mg per pellet	Inserted subcutaneously into fat in hip area 2 to 6 implants will last 3 to 4 months; 6 to 10 implants will last for 4 to 6 months

not aromatizable and may result in greater increase in LDL cholesterol and decrease in HDL cholesterol levels.[26] In addition, the 17 alpha-alkylated androgenic steroids (methyltestosterone, oxymetholone, and stanozolol) are hepatotoxic, whereas testosterone, testosterone esters, and 19-nortestosterone showed no toxic effects on the liver.[27–30] Thus, these modified 17 alpha-alkylated androgens are not recommended for testosterone replacement therapy. There are many designer synthetic androgens that are marketed over the Internet as nutritional supplements. Little is known about the pharmacologic effects of these unapproved androgens, and they should not be used as testosterone replacement, athletic or bodybuilding, nor for performance enhancement.[31,32]

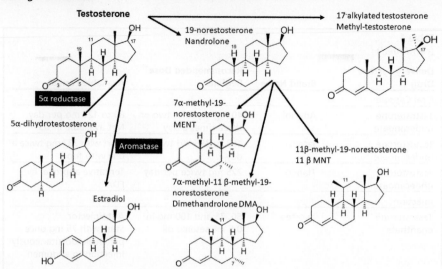

Fig. 1. Chemical structure of testosterone and its conversion to 5α-dihydrotestosterone and estradiol. Addition of a methyl group at 17α position testosterone results in methyl-testosterone that is hepatotoxic. Removal of a methyl group at the 19 position from testosterone results in 19-nortestosterone. 19-nortestosterone and its derivatives are not hepatotoxic.

- The goal of testosterone replacement is to maintain serum testosterone concentration in the midreference range of adult men (about 400–800 ng/dL; 13.9–27.8 nmol/L)
- Serum testosterone levels achieved with testosterone replacement are related to increases in lean and bone mass, sexual activity and desire, and hemoglobin and hematocrit, and decrease in fat mass
- Modified nonaromatizable androgens, in particular the 17alpha-alkylated androgens, are not recommended for testosterone replacement therapy.

Topical (Transdermal) Testosterone

Transdermal testosterone patches became available in the late 1990s and early 2000s.

Testosterone is slowly released from transdermal patches providing a state level of testosterone for more than 24 hours. The transdermal patch was introduced first as a scrotal patch[33] which requires shaving or clipping of the scrotal hair. Because of higher 5-alpha-reductase activity in the scrotal skin, the scrotal patch produced higher serum dihydrotestosterone levels.[33,34] This scrotal patch was then replaced by a large skin patch (Testoderm) which has the problem of adhesiveness to the skin. Both the scrotal and the body patch are no longer available. The only available testosterone patch is Androderm; which can be applied to the body and is available as a 2 or 4 mg testosterone patch.[35–37] The application to the skin has to be rotated and application to the same area should be avoided for at least 7 days. However, the permeation enhanced patches are a closed system with an enhancer; mild irritation at the application site occurs in over two-thirds of patients and up to 10% to 15% of men discontinue treatment because of skin irritation. The localized skin irritation can be partially mitigated by topical glucocorticoids.[38,39]

The Food and Drug Administration (FDA) approved the first testosterone gel (AndroGel) in 2003 as a new method of delivering testosterone. After application of the hydro-alcoholic gel, about 10% of the testosterone is absorbed into the subdermal area forming a reservoir whereby the testosterone is released slowly into the bloodstream providing a relatively steady serum testosterone concentration. The 1% AndroGel contains 50 mg testosterone in 5 g gel and nominally delivers about 5 mg of testosterone to the body. The gel was applied over a large area of skin over the shoulders and upper arms and over the abdomen. Steady-state levels were reached in about a week. Serum testosterone levels increase in proportion to the applied dose of the gel in hypogonadal men.[40]

The surface area of the skin to which the gel was applied had a modest effect on the bioavailability of the testosterone gel. Application to 4 different sites (shoulders and 2 sides of the abdomen) than one site (4 applications on 1 shoulder) increased mean serum testosterone levels by 23%.[41] Since both absorption through the skin and clearance of testosterone may vary from patient to patient, periodic assessment of blood levels of testosterone is recommended. It should be noted that substantial day-to-day variations of serum testosterone concentration is often seen in the same man as well as among different men after testosterone gel application. This variation was tested in a substudy of The testosterone trials, whereby hypogonadal older men administered 1% AndroGel daily for 12 months. Dose adjustment, based on a 2-h postapplication testosterone measurement, was used to maintain serum testosterone concentrations within the adult male range.[42] In the sub-study, ambulatory 2-h post-application testosterone concentrations were measured in random order at 2 ambulatory clinic visits and during a 24-h in clinic pharmacokinetics study. The ambulatory clinic 2-h postgel applications serum testosterone concentration did not correlate with the 2-h nor the average concentration of serum testosterone during a 24-h in clinic pharmacokinetics study after the same dose of testosterone gel application. Despite these variations in postgel application testosterone concentrations, more than 80% of men had their 24-h average serum testosterone concentration within the adult male reference range (300–1000 ng/dL; 10.4–34.7 nmol/L).[43] As dose adjustments may be required to keep serum testosterone in the desired range, the physician should not make major dosage decisions on a single measurement as short-term variability in blood testosterone levels may occur for unknown reasons.

Testosterone gel relieves the symptoms of low testosterone, restores sexual function and mood, increases lean mass and bone mineral density, and decreases fat mass in testosterone deficient men.[44–46] In contrast to the testosterone patches, testosterone gel causes minimal skin irritation (5.6% of patients) but has the anticipated adverse effects of androgens including acne, oiliness of skin, and urinary symptoms.[44] A 1.62% AndroGel is supplied as a pump whereby 1 actuation delivers 20.25 mg of testosterone.[47,48] The pharmacokinetic profile and safety profile are similar to the 1% gel but the recommended starting dose is 40.5 mg or 2 actuations which is less than 50 mg recommended for the 1% gel.

Several other testosterone gel preparations are available in the US including Testim (1% testosterone gel)[49], Fortesta (2% testosterone gel),[50] and the generic Vogelxo (1% testosterone gel) and Testosterone gel (1.62%). They have similar pharmacokinetics and safety profile as AndroGel. A 2% testosterone lotion (Axiron, not hydroalcoholic) was developed to be applied to the axilla. The starting dose is 60 mg/d, but the product has been discontinued because of market competition.[51]

These testosterone gel products dry rapidly within a few minutes after application. Because only about 10% of testosterone is absorbed into the subdermal tissues, the rest remains on the skin until it is washed off. On close skin contact, there may be skin-to-skin transfer of testosterone to another person, which could increase serum testosterone concentrations in women and children.[52–54] Before coming into close skin contact with another person, the area of testosterone gel application should be washed with soap and water or covered by clothing. This warning is in the prescription information for all gels (warning: secondary exposure to testosterone).

Serum testosterone concentrations reach steady state after a few days.[41] Dose adjustment can be made based on serum levels 2 to 8 hours after application. Most testosterone gels maintain serum testosterone concentrations within the adult male range for about 24 hours. The dose adjustment should aim at testosterone ranges usually within the midadult male reference range.

Transdermal testosterone

- Delivery of testosterone on the skin results in a relatively steady release of testosterone from a reservoir in the subdermal reservoir.
- Transdermal patches are a closed system and produce skin irritation that necessitates stopping application in about 10% of men.
- Transdermal testosterone gels and solutions have less skin irritation/rash but can be transferred on close skin contact resulting in secondary exposure of another person to testosterone.
- Skin transfer can be prevented by washing the application area or covering the skin with clothing.
- Dose adjustment can be accomplished by measuring testosterone concentration about 2 to 8 hours after gel application.

Buccal/Nasal Testosterone

Buccal testosterone tablets are applied twice a day to the gums whereby the tablets adhered to the gums and testosterone were absorbed into the venous system. The tablets can produce physiologic testosterone levels in hypogonadal men. Mild gum irritation is reported in about 16% of men; about 4.7% of men have dislodgement of the buccal system.[55] This product is no longer available in the United States.

Testosterone gel delivered through the nose three times a day can achieve average serum testosterone concentrations more than 24 hours within the adult male range in 73% of men. Nasal testosterone improves sexual function, body composition, and bone mineral density in hypogonadal men.[56] The medication is well tolerated and severely hypogonadal men had similar improvement than those with less severe testosterone insufficiency.[57] The dose titration from a total of 22 mg to 33 mg per day nasal testosterone can be based on the relief of symptoms of the patients.[58] Nasal administration of testosterone may have benefits on symptoms of hypogonadism while maintaining LH, FSH within the reference range in about 70% to 80% and sperm concentration more than 5 million/ml in about 90% of the treated men in a 6-month uncontrolled study suggesting that there may be less suppression of spermatogenesis with nasal testosterone.[59] Further studies may be required to be certain of this benefit in men with symptomatic low testosterone wishing to father children.

Buccal/Nasal Testosterone

- Buccal tablets dislodge from the gums and may cause gum irritation. The product has been discontinued.
- Nasal testosterone must be applied three times a day to maintain serum testosterone within the adult male range.

Oral Testosterone Capsules

As discussed above, the currently available 17 alpha-alkylated modified testosterone tablets should not be used for testosterone replacement because of possible liver toxicity[29,30] and more marked effects on lowering HDL cholesterol and increasing

LDL cholesterol concentrations.[26] Testosterone undecanoate has been available as 40 mg capsules (Andriol Testocaps) for many decades outside of the United States.[60,61] One or 2 capsules ingested 2 or 3 times per day with food result in increased blood testosterone levels.[62,63] The medication is well tolerated and has an acceptable long-term safety profile.[64] However, serum testosterone levels are frequently low before the administration of the next dose.[65]

A new oral formulation of testosterone undecanoate in self-emulsifying drug delivery system (Jatenzo) was able to increase serum testosterone concentration to the adult male range when administered with food twice a day.[66,67] This testosterone delivery system was approved in 2019 by the Food and Drug Administration based on a study that showed that the orally administered testosterone undecanoate in the self-emulsifying system was able to maintain average testosterone concentration within the adult male range in 87% of hypogonadal men comparable to transdermal testosterone lotion/gel.[68] Because of the presence of intestinal 5 alpha-reductase, serum dihydrotestosterone to testosterone ratio is increased; the clinical significance of the increased DHT levels is not known.[69] There was improvement in the sexual symptoms of hypogonadism and safety profile of this new testosterone undecanoate preparation is similar to the transdermal gels except that oral testosterone appeared to have greater increase in hematocrit, blood pressure, and greater decrease in HDL-cholesterol than the transdermal gel.[68] Ambulatory blood pressure monitoring showed that the small increase in blood pressure is most likely a class effect as it was also shown with testosterone injections. Dose adjustment is based on a serum testosterone concentration drawn 4 to 6 hours after dosing.

Another oral testosterone undecanoate absorbed also via intestinal lymphatics is administered twice a day with meals without dose adjustment (TLANDO). This oral testosterone undecanoate provides adult male range levels in 72% to 88% of hypogonadal men, and has been tentatively approved by the FDA.[70]

Oral Testosterone Capsules

- Oral testosterone undecanoate capsules had been used throughout the world except the United States with proven long-term safety.
- New testosterone undecanoate delivery systems administered twice a day with food are available and provide acceptable adult male concentrations in most hypogonadal men. Safety profile is like transdermal testosterone.

Testosterone Ester Injections

Testosterone was isolated in 1935 and chemical synthesis was completed shortly afterwards. The short-acting testosterone propionate was available in 1939 and the medium longer acting testosterone enanthate in 1954. Testosterone enanthate injection was the main testosterone preparation for therapeutic use in hypogonadal men for more than 50 years.[71] Testosterone enanthate (Delatestryl) and testosterone cypionate (Depo-Testosterone) formulated in sesame or cottonseed oil, respectively, have similar pharmacokinetics. After a single intramuscular injection of 200 to 250 mg of testosterone enanthate or cypionate, serum concentration of testosterone rise to above the physiologic level and then gradually decrease remaining in the adult reference range for about 2 weeks.[72,73] These testosterone esters are rapidly converted to testosterone in the body and are not hepatotoxic. Injectable testosterone produces higher levels about 2 days after injection and this peak may cause higher hemoglobin levels than transdermal preparations.[37] The injections are administered slowly as a deep intramuscular injection into the gluteal muscle. The patients can be trained to administer their injections, but some prefer to have the injections administered by a health professional. The starting dose of testosterone enanthate or cypionate is 200 (or 250) mg intramuscularly every 2 weeks in adult men. Dose adjustment is either based usually on the trough level of serum testosterone that should be at the lower limit of the adult male range (300 ng/dL or 10.4 nmol/L) or in the midnormal range 1 week after injection. Recent studies demonstrate that the administration of testosterone enanthate/cypionate as a weekly subcutaneous injection into the abdominal fat produced concentrations of serum testosterone within the adult male range while minimizing the peaks and troughs observed after intramuscular injections.[74] Testosterone enanthate can also be administered by a single-use autoinjector designed to eject high viscosity solution (oil) through a short 27-gauge needle (Xyosted). The autoinjector system enables patients to self-inject testosterone more easily and with less pain. The autoinjector is filled with 50, 75, or 100 mg of testosterone in sesame oil and the recommended starting dose is 75 mg every week. Steady-state pharmacokinetics of serum testosterone concentrations were attained by week 4. The injection site adverse events included erythema and induration that were transient and mild.[75] A 1-year study showed that 92.7% of hypogonadal men achieved average testosterone concentration between 300 and 1000 ng/dL (10.4–34.7 nmol/L). Dose adjustment was based on the trough testosterone level (at the lower reference range) before the next injection. Most patients reported no pain, but the common adverse events were elevated hematocrit and hemoglobin, increased blood pressure, and prostate-specific antigen levels. Testosterone enanthate administered weekly by an autoinjector may provide a viable option for some men with hypogonadism.[76]

Testosterone undecanoate in castor oil is also available as a 250 mg/mL deep intramuscular injection (Aveed) in the United States. The recommended starting dose is 750 mg (3 mL) as the initial injection, followed by a second injection 4 weeks later and subsequent injections are administered every 10 weeks. The second injection administered 4 weeks reduces the chances of subnormal serum testosterone levels after the first injection.[77,78] This recommended treatment schedule is different from that in other countries, whereby testosterone undecanoate is administered as a 1000 mg in 4 mL injection as the first dose, followed by 1000 mg in 6 weeks, and thereafter as 12 weekly injections. The use of 750 mg intramuscular injections eliminates some of the high serum testosterone levels observed with the higher dose and generates serum testosterone concentrations in the adult male range for 10 weeks.[79,80] Steady-state testosterone concentration is achieved after the third injection in hypogonadal men. The serum testosterone concentrations were inversely proportional to body weight with higher levels in men with BMI less than 30 Kg/m^2 or body weight less than 100 Kg.[81] Dose adjustment is usually based on the trough level before the next injection that should be in the lower adult male range.

The prescription information of Aveed includes warning for pulmonary oil microembolism reaction characterized by cough, dyspnea, hyperhidrosis, throat tightening, chest pain, dizziness, and syncope which occurred rarely (0.1%) in patients administered testosterone undecanoate in castor oil. Most of the adverse events resolved within 30 minutes.[82] To reduce the risks of intravascular injection of testosterone undecanoate, the injection should be administered slowly deep into the gluteal muscle ensuring that the needle is not in blood vessels. It is required that the patient remains under observation in a health care setting for at least 30 minutes after injection. Proper administration technique of the 3 mL oil injection may reduce the incidence of this side effect.

Testosterone Ester Injections

- Intramuscular testosterone enanthate and cypionate have been used since the 1950s with long-term safety data. The pharmacokinetics profile showed that there were peaks and troughs of serum testosterone after each injection.
- Weekly subcutaneous injections of testosterone enanthate provide more steady concentrations of testosterone. The patients can self-administer the injections with less pain than intramuscular injection.
- Testosterone undecanoate injections are long acting. Once steady state is reached after the third injection, the patient can administer his own injections every 10 weeks. Dose adjustment can be accomplished based on the 7-day midrange or trough serum testosterone level before the next injection when every 2-week regimen is used.

Pulmonary oil microembolism presenting usually with cough is a rare occurrence after testosterone ester injection. Injection should be administered slowly with a small gauge needle.

Testosterone Implants

Fused crystalline testosterone pellets for subcutaneous implantation require a small skin incision and insertion of the pellet through a trocar. There are problems associated with the extrusion of the implants, but the frequency of extrusions decreases as the experience of operator increases. The pellets are available as 100 or 200 mg pellets inserted into the abdomen; 4 to 6 pellets provide steady serum testosterone levels in the midadult male range for 4 to 6 months.[83] The most common adverse event is extrusion in about 8% of men that is related to physical activity. Continuation rate of use of testosterone pellets is > 90%.[84] In the United States, TESTOPEL pellets contain 75 mg of testosterone and are inserted in fat in the gluteal region. The prescription instructions indicate 2 to 6 implants will last 3 to 4 months; however, clinical studies showed that 6 to 12 pellets increased serum testosterone concentration in hypogonadal men to the adult male range within a month. Higher number of testosterone pellets produced more consistent and longer maintenance of serum testosterone concentrations for 4 to 6 months. There is a low frequency of extrusion and hematoma formation that may be related to the number of pellets inserted. They are often favored by clinicians comfortable with the insertion process.[85,86] Increased hematocrit and hemoglobin have been reported with testosterone pellets, which is directly related to dose.[87,88] Monitoring of symptoms and serum testosterone concentrations will determine when and how many pellets should be implanted to maintain testosterone within the adult male range.

Testosteorne implants

- Testosterone pellets are available in the United States as 75 mg testosterone per implant.
- Insertion of 10 to 12 pellets will maintain testosterone concentrations in the adult male range for 4 to 6 weeks with relief of symptoms
- Extrusions can occur that may depend on the number of the pellets inserted and work activity

TREATMENT OF TESTOSTERONE DEFICIENCY IN MEN USING METHODS OTHER THAN TESTOSTERONE

We describe here the use of agents other than testosterone for the treatment of hypogonadism. These include nonhepatotoxic androgens and compounds that stimulate the production of testosterone by the Leydig cells in the testis.[89,90]

Modified Androgens

Although 17alpha-alkylated androgens are not recommended for androgen replacement for hypogonadal men, there are modified androgens with higher potency than testosterone that has been tested in men. Clinical studies of dihydrotestosterone formulated as a gel have been performed in hypogonadal men.[91-93] This formulation is only marketed in a few countries in Europe and has not undergone further development. Nandrolone, 19-nortestosterone (see **Fig.1**), and its derivatives are not hepatotoxic.[28] Modified 19-nortestosterone derivatives with methyl groups at the 7 or 11 position of the steroid ring have been studied (see **Fig. 1**). Esters of these compounds have been investigated in hypogonadal men for androgen replacement and eugonadal men as a potential male contraceptive (7α-methyl-19-norestosterone, MENT[94,95]; 7α-methyl-11 β-methyl-19-norestosterone, Dimethandrolone DMA[96-98]; and 11β-methyl-19-norestosterone, 11 β MNT[98,99]). These modified androgens did not exhibit hepatotoxicity in early phase clinical studies and are being formulated as oral capsules (to be taken with food), injections, and implants. Because these modified androgens may not aromatize to estrogenic compounds, longer-term studies are required to demonstrate the lack of adverse effects on bone health.[93,100]

Selective Androgen Receptor Modulators

Nonsteroidal, orally bioavailable, selective androgen receptor modulators (SARMs) with tissue-specific action that promote muscle and bone health without affecting prostate growth have also been tested (see Harrison G. Pope and Gen Kanayama's artcile, "Body Image Disorders and Anabolic Steroid Withdrawal Hypogonadism in Men," in this issue). Nonsteroidal SARMS have been tested for safety and tolerability. Certain SARMs suppressed endogenous production of testosterone with an increase in lean mass, no change in fat mass, and decreased HDL-cholesterol and triglycerides.[101] SARMs are being developed for the prevention and treatment of frailty in older men and women with impaired ability to do their daily activity and or those with cancer cachexia.[102-104] Clinical studies showed that treatment with a SARM of men and postmenopausal women with frailty or cancer cachexia for 12 weeks significantly increased lean mass and physical function.[105-107] Other studies are in progress whereby a SARM is used to treat cancer cachexia associated with nonsmall cell lung cancer.[108] The Food and Drug Administration has not yet approved a SARM for treatment of cachexia.[109] This may be related to concern about the potential abuse of anabolic agents for enhancement of athletic performance and bodybuilding. Recreational users of SARMs can obtain these compounds without quality control via the Internet; there is a risk that inappropriate off-label use could result in deleterious effects.[110]

Human Chorionic Gonadotropin

Human chorionic gonadotropin (hCG, Pregnyl) and recombinant human luteinizing hormone (Lutropin alfa, Luveris) are administered as intramuscular or subcutaneous injections in men to stimulate Leydig cells in the testis to produce endogenous testosterone. Because these hormones rely on relatively normal Leydig cells to produce testosterone, they are effective in the treatment of men with hypogonadotropic hypogonadism but not in men with primary testicular dysfunction. Human recombinant LH is available only for ovulation induction in females. The dose of hCG for off-label use in hypogonadotropic men is between 500 to 2000 IU 2 or 3 times a week.[111] Serum testosterone after hCG administration should be in the midadult male range and the dose can be adjusted to keep testosterone within this range.

In males with delayed puberty, hCG is used to induce puberty and to assess the testicular responsiveness to this gonadotropin.[112] In males with postpubertal hypogonadotropic hypogonadism, hCG alone is usually adequate for stimulating Leydig cells to produce testosterone and maintaining adequate intratesticular testosterone concentrations to stimulate spermatogenesis.[113,114] Chronic administration of hCG may increase serum levels of estradiol; it is thought that this is due to increased serum levels of testosterone and increased aromatization of testosterone and androstenedione in the testes.[115]

Because of cost and the frequency of injections, men with hypogonadotropic hypogonadism are usually treated with testosterone until the patient and his partner desire fertility. Then hCG with or without recombinant hFSH can be used to initiate or re-initiate spermatogenesis.[111,116,117] Studies have shown that prior testosterone treatment of hypogonadal men does not adversely affect responsiveness to hCG although the recovery of spermatogenesis may take longer time.[118–120] In contrast, others have reported that testosterone replacement in hypogonadal men may adversely affect spermatogenesis after testosterone is withdrawn.[121] Recovery of spermatogenesis after testosterone treatment in healthy adult men has been documented in male hormonal contraceptive studies[122] and in men after androgen abuse.[123,124] Measurement of intratesticular testosterone showed that hCG treatment at relatively low doses was able to maintain intratesticular testosterone concentration when gonadotropins were suppressed by exogenous testosterone injections.[111] Based on this observation, hCG has been proposed to be used with testosterone injections for more rapid recovery of spermatogenesis[125] as well as preventing the suppression of spermatogenesis[126] induced by exogenous testosterone administration. These studies should be verified in multicenter, larger, controlled studies. Fertility induction in hypogonadal men is described in greater detail in Anna Goldman and Martin Kathrins' artcile, "Optimized use of the Electronic Medical Record and Other Clinical Resources to Enhance the Management of Hypogonadal Men," in this issue.

Estrogen Antagonists and Aromatase Inhibitors

Partial estrogen antagonists (eg, clomiphene) and selective estrogen receptor modulators (SERMs, eg, tamoxifen) bind to the estrogen receptors and decrease the effects of estrogens on target tissues. Aromatase inhibitors (eg, Anastrozole, Letrozole) decrease estrogen concentrations by preventing the conversion of androgens to estrogens. These agents remove the negative feedback of estrogens on the hypothalamus and pituitary and stimulate the secretion of both gonadotropins LH and FSH. LH stimulates testosterone production by the Leydig cells in the testis and together with FSH stimulates spermatogenesis. These agents have no effect in patients with complete deficiency of LH and FSH or those with primary testicular failure causing testosterone deficiency. Estrogen antagonists such as clomiphene have been used in men with testosterone insufficiency with symptomatic improvement and increased bone mineral density.[127,128] Aromatase inhibitors have been used to stimulate endogenous testosterone production.[129,130] For these agents, the increase in LH and FSH and serum testosterone can be monitored and dose adjusted to attain serum testosterone levels in the midadult range. Adverse effects with bone health occur when aromatase inhibitors are administered for months because of decreased bone mineral density associated with decreased estradiol concentrations.[119] Aromatase inhibitors are also used in uncontrolled studies in hypogonadal infertile men with and without concomitant testosterone therapy to improve testicular sperm retrieval for intracytoplasmic sperm injection.[131,132]

Nontestosterone Treatment for Testosterone Deficiency

- There are modified androgens that are not hepatotoxic and more potent than testosterone, but the efficacy and safety of these compounds have yet to be verified in hypogonadal men.
- Selective androgen receptor modulators are not usually designed for testosterone deficiency but for the treatment of sarcopenia and frailty.
- Human chorionic gonadotropin is used in boys with hypogonadotropic hypogonadism and delayed puberty to initiate puberty and spermatogenesis. Because of the cost and frequency of injections, they are not generally used for testosterone replacement in hypogonadal men unless fertility is desired.
- Estrogen receptor antagonists and aromatase inhibitors increase LH and FSH and testosterone production. These agents are not useful in men with primary hypogonadism and patients with anatomically deficient FSH and LH. Aromatase

SUMMARY

Men with testosterone deficiency should be replaced with testosterone unless there are contraindications or near-term fertility is desired. Testosterone ester injections have proven safety and efficacy for more than 70 years. Since 2000, many options are available to deliver testosterone to correct testosterone deficiency. All testosterone replacement methods have been shown to be efficacious as shown by the normalization of serum testosterone levels. These methods include transdermal patches and gels, oral capsules, intranasal testosterone, long-acting intramuscular injections, subcutaneous injections, and testosterone implants. Dose adjustment strategies to achieve serum testosterone in the midadult male range and relief of symptoms depend on the method used. Human chorionic gonadotropin, SERMs, estrogen antagonists, and aromatase inhibitors stimulate the endogenous production of testosterone and improve symptoms of hypogonadism when the testis can respond. Nonaromatizable potent modified androgens and aromatase inhibitors may cause bone loss, long-term use may not be advisable in hypogonadal men.

CLINICS CARE POINTS

- Men with testosterone deficiency should be treated with testosterone.
- Selection of the method of delivering testosterone depends on the needs of the patient and his preference.
- Some modified androgens such as the 17 alpha-alkylated androgens are hepatotoxic and nonaromatizable androgens may cause bone loss that needs to be monitored.
- All existing approved testosterone formulations achieve serum testosterone in the adult male range and improve symptoms in most hypogonadal men.
- Dose adjustment should be individualized depending on the method used and treatment goals.
- Stimulators of endogenous testosterone production are usually used for limited periods of time mainly during puberty and when the man desires fertility.
- Prior long-term treatment with testosterone products will suppress spermatogenesis that is reversible on discontinuation of treatment and human chorionic gonadotropin may accelerate the recovery of spermatogenesis.

DISCLOSURE

Drs. C. Wang and R.S. Swerdloff received research support from the Testosterone Replacement Therapy Manufacturers Consortium, Clarus Therapeutics, Chiasma, Crinetics Pharmaceuticals, and Corcept Therapeutics.

REFERENCES

1. Bhasin S, Brito JP, Cunningham GR, et al. Testosterone therapy in men with hypogonadism: an endocrine society clinical practice guideline. J Clin Endocrinol Metab 2018;103(5):1715–44.
2. Baillargeon J, Urban RJ, Ottenbacher KJ, et al. Trends in androgen prescribing in the United States, 2001 to 2011. JAMA Intern Med 2013;173(15):1465–6.
3. Layton JB, Li D, Meier CR, et al. Testosterone lab testing and initiation in the United Kingdom and the United States, 2000 to 2011. J Clin Endocrinol Metab 2014;99(3):835–42.
4. Handelsman DJ. Global trends in testosterone prescribing, 2000-2011: expanding the spectrum of prescription drug misuse. Med J Aust 2013;199(8):548–51.
5. Bandari J, Ayyash OM, Emery SL, et al. Marketing and testosterone treatment in the USA: A Systematic Review. Eur Urol focus 2017;3(4–5):395–402.
6. Baillargeon J, Kuo YF, Westra JR, et al. Testosterone prescribing in the United States, 2002-2016. JAMA 2018;320(2):200–2.
7. Ory J, White JT, Moore J, et al. Canadian trends in testosterone therapy. Can Urol Assoc J 2021;15(6):210–2.
8. Nguyen CP, Hirsch MS, Moeny D, et al. Testosterone and "Age-Related Hypogonadism"–FDA Concerns. N Engl J Med 2015;373(8):689–91.
9. Vigen R, O'Donnell CI, Baron AE, et al. Association of testosterone therapy with mortality, myocardial infarction, and stroke in men with low testosterone levels. JAMA 2013;310(17):1829–36.
10. Basaria S, Coviello AD, Travison TG, et al. Adverse events associated with testosterone administration. N Engl J Med 2010;363(2):109–22.
11. Xu L, Freeman G, Cowling BJ, et al. Testosterone therapy and cardiovascular events among men: a systematic review and meta-analysis of placebo-controlled randomized trials. BMC Med 2013;11:108.
12. Corona G, Maseroli E, Rastrelli G, et al. Cardiovascular risk associated with testosterone-boosting medications: a systematic review and meta-analysis. Expert Opin Drug Saf 2014;13(10):1327–51.
13. Rosner W, Auchus RJ, Azziz R, et al. Position statement: utility, limitations, and pitfalls in measuring testosterone: an endocrine society position statement. J Clin Endocrinol Metab 2007;92(2):405–13.
14. Travison TG, Vesper HW, Orwoll E, et al. Harmonized reference ranges for circulating testosterone levels in men of four cohort studies in the United States and Europe. J Clin Endocrinol Metab 2017;102(4):1161–73.
15. Wilson JD. The role of 5alpha-reduction in steroid hormone physiology. Reprod Fertil Dev 2001;13(7–8):673–8.
16. Peterson RE, Imperato-McGinley J, Gautier T, et al. Male pseudohermaphroditism due to steroid 5-alpha-reductase deficiency. Am J Med 1977;62(2):170–91.
17. Imperato-McGinley J, Zhu YS. Androgens and male physiology the syndrome of 5alpha-reductase-2 deficiency. Mol Cell Endocrinol 2002;198(1–2):51–9.
18. Carani C, Qin K, Simoni M, et al. Effect of testosterone and estradiol in a man with aromatase deficiency. N Engl J Med 1997;337(2):91–5.

19. Bhasin S, Woodhouse L, Casaburi R, et al. Testosterone dose-response relationships in healthy young men. Am J Physiol Endocrinol Metab 2001;281(6):E1172–81.

20. Bhasin S, Woodhouse L, Casaburi R, et al. Older men are as responsive as young men to the anabolic effects of graded doses of testosterone on the skeletal muscle. J Clin Endocrinol Metab 2005;90(2):678–88.

21. Bhasin S, Storer TW, Berman N, et al. The effects of supraphysiologic doses of testosterone on muscle size and strength in normal men. N Engl J Med 1996;335(1):1–7.

22. Finkelstein JS, Lee H, Burnett-Bowie SA, et al. Gonadal steroids and body composition, strength, and sexual function in men. N Engl J Med 2013;369(11):1011–22.

23. Finkelstein JS, Lee H, Leder BZ, et al. Gonadal steroid-dependent effects on bone turnover and bone mineral density in men. J Clin Invest 2016;126(3):1114–25.

24. Cunningham GR, Stephens-Shields AJ, Rosen RC, et al. Testosterone treatment and sexual function in older men with low testosterone levels. J Clin Endocrinol Metab 2016;101(8):3096–104.

25. Wang C, Swerdloff RS. Should the nonaromatizable androgen dihydrotestosterone be considered as an alternative to testosterone in the treatment of the andropause? J Clin Endocrinol Metab 2002;87(4):1462–6.

26. Friedl KE, Hannan CJ Jr, Jones RE, et al. High-density lipoprotein cholesterol is not decreased if an aromatizable androgen is administered. Metabolism 1990;39(1):69–74.

27. Foss GL, Simpson SL. Oral methyltestosterone and jaundice. Br Med J 1959;1(5117):259–63.

28. Welder AA, Robertson JW, Melchert RB. Toxic effects of anabolic-androgenic steroids in primary rat hepatic cell cultures. J Pharmacol Toxicol Methods 1995;33(4):187–95.

29. Boyer JL, Preisig R, Zbinden G, et al. Guidelines for assessment of potential hepatotoxic effects of synthetic androgens, anabolic agents and progestagens in their use in males as antifertility agents. Contraception 1976;13(4):461.

30. Westaby D, Ogle SJ, Paradinas FJ, et al. Liver damage from long-term methyltestosterone. Lancet 1977;2(8032):262.

31. Joseph JF, Parr MK. Synthetic androgens as designer supplements. Curr Neuropharmacol 2015;13(1):89–100.

32. Rahnema CD, Crosnoe LE, Kim ED. Designer steroids - over-the-counter supplements and their androgenic component: review of an increasing problem. Andrology 2015;3(2):150–5.

33. Cunningham GR, Cordero E, Thornby JI. Testosterone replacement with transdermal therapeutic systems. Physiological serum testosterone and elevated dihydrotestosterone levels. JAMA 1989;261(17):2525–30.

34. Findlay JC, Place V, Snyder PJ. Treatment of primary hypogonadism in men by the transdermal administration of testosterone. J Clin Endocrinol Metab 1989;68(2):369–73.

35. Meikle AW, Arver S, Dobs AS, et al. Pharmacokinetics and metabolism of a permeation-enhanced testosterone transdermal system in hypogonadal men: influence of application site- -a clinical research center study. J Clin Endocrinol Metab 1996;81(5):1832–40.

36. Meikle AW, Mazer NA, Moellmer JF, et al. Enhanced transdermal delivery of testosterone across nonscrotal skin produces physiological concentrations of

testosterone and its metabolites in hypogonadal men. J Clin Endocrinol Metab 1992;74(3):623–8.

37. Dobs AS, Meikle AW, Arver S, et al. Pharmacokinetics, efficacy, and safety of a permeation-enhanced testosterone transdermal system in comparison with bi-weekly injections of testosterone enanthate for the treatment of hypogonadal men. J Clin Endocrinol Metab 1999;84(10):3469–78.

38. Jordan WP Jr. Allergy and topical irritation associated with transdermal testos-terone administration: a comparison of scrotal and nonscrotal transdermal sys-tems. Am J Contact Dermat 1997;8(2):108–13.

39. Jordan WP Jr, Atkinson LE, Lai C. Comparison of the skin irritation potential of two testosterone transdermal systems: an investigational system and a mar-keted product. Clin Ther 1998;20(1):80–7.

40. Swerdloff RS, Wang C, Cunningham G, et al. Long-term pharmacokinetics of transdermal testosterone gel in hypogonadal men. J Clin Endocrinol Metab 2000;85(12):4500–10.

41. Wang C, Berman N, Longstreth JA, et al. Pharmacokinetics of transdermal testosterone gel in hypogonadal men: application of gel at one site versus four sites: a General Clinical Research Center Study. J Clin Endocrinol Metab 2000;85(3):964–9.

42. Snyder PJ, Bhasin S, Cunningham GR, et al. Effects of Testosterone Treatment in Older Men. N Engl J Med 2016;374(7):611–24.

43. Swerdloff RS, Pak Y, Wang C, et al. Serum Testosterone (T) Level Variability in T Gel-Treated Older Hypogonadal Men: Treatment Monitoring Implications. J Clin Endocrinol Metab 2015;100(9):3280–7.

44. Wang C, Swedloff RS, Iranmanesh A, et al. Transdermal testosterone gel im-proves sexual function, mood, muscle strength, and body composition param-eters in hypogonadal men. Testosterone Gel Study Group. J Clin Endocrinol Metab 2000;85(8):2839–53.

45. Wang C, Cunningham G, Dobs A, et al. Long-term testosterone gel (AndroGel) treatment maintains beneficial effects on sexual function and mood, lean and fat mass, and bone mineral density in hypogonadal men. J Clin Endocrinol Metab 2004;89(5):2085–98.

46. Wang C, Swerdloff RS, Iranmanesh A, et al. Effects of transdermal testosterone gel on bone turnover markers and bone mineral density in hypogonadal men. Clin Endocrinol (Oxf) 2001;54(6):739–50.

47. Kaufman JM, Miller MG, Fitzpatrick S, et al. One-year efficacy and safety study of a 1.62% testosterone gel in hypogonadal men: results of a 182-day open-label extension of a 6-month double-blind study. J Sex Med 2012;9(4):1149–61.

48. Kaufman JM, Miller MG, Garwin JL, et al. Efficacy and safety study of 1.62% testosterone gel for the treatment of hypogonadal men. J Sex Med 2011;8(7):2079–89.

49. Steidle C, Schwartz S, Jacoby K, et al. AA2500 testosterone gel normalizes androgen levels in aging males with improvements in body composition and sexual function. J Clin Endocrinol Metab 2003;88(6):2673–81.

50. Dobs AS, McGettigan J, Norwood P, et al. A novel testosterone 2% gel for the treatment of hypogonadal males. J Androl 2012;33(4):601–7.

51. Wang C, Ilani N, Arver S, et al. Efficacy and safety of the 2% formulation of testosterone topical solution applied to the axillae in androgen-deficient men. Clin Endocrinol (Oxf) 2011;75(6):836–43.

52. Stahlman J, Britto M, Fitzpatrick S, et al. Serum testosterone levels in non-dosed females after secondary exposure to 1.62% testosterone gel: effects of clothing barrier on testosterone absorption. Curr Med Res Opin 2012a;28(2):291–301.

53. Stahlman J, Britto M, Fitzpatrick S, et al. Effect of application site, clothing barrier, and application site washing on testosterone transfer with a 1.62% testosterone gel. Curr Med Res Opin 2012b;28(2):281–90.

54. Stahlman J, Britto M, Fitzpatrick S, et al. Effects of skin washing on systemic absorption of testosterone in hypogonadal males after administration of 1.62% testosterone gel. Curr Med Res Opin 2012c;28(2):271–9.

55. Wang C, Swerdloff R, Kipnes M, et al. New testosterone buccal system (Striant) delivers physiological testosterone levels: pharmacokinetics study in hypogonadal men. J Clin Endocrinol Metab 2004;89(8):3821–9.

56. Rogol AD, Tkachenko N, Bryson N. Natesto™ , a novel testosterone nasal gel, normalizes androgen levels in hypogonadal men. Andrology 2016;4(1):46–54.

57. Gronski MA, Grober ED, Gottesman IS, et al. Efficacy of nasal testosterone gel (Natesto(®)) Stratified by Baseline Endogenous Testosterone Levels. J Endocr Soc 2019;3(9):1652–62.

58. Lee J, Brock G, Barkin J, et al. Symptom-based titration decisions when using testosterone nasal gel, Natesto(®). Can Urol Assoc J 2019;13(10):301–6.

59. Ramasamy R, Masterson TA, Best JC, et al. Effect of natesto on reproductive hormones, semen parameters and hypogonadal symptoms: a single center, open label, single arm trial. J Urol 2020;204(3):557–63.

60. Skakkebaek NE, Bancroft J, Davidson DW, et al. Androgen replacement with oral testosterone undecanoate in hypogonadal men: a double blind controlled study. Clin Endocrinol (Oxf) 1981;14(1):49–61.

61. Nieschlag E, Mauss J, Coert A, et al. Plasma androgen levels in men after oral administration of testosterone or testosterone undecanoate. Acta Endocrinol (Copenh) 1975;79(2):366–74.

62. Horst HJ, Holtje WJ, Dennis M, et al. Lymphatic absorption and metabolism of orally administered testosterone undecanoate in man. Klin Wochenschr 1976; 54(18):875–9.

63. Schnabel PG, Bagchus W, Lass H, et al. The effect of food composition on serum testosterone levels after oral administration of Andriol Testocaps. Clin Endocrinol (Oxf) 2007;66(4):579–85.

64. Gooren LJ. A ten-year safety study of the oral androgen testosterone undecanoate. J Androl 1994;15(3):212–5.

65. Legros JJ, Meuleman EJ, Elbers JM, et al. Oral testosterone replacement in symptomatic late-onset hypogonadism: effects on rating scales and general safety in a randomized, placebo-controlled study. Eur J Endocrinol 2009; 160(5):821–31.

66. Yin A, Alfadhli E, Htun M, et al. Dietary fat modulates the testosterone pharmacokinetics of a new self-emulsifying formulation of oral testosterone undecanoate in hypogonadal men. J Androl 2012;33(6):1282–90.

67. Yin AY, Htun M, Swerdloff RS, et al. Reexamination of pharmacokinetics of oral testosterone undecanoate in hypogonadal men with a new self-emulsifying formulation. J Androl 2012;33(2):190–201.

68. Swerdloff RS, Wang C, White WB, et al. A new oral testosterone undecanoate formulation restores testosterone to normal concentrations in hypogonadal men. J Clin Endocrinol Metab 2020;105(8):2515–31.

69. Swerdloff RS, Dudley RE, Page ST, et al. Dihydrotestosterone: biochemistry, physiology, and clinical implications of elevated blood levels. Endocr Rev 2017;38(3):220–54.

70. DelConte A, Patel MV, Papangkorn K, et al. SAT-052 A Novel Oral Testosterone Therapy (TLANDO) Safely Restores Testosterone to Eugonadal Levels with Fixed Dose Treatment. J Endocr Soc 2020;4(Supplement_1).

71. Nieschlag E, Nieschlag S. Testosterone deficiency: a historical perspective. Asian J Androl 2014;16(2):161–8.

72. Snyder PJ, Lawrence DA. Treatment of male hypogonadism with testosterone enanthate. J Clin Endocrinol Metab 1980;51(6):1335–9.

73. Sokol RZ, Palacios A, Campfield LA, et al. Comparison of the kinetics of injectable testosterone in eugonadal and hypogonadal men. Ferti Steril 1982;37(3):425–30.

74. McFarland J, Craig W, Clarke NJ, et al. Serum testosterone concentrations remain stable between injections in patients receiving subcutaneous testosterone. J Endocr Soc 2017;1(8):1095–103.

75. Kaminetsky J, Jaffe JS, Swerdloff RS. Pharmacokinetic profile of subcutaneous testosterone enanthate delivered via a novel, prefilled single-use autoinjector: a phase ii study. Sex Med 2015;3(4):269–79.

76. Kaminetsky JC, McCullough A, Hwang K, et al. A 52-Week Study of Dose-Adjusted Subcutaneous Testosterone Enanthate in Oil Self-Administered via Disposable Auto-injector. J Urol 2018;201(3):587–94.

77. Morgentaler A, Dobs AS, Kaufman JM, et al. Long acting testosterone undecanoate therapy in men with hypogonadism: results of a pharmacokinetic clinical study. J Urol 2008;180(6):2307–13.

78. Wang C, Harnett M, Dobs AS, et al. Pharmacokinetics and safety of long-acting testosterone undecanoate injections in hypogonadal men: an 84-week phase III clinical trial. J Androl 2010;31(5):457–65.

79. von Eckardstein S, Nieschlag E. Treatment of male hypogonadism with testosterone undecanoate injected at extended intervals of 12 weeks: a phase II study. J Androl 2002;23(3):419–25.

80. Nieschlag E, Buchter D, von Eckardstein S, et al. Repeated intramuscular injections of testosterone undecanoate for substitution therapy in hypogonadal men. Clin Endocrinol (Oxf) 1999;51(6):757–63.

81. Behre HM, Abshagen K, Oettel M, et al. Intramuscular injection of testosterone undecanoate for the treatment of male hypogonadism: phase I studies. Eur J Endocrinol 1999;140(5):414–9.

82. Pastuszak AW, Hu Y, Freid JD. Occurrence of pulmonary oil microembolism after testosterone undecanoate injection: a postmarketing safety analysis. Sex Med 2020;8(2):237–42.

83. Handelsman DJ, Conway AJ, Boylan LM. Pharmacokinetics and pharmacodynamics of testosterone pellets in man. J Clin Endocrinol Metab 1990;71(1):216–22.

84. Handelsman DJ, Mackey MA, Howe C, et al. An analysis of testosterone implants for androgen replacement therapy. Clin Endocrinol (Oxf) 1997;47(3):311–6.

85. McCullough AR, Khera M, Goldstein I, et al. A multi-institutional observational study of testosterone levels after testosterone pellet (Testopel((R))) insertion. J Sex Med 2012;9(2):594–601.

86. McMahon CG, Shusterman N, Cohen B. Pharmacokinetics, clinical efficacy, safety profile, and patient-reported outcomes in patients receiving

subcutaneous testosterone pellets 900 mg for treatment of symptoms associated with androgen deficiency. J Sex Med 2017;14(7):883–90.

87. Hayden RP, Bennett NE, Tanrikut C. Hematocrit response and risk factors for significant hematocrit elevation with implantable testosterone pellets. J Urol 2016;196(6):1715–20.

88. Ip FF, di Pierro I, Brown R, et al. Trough serum testosterone predicts the development of polycythemia in hypogonadal men treated for up to 21 years with subcutaneous testosterone pellets. Eur J Endocrinol 2010;162(2):385–90.

89. Krzastek SC, Smith RP. Non-testosterone management of male hypogonadism: an examination of the existing literature. Translational Androl Urol 2020;9(Suppl 2):S160–70.

90. Aydogdu A, Swerdloff RS. Emerging medication for the treatment of male hypogonadism. Expert Opin Emerg Drugs 2016;21(3):255–66.

91. Wang C, Iranmanesh A, Berman N, et al. Comparative pharmacokinetics of three doses of percutaneous dihydrotestosterone gel in healthy elderly men–a clinical research center study. J Clin Endocrinol Metab 1998;83(8):2749–57.

92. de Lignieres B. Transdermal dihydrotestosterone treatment of 'andropause. Ann Med 1993;25(3):235–41.

93. Ly LP, Jimenez M, Zhuang TN, et al. A double-blind, placebo-controlled, randomized clinical trial of transdermal dihydrotestosterone gel on muscular strength, mobility, and quality of life in older men with partial androgen deficiency. J Clin Endocrinol Metab 2001;86(9):4078–88.

94. von Eckardstein S, Noe G, Brache V, et al. A clinical trial of 7 alpha-methyl-19-nortestosterone implants for possible use as a long-acting contraceptive for men. J Clin Endocrinol Metab 2003;88(11):5232–9.

95. Anderson RA, Wallace AM, Sattar N, et al. Evidence for tissue selectivity of the synthetic androgen 7{alpha}-Methyl-19-Nortestosterone in Hypogonadal Men. J Clin Endocrinol Metab 2003;88(6):2784–93.

96. Surampudi P, Page ST, Swerdloff RS, et al. Single, escalating dose pharmacokinetics, safety and food effects of a new oral androgen dimethandrolone undecanoate in man: a prototype oral male hormonal contraceptive. Andrology 2014; 2(4):579–87.

97. Ayoub R, Page ST, Swerdloff RS, et al. Comparison of the single dose pharmacokinetics, pharmacodynamics, and safety of two novel oral formulations of dimethandrolone undecanoate (DMAU): a potential oral, male contraceptive. Andrology 2017;5(2):278–85.

98. Wu S, Yuen F, Swerdloff RS, et al. Safety and pharmacokinetics of single-dose novel oral androgen 11beta-Methyl-19-Nortestosterone-17beta-Dodecylcarbonate in Men. J Clin Endocrinol Metab 2019;104(3):629–38.

99. Yuen F, Thirumalai A, Pham C, et al. Daily oral administration of the novel androgen 11β-MNTDC markedly suppresses serum gonadotropins in healthy men. J Clin Endocrinol Metab 2020;105(3):e835–47.

100. Thirumalai A, Yuen F, Amory JK, et al. Dimethandrolone Undecanoate, a Novel, Nonaromatizable Androgen, Increases P1NP in Healthy Men Over 28 Days. J Clin Endocrinol Metab 2021;106(1):e171–81.

101. Basaria S, Collins L, Dillon EL, et al. The safety, pharmacokinetics, and effects of LGD-4033, a novel nonsteroidal oral, selective androgen receptor modulator, in healthy young men. J Gerontol A Biol Sci Med Sci 2013;68(1):87–95.

102. Bhasin S, Jasuja R. Selective androgen receptor modulators as function promoting therapies. Curr Opin Clin Nutr Metab Care 2009;12(3):232–40.

103. Narayanan R, Coss CC, Dalton JT. Development of selective androgen receptor modulators (SARMs). Mol Cell. Endocrinol. 2018;465:134–42.

104. Solomon ZJ, Mirabal JR, Mazur DJ, et al. Selective androgen receptor modulators: current knowledge and clinical applications. Sex Med Rev 2019;7(1): 84–94.

105. Dalton JT, Barnette KG, Bohl CE, et al. The selective androgen receptor modulator GTx-024 (enobosarm) improves lean body mass and physical function in healthy elderly men and postmenopausal women: results of a double-blind, placebo-controlled phase II trial. J cachexia, sarcopenia Muscle 2011;2(3):153–61.

106. Dalton JT, Taylor RP, Mohler ML, et al. Selective androgen receptor modulators for the prevention and treatment of muscle wasting associated with cancer. Curr Opin Support Palliat Care 2013;7(4):345–51.

107. Dobs AS, Boccia RV, Croot CC, et al. Effects of enobosarm on muscle wasting and physical function in patients with cancer: a double-blind, randomised controlled phase 2 trial. Lancet Oncol 2013;14(4):335–45.

108. Crawford J, Prado CM, Johnston MA, et al. Study design and rationale for the phase 3 clinical development program of enobosarm, a selective androgen receptor modulator, for the prevention and treatment of muscle wasting in cancer patients (POWER Trials). Curr Oncol Rep 2016;18(6):37.

109. Srinath R, Dobs A. Enobosarm (GTx-024, S-22): a potential treatment for cachexia. Future Oncol (London, England) 2014;10(2):187–94.

110. Machek SB, Cardaci TD, Wilburn DT, et al. Considerations, possible contraindications, and potential mechanisms for deleterious effect in recreational and athletic use of selective androgen receptor modulators (SARMs) in lieu of anabolic androgenic steroids: A narrative review. Steroids 2020;164:108753.

111. Coviello AD, Matsumoto AM, Bremner WJ, et al. Low-dose human chorionic gonadotropin maintains intratesticular testosterone in normal men with testosterone-induced gonadotropin suppression. J Clin Endocrinol Metab 2005;90(5):2595–602.

112. Rohayem J, Hauffa BP, Zacharin M, et al. Testicular growth and spermatogenesis: new goals for pubertal hormone replacement in boys with hypogonadotropic hypogonadism? -a multicentre prospective study of hCG/rFSH treatment outcomes during adolescence. Clin Endocrinol (Oxf) 2017;86(1): 75–87.

113. Matsumoto AM, Paulsen CA, Bremner WJ. Stimulation of sperm production by human luteinizing hormone in gonadotropin-suppressed normal men. J Clin Endocrinol Metab 1984;59(5):882–7.

114. Finkel DM, Phillips JL, Snyder PJ. Stimulation of spermatogenesis by gonadotropins in men with hypogonadotropic hypogonadism. N Engl J Med 1985;313(11): 651–5.

115. Liu PY, Wishart SM, Handelsman DJ. A double-blind, placebo-controlled, randomized clinical trial of recombinant human chorionic gonadotropin on muscle strength and physical function and activity in older men with partial age-related androgen deficiency. J Clin Endocrinol Metab 2002;87(7):3125–35.

116. Liu PY, Turner L, Rushford D, et al. Efficacy and safety of recombinant human follicle stimulating hormone (Gonal-F) with urinary human chorionic gonadotrophin for induction of spermatogenesis and fertility in gonadotrophin-deficient men. Hum Reprod 1999;14(6):1540–5.

117. Liu PY, Gebski VJ, Turner L, et al. Predicting pregnancy and spermatogenesis by survival analysis during gonadotrophin treatment of gonadotrophin-deficient infertile men. Hum Reprod 2002;17(3):625–33.

118. Liu PY, Baker HW, Jayadev V, et al. Induction of spermatogenesis and fertility during gonadotropin treatment of gonadotropin-deficient infertile men: predictors of fertility outcome. J Clin Endocrinol Metab 2009;94(3):801–8.

119. Burger HG, de Kretser DM, Hudson B, et al. Effects of preceding androgen therapy on testicular response to human pituitary gonadotropin in hypogonadotropic hypogonadism: a study of three patients. Ferti Steril 1981;35(1):64–8.

120. Ley SB, Leonard JM. Male hypogonadotropic hypogonadism: factors influencing response to human chorionic gonadotropin and human menopausal gonadotropin, including prior exogenous androgens. J Clin Endocrinol Metab 1985;61(4):746–52.

121. Ohlander SJ, Lindgren MC, Lipshultz LI. Testosterone and male infertility. Urol Clin North Am 2016;43(2):195–202.

122. Liu PY, Swerdloff RS, Christenson PD, et al. Rate, extent, and modifiers of spermatogenic recovery after hormonal male contraception: an integrated analysis. Lancet 2006;367(9520):1412–20.

123. McBride JA, Coward RM. Recovery of spermatogenesis following testosterone replacement therapy or anabolic-androgenic steroid use. Asian J Androl 2016;18(3):373–80.

124. Handelsman D, Shankara-Narayana N, Yu C, et al. Rate and extent of recovery from reproductive and cardiac dysfunction due to androgen abuse in men. J Clin Endocrinol Metab 2020;105(6):dgz324.

125. Wenker EP, Dupree JM, Langille GM, et al. The Use of HCG-Based Combination Therapy for Recovery of Spermatogenesis after Testosterone Use. J Sex Med 2015;12(6):1334–7.

126. Hsieh TC, Pastuszak AW, Hwang K, et al. Concomitant intramuscular human chorionic gonadotropin preserves spermatogenesis in men undergoing testosterone replacement therapy. J Urol 2013;189(2):647–50.

127. Guay AT, Jacobson J, Perez JB, et al. Clomiphene increases free testosterone levels in men with both secondary hypogonadism and erectile dysfunction: who does and does not benefit? Int J Impot Res 2003;15(3):156–65.

128. Moskovic DJ, Katz DJ, Akhavan A, et al. Clomiphene citrate is safe and effective for long-term management of hypogonadism. BJU Int 2012;110(10):1524–8.

129. Leder BZ, Rohrer JL, Rubin SD, et al. Effects of aromatase inhibition in elderly men with low or borderline-low serum testosterone levels. J Clin Endocrinol Metab 2004;89(3):1174–80.

130. Dias JP, Shardell MD, Carlson OD, et al. Testosterone vs. aromatase inhibitor in older men with low testosterone: effects on cardiometabolic parameters. Andrology 2017;5(1):31–40.

131. Mehta A, Bolyakov A, Roosma J, et al. Successful testicular sperm retrieval in adolescents with Klinefelter syndrome treated with at least 1 year of topical testosterone and aromatase inhibitor. Fertil Steril 2013;100(4):970–4.

132. Punjani N, Bernie H, Salter C, et al. The Utilization and Impact of Aromatase Inhibitor Therapy in Men With Elevated Estradiol Levels on Testosterone Therapy. Sex Med 2021;9(4):100378.

Monitoring of Testosterone Replacement Therapy to Optimize the Benefit-to-Risk Ratio

Frances J. Hayes, MB, BCh, BAO, FRCPI

KEYWORDS

- Testosterone • Monitoring • Side effects • Hypogonadism

KEY POINTS

- To optimize the benefit-to-risk ratio of testosterone therapy, it is important that the patients selected for treatment meet established criteria for hypogonadism and have symptoms and/or conditions that could reasonably be expected to improve with testosterone replacement.
- For patients with contraindications to treatment, alternative approaches should be discussed, if available.
- Hypogonadal men who have initiated treatment with testosterone should be assessed to see if symptoms have improved, if they are compliant with therapy, and if they are experiencing any adverse effects.
- All patients treated with testosterone should have measurement of testosterone and hematocrit at 3 to 6 months, 12 months, and then annually thereafter.
- Shared decision making should be used to determine whether to screen for prostate cancer and informed by age, baseline cancer risk, and patient preference.

INTRODUCTION

The past 2 decades have seen a surge in the use of testosterone replacement therapy for the treatment of male hypogonadism.[1] There has also been a substantial increase in the number of formulations approved by the Food and Drug Administration (FDA) to treat hypogonadal patients. Available options now include the traditional intramuscular injections of testosterone esters (enanthate and cypionate), gels of different concentrations (1%, 1.62%, 2%), patches, oral and depot formulations of testosterone undecanoate, nasal testosterone, and pellets.[2] It is therefore important for endocrinologists to know how to manage these patients appropriately. Several clinical practice recommendations have been published to guide physicians on the optimal

Reproductive Endocrine Unit, BHX5, Harvard Medical School, Massachusetts General Hospital, 55 Fruit Street, Boston, MA 02114, USA
E-mail address: fhayes@mgh.harvard.edu

Endocrinol Metab Clin N Am 51 (2022) 99–108
https://doi.org/10.1016/j.ecl.2021.11.013
0889-8529/22/© 2021 Elsevier Inc. All rights reserved.

management of men with androgen deficiency.[2–4] However, evidence suggests that adherence to these guidelines is variable[5,6] with 1 study suggesting that fewer than 50% of men treated with testosterone received the appropriate monitoring after treatment initiation.[6] The goal of this article is to provide a framework for monitoring patients treated with testosterone to ensure that benefits are optimized, risks are minimized, and any side effects are both identified early and managed appropriately.

STRATEGIES TO OPTIMIZE BENEFIT

In hypogonadal patients, testosterone replacement has a multitude of benefits, including an improvement in energy levels, sexual function, body composition, and bone mass.[2] However, testosterone is a schedule 3 controlled substance with potential for harm if used either without the appropriate monitoring or for an inappropriate indication. The following approach can help to ensure that optimal benefit is achieved from testosterone therapy.

Select the Right Patient and Formulation

In order to optimize the benefit-to-risk ratio, it is important that the patients selected for testosterone therapy meet established criteria for hypogonadism and have symptoms and/or conditions that could reasonably be expected to improve with testosterone replacement, for example, decreased libido. During the initial consultation, physicians should set appropriate expectations in terms of both the magnitude and expected timeline of benefit so that patients do not terminate treatment prematurely. This discussion is especially important in middle-aged and older patients in whom the benefits derived may be more modest than expected by patients based on data obtained from the T trials.[7,8] This coordinated set of 7 placebo-controlled, double-blind trials in 788 hypogonadal men with a mean age of 72 years showed a moderate improvement in sexual function overall (effect size of 0.45), with a greater improvement in libido than erectile function such that ~20% of men treated with testosterone reported that their sexual desire was "much better" than before treatment compared with less than 10% of men treated with placebo.[7] A significant improvement in walking distance was seen in 20.5% of men treated with testosterone compared with 12.6% of men who received placebo, but there was no improvement in vitality or cognitive function.[7,8]

The pros and cons of the different testosterone formulations should be discussed with the patient. Many factors can influence treatment choice, including patient preference, ease of use, insurance coverage, and side-effect profile. Although some patients may have a fear of needles that precludes use of testosterone injections, others may dislike the need for daily application of transdermal preparations. Given the many different options from which to choose, the physician should be able to identity the best fit for each individual and thus facilitate optimal adherence.

Assess Symptoms and Testosterone Levels

Once therapy with testosterone has been initiated, the patient should be reevaluated to ensure that symptoms of hypogonadism have been alleviated and that testosterone levels have been restored to the physiologic range (**Box 1**). For most patients, the goal is to maintain testosterone levels in the mid-normal range for young, healthy men, which is typically 400 to 600 ng/dL. Subtherapeutic levels may result in lack of efficacy and self-discontinuation of treatment.

Testosterone levels should be measured 3 to 6 months after starting treatment by which time a steady state will have been achieved (see **Box 1**). The pharmacokinetics

---

Box 1
Monitoring of men receiving testosterone therapy

All patients:
  Patient history
  - At 3 to 12 months, assess if:
    ○ Symptoms have improved
    ○ Patient is compliant with therapy
    ○ Patient has experienced any adverse effects
  Biochemical evaluation
  - Measure testosterone concentrations 3 to 6 months after starting therapy; see text for timing of measurement depending on the formulation used.
  - Check hematocrit at baseline, 3 to 6 months after starting treatment and then annually. If hematocrit is greater than 54%, stop therapy until it decreases to a safe level, evaluate for other causes of erythrocytosis (sleep apnea, chronic obstructive pulmonary disease), and reinitiate therapy at a lower dose.

Patients who opt for prostate monitoring
  - For men aged 55 to 69 years and for those 40 to 69 years who are at increased risk of prostate cancer and choose prostate monitoring, perform DRE, and measure PSA at baseline, 3 to 12 months after starting treatment and then in accordance with guidelines for prostate cancer screening based on age and sex of the patient.
  - Obtain urologic consultation in the following situations:
    ○ An increase in serum PSA level greater than 1.4 ng/mL within 12 months of starting testosterone
    ○ A confirmed PSA level greater than 4 ng/mL at any time
    ○ Detection of a prostate abnormality on DRE
    ○ Significant worsening of lower urinary tract symptoms

---

of the formulation used should guide the timing of therapeutic level monitoring (**Table 1**). In patients using transdermal preparations, testosterone levels have been shown to vary considerably from day to day.[9] Given this high intraindividual variability, one should be cautious about making dose adjustments based on a single measurement. In patients receiving injections of testosterone cypionate or enanthate, there is the option to alter either the dose or the frequency of the testosterone injection depending on the level obtained.

Table 1
Optimal time to measure testosterone for different formulations

Formulations	Optimal Timing
Injectables	
T enanthate or cypionate	Midway between injections aiming for level in mid-normal range or before injection is due, aiming for level at lower end of normal
T undecanoate	At end of dosing interval just before the next injection, aiming for level at lower end of normal
Transdermal	
T gels	Assess 2–8 h after applying the gel in the morning
T patches	Assess in the morning, having applied the patch the previous evening
Oral	
T undecanoate	Assess 6 h after the morning dose
Subdermal	
T pellets	Measure at the end of the dosing interval

STRATEGIES TO MINIMIZE RISK
Patient Selection

Given the known adverse effects of testosterone therapy, there are many situations where its use is contraindicated (**Box 2**), and other therapeutic options should be offered. In other situations, it should be used cautiously, and efforts should be made to address any modifiable risk factors.

For hypogonadal patients desiring fertility in the near future, testosterone therapy is not the optimal choice given the likelihood that it will suppress endogenous follicle-stimulating hormone secretion and spermatogenesis. Studies from male contraceptive trials show that approximately two-thirds of men have recovery of spermatogenesis within 6 months of discontinuing testosterone therapy.[10] However, both the time course and the extent of recovery of spermatogenesis after treatment cessation are variable.[10] Although the doses of testosterone used in male contraceptive regimens are considerably higher than those used to treat hypogonadism, it is nonetheless prudent to counsel patients with plans to start a family about implications for fertility. Patients with hypogonadotropic hypogonadism can be offered gonadotropin injections, which would stimulate both testosterone secretion and spermatogenesis.[11] However, it is also important to bear in mind that depending on the degree of hypogonadism and the extent to which intratesticular testosterone concentrations are preserved, sperm production may not be suppressed. Thus, an alternative approach for those patients is to obtain a pretreatment semen analysis and bank any sperm that are obtained. Selective estrogen receptor modulators, such as clomiphene, are sometimes prescribed in hypogonadal men seeking fertility.[12] However, they are not approved for this indication, and there are no randomized, placebo-controlled trials to support their efficacy or safety.

Hormone-sensitive tumors, such as prostate cancer and breast cancer, are also contraindications to testosterone use. For patients with a history of localized prostate cancer, the discussion is more nuanced, and potential benefits in terms of quality of life need to be weighed against uncertainty regarding long-term safety. Based on quite limited data, administration of testosterone to patients who have had a radical prostatectomy and have undetectable prostate-specific antigen (PSA) levels with no evidence of residual disease 2 years from surgery, does not appear to be associated

---

Box 2

Situations whereby testosterone therapy should be avoided or used with caution

Very high risk of serious outcomes
  Prostate cancer
  Breast cancer

Moderate to high risk of adverse outcomes
  Desire for fertility in the near future
  Unevaluated prostate nodule or induration
  Baseline PSA greater than 4 ng/mL or greater than 3 ng/mL in men at high risk of prostate cancer
  Severe lower urinary tract symptoms
  Uncontrolled or poorly controlled heart failure
  Myocardial infarction or stroke within the previous 6 months
  Hematocrit greater than 48% (>50% for men living at high altitude)
  Untreated severe obstructive sleep apnea

Adapted from Bhasin S, Brito JP, Cunningham GR, Hayes FJ, Hodis HN, Matsumoto AM, Snyder PJ, Swerdloff RS, Wu FC, Yialamas MA. Testosterone Therapy in Men With Hypogonadism: An Endocrine Society Clinical Practice Guideline. J Clin Endocrinol Metab. 2018 May 1;103(5):1715-1744.

with an increased risk of disease recurrence.[13] A recent systematic review and meta-analysis confirmed the apparent lack of increased risk of recurrence but emphasized that the quality of the evidence is low and that use of testosterone replacement in this patient population remains investigational.[14]

With regard to prostate health, testosterone therapy is not recommended for men with severe lower urinary tract symptoms or for those with a palpable prostate nodule or induration, baseline PSA greater than 4 ng/mL or greater than 3 ng/mL in men at increased risk of prostate cancer (African American men and men with a first-degree relative with prostate cancer) until they have been evaluated and cleared by a urologist.[2] Given that testosterone therapy can cause erythrocytosis and promote fluid retention, there are concerns about its use in men with baseline hematocrit levels greater than 48% (>50% for men living at high altitude) and those with uncontrolled heart failure. In addition, the Endocrine Society clinical practice guideline recommends against testosterone use in men with untreated severe obstructive sleep apnea, men who have had a major adverse cardiovascular event (stroke or myocardial infarction) in the previous 6 months, or men who are at increased risk of venous thromboembolism owing to an inherited thrombophilia.[2]

For patients perceived to be high risk, alternatives to testosterone therapy should be discussed, such as use of phosphodiesterase-5 inhibitors for erectile dysfunction. In patients with functional hypogonadism with no demonstrable organic pathologic condition, a more holistic approach could be considered focused on lifestyle intervention, management of comorbid illnesses, and discontinuation of offending medications.[15] In some cases, it may be possible to correct modifiable risk factors, such as smoking cessation or instituting CPAP (continuous positive airway pressure) therapy in those with obstructive sleep apnea and a high baseline hematocrit level.

Monitoring

In addition to assessing the effect of testosterone on symptoms of hypogonadism, follow-up evaluation should also focus on assessing the presence of side effects, which can be both formulation-specific and a class effect. If a patient has derived significant benefit from testosterone replacement but is experiencing a formulation-specific side effect, an alternative preparation should be prescribed, and levels should be reassessed on the new agent.

Intramuscular injections of testosterone enanthate and cypionate were the mainstay of treatment for male hypogonadism for decades because of their low cost and relatively infrequent dosing. However, their disadvantages include the discomfort of an intramuscular injection, and fluctuations in serum testosterone during the dosing interval. Given the unfavorable pharmacokinetics of these formulations, the resultant peaks and troughs of testosterone levels after administration may cause patients to experience undesirable swings in mood, libido, and energy levels. There is also evidence of a greater increase in hematocrit levels when testosterone is administered by the intramuscular as opposed to the transdermal route.[16] The longer-acting depot formulation of testosterone called testosterone undecanoate, which was approved for use in the United States in 2014, has more favorable pharmacokinetics requiring administration every 10 weeks.[17] However, it has the potential to cause pulmonary oil microembolism and anaphylaxis. Although both side effects are rare with an incidence of 1.5 cases per 10,000 and 0.4 cases per 10,000 injections, respectively, the FDA stipulated that the injection be administered in an office or hospital setting by a registered health care provider and the patient monitored for 30 minutes because of this potential risk.

Patients who initiated treatment with injections but experience any of the adverse effects discussed should be offered alternative treatment modalities, such as a gel or patch, which are popular because of their ease of use. However, many patients experience skin irritation from testosterone patches because of ingredients that are added to facilitate absorption of testosterone. In about 10% of patients, these skin reactions are sufficiently severe to warrant discontinuation of therapy. By contrast, risk of skin irritation with gels is low. However, there is the potential for transfer during intimate contact with a female partner or a child, which could result in virilization of the female partner and precocious puberty in the child. When appropriate precautions, such as washing hands after application and covering the application site with clothing, are followed, the incidence of secondary exposure with gels is rare, estimated at 8 cases per 1.8 million prescriptions. Testosterone pellets have the advantage of a long duration of action, but there is a risk of extrusion and infection as well as the need for a minor surgical procedure.

In addition to the formulation-specific side effects described above, there are well-known class effects of androgens, which are dose dependent and can vary in their impact depending on the age of the patient.[2] In younger patients, acne is a relatively common side effect, which patients should be alerted to in advance. Many patients will also experience a modest decrease in high-density lipoprotein cholesterol. Hypogonadal men may have a normochromic, normocytic anemia, and testosterone replacement increases hemoglobin and hematocrit levels.[18] However, in older patients, especially those with underlying lung disease, obstructive sleep apnea or those who live at high altitudes, significant erythrocytosis can occur and is the most common adverse event observed in clinical trials.[19,20] Although the actual hematocrit level at which the risk of cardiovascular and cerebrovascular events increases is not known, a hematocrit greater than 54% is an indication to stop testosterone therapy until the level decreases and an evaluation for secondary causes has been performed. In cases where the testosterone level is already in the lower end of the normal range and dose reduction is therefore not appropriate, therapeutic phlebotomy can be considered.

The relationship between testosterone replacement and cardiovascular disease has generated considerable controversy based largely on the results of cross-sectional epidemiologic studies, which have given conflicting results.[21] There have been no randomized controlled clinical trials that were adequately powered or followed patients for long enough duration to determine if testosterone replacement increases risk of cardiovascular events. Most meta-analyses have not shown a statistically significant association between the use of testosterone and major adverse cardiovascular events. Nonetheless, in 2014, the FDA mandated a labeling change to testosterone formulations about a possible increased risk of cardiovascular events. A warning about an increased risk of venous thromboembolic events was also issued by the FDA based on case reports of deep vein thrombosis in patients with an inherited thrombophilia as well as 1 case control study.[22,23] The number of thromboembolic events in randomized trials has been too low to draw any firm conclusions, but a large case control study of men treated with testosterone failed to show an increased risk of venous thromboembolism.[24]

Recommendations regarding whom to screen for prostate cancer should be based on the principle of shared decision making and informed by age, baseline risk of prostate cancer, and patient preference.[2,25-28] For men aged 55 to 69 years of age, who are at average risk of prostate cancer and choose prostate monitoring, digital rectal examination (DRE) and PSA measurement should be done at baseline and then 3 to 12 months after starting treatment. In men who are at increased risk of prostate cancer by virtue of their race (African American) or family history (first-degree relative with prostate cancer), screening is recommended at age 40. Referral to urology is recommended in the following situations: (1) An increase in PSA of greater than 1.4 ng/mL above baseline within 12 months of starting testosterone therapy; (2) An absolute PSA level of greater than 4 ng/mL at any time; (3) Detection of a prostate abnormality on DRE; and (4) Significant worsening of lower urinary tract symptoms.

Testosterone therapy increases bone mineral density (BMD) and strength, especially in trabecular bone.[29,30] However, there are no data on the impact of testosterone replacement on fracture risk in hypogonadal men, and it is not an approved therapy for osteoporosis. The cost-effectiveness of measuring BMD and the frequency at which it should be performed in this patient population have not been established. Pending further evidence, assessment of BMD by a dual-energy x-ray absorptiometry scan should be considered in men with congenital causes of hypogonadism, who tend not to achieve their peak bone mass,[31] those with severe hypogonadism,[32] and men with other risk factors for bone loss, such as use of glucocorticoids. In hypogonadal men found to have osteoporosis during their baseline evaluation but who are not considered to be at high risk of fracture, it is reasonable to evaluate the response to testosterone replacement by repeat bone density imaging 2 years after initiating treatment. For patients whose bone density remains in the osteoporosis range, treatment with an approved osteoporosis medication should then be considered.

REVIEW NEED FOR ONGOING THERAPY

For many hypogonadal men, treatment with testosterone is lifelong. However, if a patient with no identifiable cause of hypogonadism despite the appropriate workup remains symptomatic after normal testosterone levels have been maintained for several months, consideration should be given to discontinuing therapy given the absence of long-term safety data in this population. Similarly, if a patient has a reversible cause of hypogonadism, for example, prior opiate use, it is reasonable to recommend a trial off testosterone treatment to allow the hypothalamic-pituitary-gonadal axis to be reevaluated.

Patients with congenital hypogonadotropic hypogonadism typically present with profoundly low testosterone levels and failure to develop the secondary sex characteristics of puberty. However, even in this population, evidence suggests that 10% to 22% undergo a spontaneous reversal following normalization of the sex steroid milieu.[33,34] Neither severity of GnRH deficiency nor the phenotypic presentation predicts those who will undergo reversal, although the cohort of patients who reverse appears to be enriched for rare variants that disrupt neurokinin signaling.[33] A common sign of reversal in men is increased testicular growth while on testosterone replacement, thus underscoring the importance of assessing testicular volume while on treatment. To date, there are no evidence-based guidelines supporting the frequency and interval of periodic treatment washouts to assess for reversal. It is strongly recommended that any cessation of treatment be medically supervised to ensure that patients not exhibiting biochemical signs of reversal resume treatment in a timely manner.[34]

CLINICS CARE POINTS

- For patients receiving intramuscular testosterone injections, it is important to know when the last injection was administered, and it is most helpful to measure testosterone either midway between injections when the goal is to have it in the mid-normal range or just before the injection is due when the target is the lower end of normal.

- For patients being treated with transdermal formulations of testosterone, the testosterone level should be drawn at least 2 hours after gel application after confirming that the gel was not applied over the antecubital fossa from which the blood sample will be drawn.

- Remember to screen for secondary causes of erythrocytosis in hypogonadal men who have a high hematocrit at baseline or following testosterone treatment when levels are in the target range.
- Given the significant intrapatient variability in prostate-specific antigen levels, the level should always be repeated before taking any additional diagnostic or therapeutic steps.
- If a patient has a potentially reversible cause of hypogonadism, such as obesity, and is successful in losing weight, consideration should be given to having a trial off treatment to allow the hypothalamic-pituitary-gonadal axis to be reevaluated.
- In patients with congenital hypogonadism, testicular growth should be monitored on treatment, as its occurrence on testosterone is a clue to reversal and merits a supervised trial off therapy.

DISCLOSURE

The author has nothing to disclose.

REFERENCES

1. Layton JB, Li D, Meier CR, et al. Testosterone lab testing and initiation in the United Kingdom and the United States, 2000 to 2011. J Clin Endocrinol Metab 2014;99:835–42.
2. Bhasin S, Brito JP, Cunningham GR, et al. Testosterone therapy in men with hypogonadism: an Endocrine Society clinical practice guideline. J Clin Endocrinol Metab 2018;103:1715–44.
3. Wang C, Nieschlag E, Swerdloff R, et al. Investigation, treatment and monitoring of late-onset hypogonadism in males: ISA, ISSAM, EAU, EAA and ASA recommendations. Eur J Endocrinol 2008;159:507–14.
4. Mulhall JP, Trost LW, Brannigan RE, et al. Evaluation and management of testosterone deficiency: AUA guideline. J Urol 2018;200:423–32.
5. Grossmann M, Anawalt BD, Wu FCW. Clinical practice patterns in the assessment and management of low testosterone in men: an international survey of endocrinologists. Clin Endocrinol 2015;82:234–41.
6. Malik RD, Wang CE, Lapin B, et al. Characteristics of men undergoing testosterone replacement therapy and adherence to follow-up recommendations in metropolitan, multicenter healthcare system. Urology 2015;85:1382–8.
7. Snyder PJ, Bhasin S, Cunningham GR, et al. Lessons from the testosterone trials. Endocr Rev 2018;39:369–86.
8. Snyder PJ, Bhasin S, Cunningham GR, et al. Lessons from the T trials. Endocr Rev 2018;39:369–86.
9. Swerdloff RS, Pak Y, Wang C, et al. Serum testosterone (T) level variability in T gel-treated older hypogonadal men: treatment monitoring implications. J Clin Endocrinol Metab 2015;100:3280–7.
10. Liu PY, Swerdloff RS, Christenson PD, et al. Hormonal male contraception summit group. Rate, extent and modifiers of spermatogenic recovery after hormonal male contraception: an integrated analysis. Lancet 2006;367:1412–20.
11. King TF, Hayes FJ. Long-term outcome of idiopathic hypogonadotropic hypogonadism. Curr Opin Endocrinol Diabetes Obes 2012;19:204–10.
12. Krzastek SC, Sharma D, Adullah N, et al. Long-term safety and efficacy of clomiphene citrate for the treatment of hypogonadism. J Urol 2019;202:1029–35.

13. Pastuszak AW, Pearlman AM, Shun Lai W, et al. Testosterone replacement therapy in patients with prostate cancer after radical prostatectomy. J Urol 2013;190:639.

14. Teeling F, Raison N, Shabbir M, et al. Testosterone therapy for high-risk prostate cancer survivors: a systematic review and meta-analysis. Urology 2019;126: 16–23.

15. Grossmann M, Matsumoto AM. A perspective on middle-aged and older men with functional hypogonadism: focus on holistic management. J Clin Endocrinol Metab 2017;102:1067–75.

16. Dobs AS, Meikle AW, Arver S, et al. Pharmacokinetics, efficacy, and safety of a permeation-enhanced testosterone transdermal system in comparison with bi-weekly injections of testosterone enanthate for the treatment of hypogonadal men. J Clin Endocrinol Metab 1999;84:3469–78.

17. Schubert M, Minnemann T, Hübler D, et al. Intramuscular testosterone undeca-noate: pharmacokinetic aspects of a novel testosterone formulation during long-term treatment of men with hypogonadism. J Clin Endocrinol Metab 2004; 89:5429–34.

18. Roy CN, Snyder PJ, Stephens-Shields AJ, et al. Association of testosterone levels with anemia in older men–a controlled clinical trial. JAMA Intern Med 2017;177: 480–90.

19. Coviello AD, Kaplan B, Lakshman KM, et al. Effects of graded doses of testos-terone on erythropoiesis in healthy young and older men. J Clin Endocrinol Metab 2008;93:914–9.

20. Fernandez-Balsells MM, Murad MH, Lane M, et al. Clinical review 1: adverse ef-fects of testosterone therapy in adult men: a systematic review and meta-anal-ysis. J Clin Endocrinol Metab 2010;95:2560–75.

21. Gagliano-Jucá T, Basaria S. Testosterone replacement therapy and cardiovascu-lar risk. Nat Rev Cardiol 2019;16:555–74.

22. Glueck CJ, Prince M, Patel N, et al. Thrombophilia in 67 patients with thrombotic events after starting testosterone therapy. Clin Appl Thromb Hemost 2016; 22:548.

23. Martinez C, Suissa S, Rietbrock S, et al. Testosterone treatment and risk of venous thromboembolism; population based case-control study. BMJ 2016; 355:5968.

24. Baillargeon J, Urban RJ, Morgentaler A, et al. Risk of venous thromboembolism in men receiving testosterone therapy. Mayo Clin Proc 2015;90:1038–45.

25. Catalona WJ, Hudson MA, Scardino PT, et al. Selection of optimal prostate spe-cific antigen cutoffs for early detection of prostate cancer: receiver operating characteristic curves. J Urol 1994;152:2037–42.

26. Thompson IM, Pauler DK, Goodman PJ, et al. Prevalence of prostate cancer among men with a prostate-specific antigen level >4.0 ng per milliliter. N Engl J Med 2004;350:2239–46.

27. Ankerst DP, Hoefler J, Bock S, et al. Prostate cancer prevention trial risk calcu-lator 2.0 for the prediction of low- vs high-grade prostate cancer. Urology 2014; 83:1362–8.

28. Pinsky PF, Prorok PC, Kramer BS. Prostate cancer screening—a perspective on the current state of the evidence. N Engl J Med 2017;376:1285–9.

29. Aminorroaya A, Kelleher S, Conway AJ, et al. Adequacy of androgen replace-ment influences bone density response to testosterone in androgen-deficient men. Eur J Endocrinol 2005;152:881–6.

30. Snyder PJ, Kopperdahl DL, Stephens-Shields AJ, et al. Effect of testosterone treatment on volumetric bone density and strength in older men with low testosterone: a controlled clinical trial. JAMA Intern Med 2017;177:471–9.
31. Finkelstein JS, Klibanski A, Neer RM. A longitudinal evaluation of bone mineral density in adult men with histories of delayed puberty. J Clin Endocrinol Metab 1996;81:1152–5.
32. Greenspan SL, Coates P, Sereika SM, et al. Bone loss after initiation of androgen deprivation therapy in patients with prostate cancer. J Clin Endocrinol Metab 2005;90:6410–7.
33. Raivio T, Falardeau J, Dwyer A, et al. Reversal of idiopathic hypogonadotropic hypogonadism. N Engl J Med 2007;357:863–73.
34. Dwyer AA, Raivio T, Pitteloud N. Management of endocrine disease: reversible hypogonadotropic hypogonadism. Eur J Endocrinol 2016;174:R267–74.

The Effects of Testosterone Treatment on Cardiovascular Health

Channa N. Jayasena, MA, PhD, MRCP, FRCPath[a],*,
Carmen Lok Tung Ho, BSc[a], Shalender Bhasin, MB, BS[b]

KEYWORDS

- Testosterone • Hypogonadism • Cardiovascular • Hypertension • Diabetes

KEY POINTS

- Testosterone has complex, direct effects on myocardial function.
- Some studies have observed minor reductions in total cholesterol and HDL cholesterol during testosterone replacement therapy.
- Clinical trials evidence on the cardiovascular safety of testosterone therapy is contradictory, owing to design, and/or lack of statistical power.

INTRODUCTION

The prescription rates for testosterone products have risen markedly over the last 20 years, due to multiple factors, including heighted awareness about TRT because of direct-to-consumer pharmaceutical marketing, media coverage, and increased off-label use of testosterone for middle-aged and older men with age-related conditions, such as obesity and type 2 diabetes mellitus. However, the cardiovascular safety of long-term TRT remains unknown because of insufficient RCT data and conflicting evidence from epidemiologic, pharmacovigilance, and retrospective studies and small trials. This has affected prescribing behavior among clinicians, leading to disparities in the treatment of men with hypogonadism. This article will provide a critical summary of the available evidence of the cardiovascular effects and safety of TRT. Areas of controversy and gaps in our current evidence are highlighted along with a synthesis of the available evidence.

[a] Section of Endocrinology and Investigative Medicine, Imperial College London, W12 0HS, UK;
[b] Boston Claude D. Pepper Older Americans Independence Center, Research Program in Men's Health: Aging and Metabolism, Brigham and Women's Hospital, Harvard Medical School, 221 Longwood Avenue, Boston, MA 02115, USA
* Corresponding author.
E-mail address: c.jayasena@imperial.ac.uk

Endocrinol Metab Clin N Am 51 (2022) 109–122
https://doi.org/10.1016/j.ecl.2021.11.006
0889-8529/22/© 2021 Elsevier Inc. All rights reserved.

PHYSIOLOGIC EFFECTS OF TESTOSTERONE ON CARDIOVASCULAR HEALTH

Testosterone exerts several diverse effects on cardiovascular physiology; some of these physiologic effects may increase the risk of cardiovascular events while others may reduce cardiovascular risk. Androgen receptors (ARs) are located in cardiac myocytes, vascular smooth muscle, and vascular endothelial cells.[1–4]

Testosterone exerts some potentially beneficial effects on the cardiovascular system. Testosterone is a potent vasodilator; it inhibits L-type calcium channels, resulting in coronary vasodilatation and increased coronary blood flow.[5,6] DHT is more potent than testosterone in mediating these nongenomic effects on vascular smooth muscle relaxation. Testosterone improves endothelial function, reduces vascular reactivity,[7] and shortens QTc interval.[8] Furthermore, testosterone administration decreases whole body, subcutaneous, and intraabdominal fat.[9,10]

In mice, orchiectomy increases sarcoplasmic reticulum (SR) calcium load within ventricular myocytes and the expression of SERCA-2a which is implicated in the preservation of ventricular function after myocardial infarction.[11] Testosterone supplementation was associated with left ventricle dysfunction in orchiectomised mice. Testosterone administration by downregulating SERCA-2a expression causes reduced SR calcium accumulation[11] thereby attenuating the cardiac inotropic response.[12]

Several physiologic effects of testosterone could potentially increase the risk of cardiovascular events. As discussed later, testosterone administration reduces plasma HDL cholesterol depending on the administered dose, the route of administration.[13,14] Testosterone induces platelet aggregation by stimulating thromboxane A2[15] and promotes sodium and water retention,[16] which can contribute to edema formation and worsen preexisting heart failure. In preclinical models, testosterone promotes smooth muscle proliferation[17] and increases the expression of vascular cell adhesion molecule.[18] Testosterone increases hematocrit[19] by stimulating iron-dependent erythropoiesis by suppressing hepcidin,[20,21] increasing erythropoietin,[22] and by direct effects on the bone marrow to increase the numbers of erythropoietic progenitors. Older men experience greater increments in hematocrit than younger men.[23]

Testosterone administration increases the levels of prothrombotic as well as antithrombotic factors. It does not significantly affect myocardial infarct size in preclinical models of myocardial infarction.[24] Testosterone has been shown to retard atherosclerosis in some preclinical models[25] but not in others,[26] and induce myocardial hypertrophy in some mouse strains,[4,24] but not in others.

EFFECTS OF TESTOSTERONE ON BLOOD PRESSURE

Blood pressure is higher in men when compared with women.[27–29] Testosterone may play a role in the sex differences in BP, which only appears in boys and girls after puberty.[30] Orchiectomy or administration of the AR antagonist, flutamide, attenuates the development of salt-induced hypertension has been observed in the male rats.[31] However, the 5-alpha-reductase inhibitor, finasteride, does not affect the onset of hypertension, suggesting that testosterone's conversion to DHT may not be implicated in the development of hypertension in this model.[30] Female rats treated with testosterone during the neonatal period, develop higher blood pressures than control animals.[31] Furthermore, women with elevated androgens due to virilising tumors or polycystic ovarian syndrome (PCOS) have higher BP when compared with age-matched women without PCOS.[30] AR signaling increases the activity of the renin angiotensin aldosterone (RAA) system; male rats have higher plasma renin activity versus females, and castration reduces plasma renin activity in male rats.[30] Testosterone exposure also increases renal angiotensinogen mRNA.[25] Testosterone administration is associated with transient sodium and water retention in men and women in the first few weeks after starting testosterone treatment and some men, especially older men, with hypogonadism experience edema during TRT.[32] However, clinical data suggest that the effects of testosterone on BP are complex; hypogonadal men have been observed to have higher systolic blood pressures than eugonadal men.[33] Although most testosterone studies have not reported an increase in BP during testosterone treatment,[32,34] recent studies of oral testosterone undecanoate that performed standardized measurements of blood pressure during the clinic visits as well as ambulatory blood pressure measurement found that the BP more than 24 hours was higher following 120 and 180 days of treatment with oral testosterone undecanoate than at baseline; the effects on diastolic BP more than 24 h were less than for the systolic BP.[35–37] The US Food and Drug Administration has required a boxed warning on oral testosterone undecanoate labeling stating that the drug can cause blood pressure to rise.[38]

EFFECTS OF TESTOSTERONE ON SERUM LIPID PARAMETERS

In epidemiologic studies, low testosterone levels are generally associated with a proatherogenic lipid profile and higher HDL cholesterol[39–42]; some studies have also reported a negative association between circulating testosterone and VLDL cholesterol.[43] Testosterone levels are positively associated with smaller or less atherogenic VLDL particles[44] and higher testosterone levels have also been associated with a lower apoB to apo A-1 ratio.[45]

The intervention studies generally have reported modest reductions in total and high-density lipoprotein (HDL) cholesterol during TRT[32,34,46,47] in men with hypogonadism; 2 of these studies reported significant reductions in low-density lipoprotein (LDL) cholesterol in hypogonadal men with T2DM.[34,46] However, some RCTs have failed to observe any significant changes in total, LDL or HDL cholesterol during treatment with transdermal testosterone.[48–52] Nonaromatizable oral androgens suppress HDL cholesterol substantially more than transdermal or injectable testosterone esters. Testosterone-induced suppression of HDL cholesterol is associated with the upregulation of hepatic triacylglycerol lipase, changes in HDL proteome, and suppression of apolipoprotein A1,[53] but does not seem to reduce the cholesterol efflux capacity of HDL particles. TRT seems to have no significant effect on serum triglyceride levels. In summary, overall, TRT is generally associated with a modest reduction in total cholesterol and HDL cholesterol without a concomitant reduction in LDL cholesterol.

EFFECTS OF TESTOSTERONE ON VENOUS THROMBOEMBOLISM

Testosterone stimulates erythropoiesis by multiple mechanisms[20,21] and increases haematocrit.[19] Erythrocytosis is the most frequent adverse event associated with TRT in randomized trials.[54] However, there is a paucity of high-quality evidence of an association between testosterone replacement therapy and venous thromboembolism (VTE) in men with hypogonadism.[21,55] To date, no RCTs of TRT administration have captured significant numbers of events to accurately determine VTE risk in men with hypogonadism. A case-control study reported an increased risk of VTE in the first 6 months following commencement of testosterone treatment.[56] Recently, the IBM MarketScan Commercial Claims and Encounter Database and the Medicare Supplemental Database was used to compare VTE events within 39,622 men during 1, 3, and 6 months before TRT commencement versus 1, 3, and 6 months after starting TRT.[57] This study suggested that men with hypogonadism have a twofold increased risk of VTE within the 6 months following TRT commencement. However, the number of confirmed VTE events in RCTs has been exceedingly small. Most of the reported VTE events in published case reports have occurred in men with preexisting hypercoagulable condition.[58] It is prudent to consider VTE risk and counsel men with hypogonadism appropriately when considering TRT.

EFFECTS OF TESTOSTERONE ON GLUCOSE INTOLERANCE AND TYPE 2 DIABETES

In epidemiologic studies, low total testosterone levels are associated with increased visceral fat volume,[59] serum glucose concentration,[60] and increased risk of type 2 diabetes mellitus (T2DM) both cross-sectionally and longitudinally.[61] The association of free testosterone and T2DM has been inconsistent; some studies have reported a weak association[62] while others have failed to find any relation.[63] The lack of a strong correlation between free testosterone and T2DM suggests that SHBG may be the primary determinant of the observed relation between total testosterone levels and T2DM. Indeed, circulating SHBG level is an independent predictor of incident T2DM even after adjustment for free or total testosterone levels. Polymorphisms of the SHBG gene that are associated with low SHBG levels are associated with increased risk of T2DM.[64]

In Mendelian randomization studies, higher genetically determined testosterone levels are associated with the risk of T2DM in a sexually dimorphic manner; in men, higher genetically determined testosterone levels are associated with lower risk of T2DM, but in women, higher genetically determined testosterone levels are associated with increased risk of T2DM.[65]

The effects of testosterone on insulin sensitivity have been inconsistent across studies. In general studies of men in whom severe testosterone deficiency was induced rapidly by acute withdrawal of testosterone replacement therapy in men known to have hypogonadism[66] develop insulin resistance. Similarly, men receiving with prostate who receive androgen deprivation therapy are at increased risk of developing impaired glucose tolerance, insulin resistance, and T2DM.[67–69] The worsening of insulin sensitivity associated with the development of severe testosterone deficiency may be related in part to loss of skeletal muscle mass, increase in whole body and visceral fat mass, and to the effects of testosterone on lipid oxidation and mitochondrial function.[70] Dhindsa and colleagues performed euglycaemic hyperinsulinaemia clamp studies showing that 3 weeks of testosterone administration have no detectable effects on insulin sensitivity or other glucose parameters in men with type 2 diabetes; however, 24 weeks of testosterone administration were associated with significant changes in body composition and improvement in insulin sensitivity.[71] Changes in insulin sensitivity was accompanied by reductions in circulating free fatty acids (FFAs)[71] and increased adipose expression of insulin signaling markers such as insulin receptor β subunit, insulin reception substrate (IRS) 1, protein kinase B (AKT-2), and glucose transporter types 4 (GLUT-4).

However, well-controlled randomized trials of testosterone treatment that recruited men with mild testosterone deficiency or with low normal testosterone levels have failed to find consistent improvements in insulin sensitivity with testosterone treatment. For example, in the testosterone trials (TTrials),[72] testosterone treatment of older men with low testosterone levels and one or more symptoms of testosterone deficiency was associated with a small reduction in insulin but not glucose levels and only a small change in HOMA-IR. In another study, 2 years of testosterone treatment in elderly men with low or low normal testosterone levels did not improve carbohydrate tolerance, insulin secretion, insulin action, glucose effectiveness, hepatic insulin clearance, or the pattern of postprandial glucose metabolism.[73] Another placebo-controlled randomized trial also found no significant improvement in insulin sensitivity after 3 years of testosterone treatment relative to placebo in middle-aged and older men with low or low normal testosterone levels.[74]

The clinical effects of testosterone on diabetes risk and diabetes prevention are covered in detail by Yeap & Wittert elsewhere in this issue. In the T4DM Trial, testosterone treatment administered in combination with a lifestyle intervention for 2 years of men, 50 to 74 years, with impaired glucose tolerance or newly diagnosed type 2 diabetes, but without symptomatic testosterone deficiency, reduced the proportion of randomized men with type 2 diabetes beyond the effects of the lifestyle intervention.[75] However, the study participants in this large well-conducted trial were not hypogonadal. In the TIMES2 trial,[34] testosterone treatment did not consistently improve hemoglobin A_{1c} in hypogonadal men with T2DM or metabolic syndrome. Thus, in spite of strong association of low testosterone levels with increased risk of T2DM in epidemiologic studies, randomized intervention trials in hypogonadal men have not provided clear evidence of improvement in glycemic control, prevention of progression from prediabetes to diabetes, or diabetes remission.

THE EFFECTS OF TESTOSTERONE TREATMENT ON THE RISK OF MAJOR ADVERSE CARDIOVASCULAR EVENTS
Epidemiologic Studies

The relation of testosterone levels and coronary artery disease in cross-sectional and prospective cohort studies has been inconsistent. Some cross-sectional studies have shown low levels of testosterone to be associated with increased risk for coronary artery disease,[76] while others have shown no association.[77] The relationship between serum testosterone levels and the incidence of cardiovascular events also has been inconsistent in prospective epidemiologic studies.

Epidemiologic studies have found a consistent negative association between circulating testosterone concentrations and common carotid artery intima-media thickness, a measure of subclinical atherosclerosis. For example, in the Rotterdam study, the men in the lowest quartile of testosterone levels had greater progression of intima-media thickness than men in highest quartile of testosterone levels.[78] However, the same study did not identify a significant difference in the rates of change in coronary artery calcium between the group administrated with testosterone or placebo.[78]

The relation of testosterone and mortality has been heterogeneous across studies. A meta-analysis by Corona and colleagues reported an association of low testosterone levels with increased risk of cardiovascular disease. Furthermore, study participants with the lowest testosterone levels seemed to have the highest overall mortality and cardiovascular mortality.[79] Another meta-analysis of 11 randomized trials by Araujo and colleagues found that in aggregate, lower testosterone levels were associated with higher risk of all-cause mortality, especially cardiovascular mortality.[80] Epidemiologic studies can only show association but cannot prove causality; reverse causality cannot be excluded. It is possible that testosterone is a marker of health, and those who are higher risk of dying have lower testosterone levels. Ruige and colleagues found that higher testosterone levels were associated with a lower risk for cardiovascular events in men more than 70 years of age but not in men who were younger than this age group.[77]

Pharmacovigilance Studies and Retrospective Analyses of Electronic Medical Records

The pharmacovigilance studies and retrospective analyses of electronic medical records have yielded inconsistent results because of their inherent limitations. In a retrospective analysis of male veterans who underwent angiography and had low testosterone concentrations, Vigen and colleagues observed that TRT was associated with an increased risk of the composite cardiovascular outcome of myocardial infarction, stroke, and death when (hazard ratio, HR = 1.29)[81] relative to no TRT. Finkle used an insurance database and found an increased risk of nonfatal myocardial infarction during the 90 days following initial prescription for TRT when compared with the period before commencing TRT (relative risk (RR) = 1.36).[82] However, another retrospective study of men with low testosterone concluded that TRT was associated with reduced all-cause mortality when compared with no TRT (HR = 0.61).[83] Muraleedharan and colleagues retrospectively concluded that low serum testosterone may predict increased all-cause mortality in 581 men with type 2 diabetes (HR 2.3).[84] Furthermore, Boden and colleagues conducted a post hoc analysis of the AIM-HIGH trial of men with metabolic syndrome and low baseline levels of HDL cholesterol. The 643 out of 2118 men with levels of serum testosterone less than 300 ng/dL had a higher risk of the primary composite outcome (coronary heart disease, death, MI, stroke, hospitalization for acute coronary syndrome, or coronary or cerebral revascularization) when compared with the normal testosterone group (HR 1.23).[85] Taken collectively, observational studies provide little consensus on TRT safety, and have each been used to substantiate claims TRT either reduces or increases the risk of MACE outcomes.

These pharmacovigilance and retrospective studies suffer from many limitations, including heterogeneous study populations and differences in treatment indications, treatment regimens and duration, and on-treatment testosterone levels, and in other aspects of study design. These studies used variable definitions of cardiovascular outcomes that were often not prespecified, and the ascertainment methods varied across studies. They also suffered from a potential for residual confounding in that the patients assigned to testosterone therapy differed from comparators in baseline cardiovascular risk factors. Due to the inherent limitations and inconsistency of findings, these pharmacovigilance and retrospective analyses do not permit strong inferences about the relation between testosterone therapy and mortality and cardiovascular outcomes.

Randomized Controlled Trials

The testosterone replacement for older men with sarcopenia (TOM) randomized controlled trial was designed to investigate functional mobility following TRT in 209 men with hypogonadism and frailty.[32] However, the study was stopped early by its data and safety monitoring board due to an unexpected increase in cardiovascular events within the TRT versus the placebo arm, albeit with small absolute number of events (23 vs 5, respectively). However, the cardiovascular events were not prespecified nor adjudicated prospectively. The number of major adverse cardiovascular events (MACEs) was small. Subsequent RCTs have often excluded men with the increased baseline cardiovascular risk, so it is unsurprising that the number of MACE has been small in most trials. Several meta-analyses have examined the association between testosterone replacement and cardiovascular events, major cardiovascular events, and death in RCTs and overall, these meta-analyses have not shown a statistically significant association between testosterone and cardiovascular events, major cardiovascular events, or deaths.[23,86–88] These meta-analyses are limited by the heterogeneity of randomized trials included in these analyses with respect to eligibility criteria, testosterone dose and formulation, and intervention durations. The variable quality of adverse event recording in clinical trials has been well-documented, and was particularly apparent in these trials, which reported a very low frequency of all adverse events as well cardiovascular events. The small size of many trials and the inclusion of pilot studies with very small sample sizes was another

Table 1	
Key points of the biological plausibility: effects of testosterone on cardiovascular physiology	
Potential Cardiovascular Risks	**Potential Cardiovascular Benefits**
• Increase in hematocrit[19] • Suppression of HDL cholesterol[34] • Platelet aggregation[15] • Sodium retention • Smooth muscle proliferation[17] • Increased VCAM expression	• Vasodilator effect which increases coronary and penile blood flow[6] • Decreased whole body and visceral fat[59] • Improves vascular reactivity[5,7] • Shortens QTc interval[8]

constraint. Cardiovascular outcomes were not prespecified, they were often defined post hoc, and were of varying clinical significance. The major cardiovascular events were not adjudicated, not specified prospectively, and the total number of major cardiovascular events was too small to draw strong inferences. None of the trials has been large enough or long enough to determine the effects of testosterone treatment on MACE.

Two randomized trials—the Cardiovascular Trial of the TTrials[32] and the Testosterone Effects on Atherosclerosis in Aging Men (The TEAAM Trial)[78] determined the effects of testosterone treatment relative to placebo on the rate of atherogenesis progression. The rate of atherosclerosis progressed assessed using the common carotid artery -intima-media thickness or the coronary calcium scores did not differ between testosterone-treated and placebo-treated men in either of the 2 trials. However, in the Cardiovascular Trial of the TTrials,[32] testosterone treatment was associated with greater increase in the volume of noncalcified plaque in the coronary arteries, assessed using computed tomography angiography, compared with placebo.

An extensive review by the FDA concluded that *"the studies...have significant limitations that weaken their evidentiary value for confirming a causal relationship between testosterone and adverse cardiovascular outcomes."* Nevertheless, the US Food and Drug Administration (FDA) directed the pharmaceutical companies to include in the label warning about the potential cardiovascular risks of TRT.[89] The European Medicines Agency also found no conclusive link between testosterone treatment and cardiovascular risk. Fortunately, 2 ongoing studies are aiming to close the evidence gap. The National Institute for Health Research (NIHR) TestES (Testosterone Effects and Safety) consortium is currently collating individual patient data (IPD) and adverse events from published RCTs to analyze the risks of subtypes of MACE within men with hypogonadism treated with TRT when compared with placebo (https://www.imperial.ac.uk/metabolism-digestion-reproduction/research/diabetes-endocrinology-metabolism/endocrinology-and-investigative-medicine/nihr-testosterone/). Furthermore, the Phase 4, randomized placebo-controlled trial (The TRAVERSE Trial) is recruiting approximately 6000 men aged 45 to 80 years with either preexisting cardiovascular disease or at least 3 cardiovascular risk factors, with the primary objective of comparing the effect of TRT versus placebo on the incidence of MACE.

SUMMARY

Overall, TRT exerts multiple physiologic effects, both positive and negative, on cardiovascular health (**Table 1**). Finally, there are insufficient RCT data to determine whether TRT increases MACE risk. Studies are underway to clarify this important question. The Endocrine Society's testosterone treatment guideline recommends avoiding testosterone treatment in hypogonadal men who incurred a MACE in the preceding 6 months and in men with a known hypercoagulable condition, such as a mutation on anti-thrombin 3, protein C or protein S. Testosterone treatment of hypogonadal men with increased risk of cardiovascular events requires consideration and counseling of the potential risks versus benefits of testosterone replacement therapy.

CLINICS CARE POINTS

- Testosterone replacement therapy for young men with classical hypogonadism due to known diseases of the testis, pituitary, or the hypothalamus is associated with low frequency of adverse events.

- The long-term cardiovascular safety of testosterone replacement therapy remains uncertain.

- Testosterone treatment of older men with age-related decline in testosterone levels is not currently approved by the US Food and Drug Administration. The long-term benefits, as well as long term risks of testosterone treatment in older men with age related decline in testosterone levels, remain unknown.

- Testosterone treatment should be avoided in men with hypogonadism who have suffered a major adverse cardiovascular event in the preceding 6 months or who suffer from a hypercoagulable state.

- Testosterone treatment of hypogonadal men with increased risk of cardiovascular events requires consideration and counseling of the potential risks versus benefits of testosterone replacement therapy.

DISCLOSURE

Dr C.N. Jayasena is funded by an NIHR Post-Doctoral Fellowship and NIHR Health Technology Assessment Grant. Dr S. Bhasin reports receiving research grants from the National Institute on Aging, the National Institute of Child Health and Human Development, the National Institute of Nursing Research, the Patient-Centered Outcomes Research Institute (PCORI), AbbVie, Transition Therapeutics, and Metro International Biotechnology and has an equity interest in FPT, LLC. These grants are managed by the Brigham and Women's Hospital. These conflicts are overseen and managed in accordance with the policies of the Office of Industry Interactions, Massachusetts General Brigham Healthcare System, Boston MA.

REFERENCES

1. Yeh S, Tsai M-Y, Xu Q, et al. Generation and Characterization of Androgen Receptor Knockout (ARKO) Mice: An in vivo Model for the Study of Androgen Functions in Selective Tissues. Proc Natl Acad Sci U S A 2002;99(21):13498–503. Available at: https://www.jstor.org/stable/3073435.

2. Yu I, Lin H, Liu N, et al. Neuronal androgen receptor regulates insulin sensitivity via suppression of hypothalamic NF-κB—Mediated PTP1B Expression. Diabetes 2013;62(2):411–23. Available at: https://www.ncbi.nlm.nih.gov/pubmed/23139353.

3. Huang C, Lee SO, Chang E, et al. Androgen receptor (AR) in cardiovascular diseases. J Endocrinol 2016;229(1):R1–16.

4. Marsh JD, Lehmann MH, Ritchie RH, et al. Androgen Receptors Mediate Hypertrophy in Cardiac Myocytes. Circulation 1998;98(3):256–61. Available at: http://circ.ahajournals.org/cgi/content/abstract/98/3/256.

5. Herring MJ, Oskui PM, Hale SL, et al. Testosterone and the cardiovascular system: a comprehensive review of the basic science literature. J Am Heart Assoc

2013;2(4):e000271. Available at: https://onlinelibrary.wiley.com/doi/abs/10.1161/JAHA.113.000271.

6. Scragg JL, Jones RD, Channer KS, et al. Testosterone is a potent inhibitor of L-type Ca 2+ channels. Biochem Biophys Res Commun 2004;318(2):503–6.

7. Empen K, Lorbeer R, Dörr M, et al. Association of testosterone levels with endothelial function in men: results from a population-based study. Arterioscler Thromb Vasc Biol 2012;32(2):481–6. Available at: http://ovidsp.ovid.com/ovidweb.cgi?T=JS&NEWS=n&CSC=Y&PAGE=fulltext&D=ovft&AN=00043605-201202000-00041.

8. Schwartz JB, Volterrani M, Caminiti G, et al. Effects of testosterone on the Q-T Interval in older men and older women with chronic heart failure. Int J Androl 2011;34(5pt2):e415–21. Available at: https://api.istex.fr/ark:/67375/WNG-XMWPBTD2-M/fulltext.pdf.

9. Bhasin S. Effects of Testosterone Administration on Fat Distribution, Insulin Sensitivity, and Atherosclerosis Progression. Clin Infect Dis 2003;37(Supplement-2):S142–9. Available at: https://api.istex.fr/ark:/67375/HXZ-8KZGKG2P-D/fulltext.pdf.

10. Bhasin S, Parker RA, Sattler F, et al. Effects of testosterone supplementation on whole body and regional fat mass and distribution in human immunodeficiency virus-infected men with abdominal obesity. J Clin Endocrinol Metab 2007;92(3):1049–57.

11. Ribeiro Júnior RF, Ronconi KS, Jesus ICG, et al. Testosterone deficiency prevents left ventricular contractility dysfunction after myocardial infarction. Mol Cell Endocrinol 2018;460:14–23.

12. Fernandes AA, Ribeiro RF, de Moura VGC, et al. SERCA-2a is involved in the right ventricular function following myocardial infarction in rats. Life Sci (1973) 2015;124:24–30.

13. Bagatell CJ, Knopp RH, Vale WW, et al. Physiologic testosterone levels in normal men suppress high-density lipoprotein cholesterol levels. Ann Intern Med 1992;116(12):967–73. Available at: https://www.ncbi.nlm.nih.gov/pubmed/1586105.

14. Bagatell CJ, Bremner WJ. Androgen and progestagen effects on plasma lipids. Prog Cardiovasc Dis 1995;38(3):255–71.

15. Ajayi AAL, Mathur R, Halushka PV. Testosterone increases human platelet thromboxane A2 receptor density and aggregation responses. Circulation 1995;91(11):2742–7. Available at: http://circ.ahajournals.org/cgi/content/abstract/91/11/2742.

16. Johannsson G, Gibney J, Wolthers T, et al. Independent and combined effects of testosterone and growth hormone on extracellular water in hypopituitary men. J Clin Endocrinol Metab 2005;90(7):3989–94.

17. Fujimoto R, Morimoto I, Morita E, et al. Androgen receptors, 5 alpha-reductase activity and androgen-dependent proliferation of vascular smooth muscle cells. J Steroid Biochem Mol Biol 1994;50(3):169–74.

18. Death AK, McGrath KCY, Sader MA, et al. Dihydrotestosterone promotes vascular cell adhesion molecule-1 expression in male human endothelial cells via a nuclear factor-κb-dependent pathway. Endocrinology (Philadelphia) 2004;145(4):1889–97.

19. Bhasin S, Brito J, Cunningham G, et al. Testosterone therapy in men with hypogonadism: an endocrine society clinical practice guideline. J Clin Endocrinol Metab 2018;103(5):1715–44. Available at: http://ovidsp.ovid.com/ovidweb.cgi?T=JS&NEWS=n&CSC=Y&PAGE=fulltext&D=ovft&AN=00004678-201805000-00001.

20. Ohlander SJ, Varghese B, Pastuszak AW. Erythrocytosis following testosterone therapy. Sex Med Rev 2018;6(1):77–85.

21. Sharma R, Oni OA, Chen G, et al. Association Between Testosterone Replacement Therapy and the Incidence of DVT and pulmonary embolism: a retrospective cohort study of the veterans administration database. Chest 2016;150(3): 563–71. Available at: https://www.ncbi.nlm.nih.gov/pubmed/27179907.

22. Bachman E, Travison TG, Basaria S, et al. Testosterone induces erythrocytosis via increased erythropoietin and suppressed hepcidin: evidence for a new erythropoietin/hemoglobin set point. J Gerontol A Biol Sci Med Sci 2014;69(6):725–35. Available at: https://www.ncbi.nlm.nih.gov/pubmed/24158761.

23. Haddad RM, Kennedy CC, Caples SM, et al. Testosterone and cardiovascular risk in men: a systematic review and meta-analysis of randomized placebo-controlled trials. Mayo Clin Proc 2007;82(1):29–39. Available at: https://www.ncbi.nlm.nih.gov/pubmed/17285783.

24. Nahrendorf M, Frantz S, Neubauer S, et al. Effect of testosterone on post-myocardial infarction remodeling and function. Cardiovasc Res 2003;57(2): 370–8. Available at: https://www.ncbi.nlm.nih.gov/pubmed/12566109.

25. Nathan L, Shi W, Dinh H, et al. Testosterone Inhibits Early Atherogenesis by Conversion to Estradiol: Critical Role of Aromatase. Proc Natl Acad Sci U S A 2001; 98(6):3589–93. Available at: https://www.jstor.org/stable/3055279.

26. Bhasin S, Herbst K. Testosterone and atherosclerosis progression in men. Diabetes care 2003;26(6):1929–31. Available at: https://www.ncbi.nlm.nih.gov/pubmed/12766137.

27. Ganten U, Schröder G, Witt M, et al. Sexual dimorphism of blood pressure in spontaneously hypertensive rats: effects of anti-androgen treatment. J Hypertens 1989;7(9):721–6. Available at: http://ovidsp.ovid.com/ovidweb.cgi?T=JS&NEWS=n&CSC=Y&PAGE=fulltext&D=ovft&AN=00004872-198909000-00005.

28. Crofton J, Ota M, Share L. Role of vasopressin, the renin—angiotensin system and sex in Dahl salt-sensitive hypertension. J Hypertens 1993;11(10):1031–8. Available at: http://ovidsp.ovid.com/ovidweb.cgi?T=JS&NEWS=n&CSC=Y&PAGE=fulltext&D=ovft&AN=00004872-199310000-00005.

29. Chen Y, Meng Q. Sexual dimorphism of blood pressure in spontaneously hypertensive rats is androgen dependent. Life Sci (1973) 1991;48(1):85–96.

30. Reckelhoff JF. Gender Differences in the Regulation of Blood Pressure. Hypertension 2001;37(5):1199–208. Available at: http://hyper.ahajournals.org/cgi/content/abstract/37/5/1199.

31. Rowland NE, Fregly MJ. Role of gonadal hormones in hypertension in the dahl salt-sensitive rat. Clin Exp Hypertens (1993) 1992;A14(3):367–75. Available at: http://www.tandfonline.com/doi/abs/10.3109/10641969209036195.

32. Basaria S, Coviello AD, Travison TG, et al. Adverse Events Associated with Testosterone Administration. N Engl J Med 2010;363(2):109–22.

33. Rezanezhad B, Borgquist R, Willenheimer R, et al. The association between serum testosterone and risk factors for atherosclerosis. Curr Urol 2019;13(2): 101–6. Available at: https://www.karger.com/Article/FullText/499285.

34. Jones TH, Arver S, Behre HM, et al. Testosterone replacement in hypogonadal men with type 2 diabetes and/or metabolic syndrome (the TIMES2 Study). Diabetes care 2011;34(4):828–37. Available at: https://www.narcis.nl/publication/RecordID/oai:pure.atira.dk:publications%2Faae47901-c35f-4e3c-a15d-f7c3c9a599a8.

35. Swerdloff RS, Wang C, White WB, et al. A new oral testosterone undecanoate formulation restores testosterone to normal concentrations in hypogonadal men. J Clin Endocrinol Metab 2020;105(8):2515–31. Available at: http://ovidsp.ovid.com/ovidweb.cgi?

T=JS&NEWS=n&CSC=Y&PAGE=fulltext&D=ovft&AN=00004678-202008000-00003.

36. Gittelman M, Jaffe JS, Kaminetsky JC. Safety of a new subcutaneous testosterone enanthate auto-injector: results of a 26-week study. J Sex Med 2019; 16(11):1741–8.

37. White WB, Bernstein JS, Rittmaster R, et al. Effects of the oral testosterone undecanoate Kyzatrex™ on ambulatory blood pressure in hypogonadal men. J Clin Hypertens (Greenwich) 2021;23(7):1420–30. Available at: https://onlinelibrary.wiley.com/doi/abs/10.1111/jch.14297.

38. Aschenbrenner D. First oral testosterone product now available. Am J Nurs 2019; 119(8):22–3. Available at: http://ovidsp.ovid.com/ovidweb.cgi?T=JS&NEWS=n&CSC=Y&PAGE=fulltext&D=ovft&AN=00000446-201908000-00022.

39. Haffner SM, Mykkänen L, Valdez RA, et al. Relationship of sex hormones to lipids and lipoproteins in nondiabetic men. J Clin Endocrinol Metab 1993;77(6):1610–5.

40. Agledahl I, Skjærpe P, Hansen J, et al. Low serum testosterone in men is inversely associated with non-fasting serum triglycerides: The Tromsø study. Nutr Metab Cardiovasc Dis 2007;18(4):256–62. Available at: https://www.clinicalkey.es/playcontent/1-s2.0-S0939475307000348.

41. Mäkinen JI, Perheentupa A, Irjala K, et al. Endogenous testosterone and serum lipids in middle-aged men. Atherosclerosis 2007;197(2):688–93. Available at: https://www.clinicalkey.es/playcontent/1-s2.0-S0021915007003401.

42. Zmuda JM, Cauley JA, Kriska A, et al. Longitudinal relation between endogenous testosterone and cardiovascular disease risk factors in middle-aged men: a 13-year follow-up of former multiple risk factor intervention trial participants. Am J Epidemiol 1997;146(8):609–17. Available at: https://www.ncbi.nlm.nih.gov/pubmed/9345114.

43. Khaw KT, Barrett-Connor E. Endogenous sex hormones, high density lipoprotein cholesterol, and other lipoprotein fractions in men. Arterioscler Thromb Vasc Biol 1991;11(3):489–94. Available at: http://atvb.ahajournals.org/cgi/content/abstract/11/3/489.

44. Vaidya D, Dobs A, Gapstur SM, et al. The association of endogenous sex hormones with lipoprotein subfraction profile in the Multi-Ethnic Study of Atherosclerosis. Metab Clin Exp 2008;57(6):782–90. Available at: https://www.clinicalkey.es/playcontent/1-s2.0-S0026049508000528.

45. Ohlsson C, Barrett-Connor E, Bhasin S, et al. High serum testosterone is associated with reduced risk of cardiovascular events in elderly men. The MrOS (Osteoporotic Fractures in Men) study in Sweden. J Am Coll Cardiol 2011;58(16): 1674–81. Available at: https://www.ncbi.nlm.nih.gov/pubmed/21982312.

46. Gianatti EJ, Hoermann R, Lam Q, et al. Effect of testosterone treatment on cardiac biomarkers in a randomized controlled trial of men with type 2 diabetes. Clin Endocrinol (Oxford) 2016;84(1):55–62. Available at: https://api.istex.fr/ark:/67375/WNG-GPF8HBTD-R/fulltext.pdf.

47. Emmelot-Vonk MH, Verhaar HJJ, Nakhai Pour HR, et al. Effect of testosterone supplementation on functional mobility, cognition, and other parameters in older men : a randomized controlled trial. JAMA 2008;299(1):39–52.

48. Groti K, Žuran I, Antonič B, et al. The impact of testosterone replacement therapy on glycemic control, vascular function, and components of the metabolic syndrome in obese hypogonadal men with type 2 diabetes. The aging male 2018; 21(3):158–69. Available at: http://www.tandfonline.com/doi/abs/10.1080/13685538.2018.1468429.

49. Aversa A, Bruzziches R, Francomano D, et al. Effects of testosterone undeca-noate on cardiovascular risk factors and atherosclerosis in middle-aged men with late-onset hypogonadism and metabolic syndrome: results from a 24-month, randomized, double-blind, placebo-controlled study. J Sex Med 2010;7(10): 3495–503.

50. Svartberg J, Agledahl I, Figenschau Y, et al. Testosterone treatment in elderly men with subnormal testosterone levels improves body composition and BMD in the hip. Int J Impot Res 2008;20(4):378–87.

51. Paduch DA, Polzer PK, Ni X, et al. Testosterone replacement in androgen-deficient men with ejaculatory dysfunction: a randomized controlled trial. J Clin Endocrinol Metab 2015;100(8):2956–62.

52. Kenny AM, Kleppinger A, Annis K, et al. Effects of Transdermal Testosterone on Bone and Muscle in Older Men with Low Bioavailable Testosterone Levels, Low Bone Mass, and Physical Frailty. J Am Geriatr Soc 2010;58(6):1134–43. Available at: https://api.istex.fr/ark:/67375/WNG-7SR5DCSQ-4/fulltext.pdf.

53. Rubinow KB, Tang C, Hoofnagle AN, et al. Acute sex steroid withdrawal increases cholesterol efflux capacity and HDL-associated clusterin in men. Steroids 2012; 77(5):454–60.

54. Ponce OJ, Spencer-Bonilla G, Alvarez-Villalobos N, et al. The efficacy and adverse events of testosterone replacement therapy in hypogonadal men: a sys-tematic review and meta-analysis of randomized, placebo-controlled trials. J Clin Endocrinol Metab 2018;103(5):1745–54. Available at: http://ovidsp.ovid.com/ ovidweb.cgi?T=JS&NEWS=n&CSC=Y&PAGE=fulltext&D=ovft&AN=00004678-201805000-00002.

55. Baillargeon J, Urban RJ, Morgentaler A, et al. Risk of Venous Thromboembolism in Men Receiving Testosterone Therapy. Mayo Clin Proc 2015;90(8):1038–45. Available at: https://www.clinicalkey.es/playcontent/1-s2.0-S0025619615004280.

56. Martinez C, Suissa S, Rietbrock S, et al. Testosterone treatment and risk of venous thromboembolism: population based case-control study. BMJ 2016; 355:i5968.

57. Walker RF, Zakai NA, MacLehose RF, et al. Association of testosterone therapy with risk of venous thromboembolism among men with and without hypogonad-ism. JAMA Intern Med 2020;180(2):190–7.

58. Glueck CJ, Prince M, Patel N, et al. Thrombophilia in 67 patients with thrombotic events after starting testosterone therapy. Clin Appl Thromb Hemostat 2016; 22(6):548–53. Available at: https://journals.sagepub.com/doi/full/10.1177/ 1076029615619486.

59. Fui MNT, Dupuis P, Grossmann M. Lowered testosterone in male obesity: Mech-anisms, morbidity and management. Asian J Androl 2014;16(2):223–31. Avail-able at: https://www.ncbi.nlm.nih.gov/pubmed/24407187.

60. MI EP. Low testosterone level increases fasting blood glucose level in adult males. Universa Medicina 2015;31(3):200–7. Available at: https://explore. openaire.eu/search/publication?articleId=dedup_wf_001: 2129979ed51a29513d18ad3f426cecea.

61. Menéndez E, Valdés S, Botas P, et al. Glucose tolerance and plasma testosterone concentrations in men. Results of the Asturias Study. Endocrinol Nutr 2011;58(1): 3–8. Available at: https://www.ncbi.nlm.nih.gov/pubmed/21215713.

62. Haffner SM, Karhapaa P, Mykkanen L, et al. Insulin resistance, body fat distribu-tion, and sex hormones in men. Diabetes 1994;43(2):212–9. Available at: http:// diabetes.diabetesjournals.org/content/43/2/212.abstract.

63. Abate N, Haffner SM, Garg A, et al. Sex steroid hormones, upper body obesity, and insulin resistance. J Clin Endocrinol Metab 2002;87(10):4522–7.

64. Quan L, Wang L, Wang J, et al. Association between sex hormone binding globulin gene polymorphism and type 2 diabetes mellitus. Int J Clin Exp Pathol 2019; 12(9):3514–20. Available at: https://www.ncbi.nlm.nih.gov/pubmed/31934198.

65. Ruth KS, Day FR, Tyrrell J, et al. Using human genetics to understand the disease impacts of testosterone in men and women. Nat Med 2020;26(2):252–8. Available at: https://www.ncbi.nlm.nih.gov/pubmed/32042192.

66. Yialamas MA, Dwyer AA, Hanley E, et al. Acute Sex Steroid Withdrawal Reduces Insulin Sensitivity in Healthy Men with Idiopathic Hypogonadotropic Hypogonadism. J Clin Endocrinol Metab 2007;92(11):4254–9.

67. Smith MR, Lee H, Nathan DM. Insulin sensitivity during combined androgen blockade for prostate cancer. J Clin Endocrinol Metab 2006;91(4):1305–8.

68. Keating NL, O'Malley AJ, Smith MR. Diabetes and cardiovascular disease during androgen deprivation therapy for prostate cancer. J Clin Oncol 2006;24(27): 4448–56. Available at: http://jco.ascopubs.org/content/24/27/4448.abstract.

69. Keating NL, Liu P, O'Malley AJ, et al. Androgen-deprivation therapy and diabetes control among diabetic men with prostate cancer. Eur Urol 2013;65(4):816–24. Available at: https://www.clinicalkey.es/playcontent/1-s2.0-S0302283813001358.

70. Pitteloud N, Mootha VK, Hayes FJ, et al. Relationship Between Testosterone Levels, Insulin Sensitivity, and Mitochondrial Function in Men. Diabetes care 2005;28(7):1636–42. Available at: http://care.diabetesjournals.org/content/28/7/1636.abstract.

71. Dhindsa S, Ghanim H, Batra M, et al. Insulin resistance and inflammation in hypogonadotropic hypogonadism and their reduction after testosterone replacement in men with type 2 diabetes. Diabetes care 2016;39(1):82–91. Available at: https://www.ncbi.nlm.nih.gov/pubmed/26622051.

72. Mohler ER, Ellenberg SS, Lewis CE, et al. The Effect of Testosterone on Cardiovascular Biomarkers in the Testosterone Trials. J Clin Endocrinol Metab 2018; 103(2):681–8. Available at: https://www.ncbi.nlm.nih.gov/pubmed/29253154.

73. Basu R, Dalla Man C, Rizza RA, et al. Effect of 2 years of testosterone replacement on insulin secretion, insulin action, glucose effectiveness, hepatic insulin clearance, and postprandial glucose turnover in elderly men. Diabetes care 2007;30(8):1972–8. Available at: http://care.diabetesjournals.org/content/30/8/1972.abstract.

74. Huang G, Pencina KM, Li Z, et al. Long-term testosterone administration on insulin sensitivity in older men with low or low-normal testosterone levels. J Clin Endocrinol Metab 2018;103(4):1678–85. Available at: http://ovidsp.ovid.com/ovidweb.cgi?T=JS&NEWS=n&CSC=Y&PAGE=fulltext&D=ovft&AN=00004678-201804000-00052.

75. Wittert G, Bracken K, Robledo KP, et al. Testosterone treatment to prevent or revert type 2 diabetes in men enrolled in a lifestyle programme (T4DM): a randomised, double-blind, placebo-controlled, 2-year, phase 3b trial. Lancet Diabetes Endocrinol 2021;9(1):32–45.

76. Rosano GMC, Leonardo F, Pagnotta P, et al. Acute anti-ischemic effect of testosterone in men with coronary artery disease. Circulation 1999;99(13):1666–70. Available at: http://circ.ahajournals.org/cgi/content/abstract/99/13/1666.

77. Ruige JB, Mahmoud AM, De Bacquer D, et al. Endogenous testosterone and cardiovascular disease in healthy men: a meta-analysis. Heart 2011;97(11):870–5.

78. Basaria S, Harman SM, Travison TG, et al. Effects of testosterone administration for 3 years on subclinical atherosclerosis progression in older men with low or

low-normal testosterone levels: a randomized clinical trial. JAMA 2015;314(6): 570–81.

79. Corona G, Rastrelli G, Monami M, et al. Hypogonadism as a risk factor for cardiovascular mortality in men: a meta-analytic study. Eur J Endocrinol 2011;165(5): 687–701.

80. Araujo AB, Dixon JM, Suarez EA, et al. Clinical review: endogenous testosterone and mortality in men: a systematic review and meta-analysis. J Clin Endocrinol Metab 2011;96(10):3007–19. Available at: https://www.ncbi.nlm.nih.gov/pubmed/21816776.

81. Vigen R, O'Donnell CI, Barón AE, et al. Association of testosterone therapy with mortality, myocardial infarction, and stroke in men with low testosterone levels. JAMA 2013;310(17):1829–36.

82. Finkle WD, Greenland S, Ridgeway GK, et al. Increased risk of non-fatal myocardial infarction following testosterone therapy prescription in men. PLoS One 2014; 9(1):e85805. Available at: https://www.ncbi.nlm.nih.gov/pubmed/24489673.

83. Shores MM, Smith NL, Forsberg CW, et al. Testosterone Treatment and Mortality in Men with Low Testosterone Levels. J Clin Endocrinol Metab 2012;97(6):2050–8.

84. Muraleedharan V, Marsh H, Kapoor D, et al. Testosterone deficiency is associated with increased risk of mortality and testosterone replacement improves survival in men with type 2 diabetes. Eur J Endocrinol 2013;169(6):725–33.

85. Boden WE, Miller MG, McBride R, et al. Testosterone concentrations and risk of cardiovascular events in androgen-deficient men with atherosclerotic cardiovascular disease. Am Heart J 2020;224:65–76.

86. Nguyen PL, Je Y, Schutz FAB, et al. Association of androgen deprivation therapy with cardiovascular death in patients with prostate cancer: a meta-analysis of randomized trials. JAMA 2011;306(21):2359–66.

87. Calof OM, Singh AB, Lee ML, et al. Adverse events associated with testosterone replacement in middle-aged and older men: a meta-analysis of randomized, placebo-controlled trials. J Gerontol A Biol Sci Med Sci 2005;60(11):1451–7. Available at: https://api.istex.fr/ark:/67375/HXZ-TVW8H35J-6/fulltext.pdf.

88. Fernández-Balsells MM, Murad MH, Lane M, et al. Adverse effects of testosterone therapy in adult men: a systematic review and meta-analysis. J Clin Endocrinol Metab 2010;95(6):2560–75.

89. US Food and Drug Administration. FDA cautions about using testosterone products for low testosterone due to aging; requires labeling change to inform of possible increased risk of heart attack and stroke with use. FDA Drug Safety Communication. January 31, 2014.

Testosterone Treatment and the Risk of Prostate Adverse Events

Jason A. Levy, DO, MS[a], Arthur L. Burnett, MD, MBA[b],
Adrian S. Dobs, MD, MHS[c],*

KEYWORDS

- Hypogonadism • Testosterone (T) • Prostate cancer (PCa)
- Benign prostatic hyperplasia (BPH)

KEY POINTS

- Currently, there are no grounds to discourage testosterone therapy in hypogonadal patients with benign prostatic hyperplasia and/or lower urinary tract symptoms and there is evidence of limited benefit from androgen administration.
- Further studies should be conducted regarding testosterone's effect on the prostate.
- Current literature demonstrates an absence of such evidence despite concerns of the link to the development of prostate cancer.
- There remains limited evidence regarding testosterone replacement therapy in patients with previously diagnosed prostate cancer to appropriately quantify the risk versus benefits.

INTRODUCTION

Definition

Hypogonadism is a clinical syndrome that results from failure of the testis to produce physiologic concentrations of testosterone (T).[1] Various thresholds exist to define low total T ranging from 230 to 350 ng/dL. Peak T levels typically are measured between 3 and 8 AM with total T level decreasing during the first 30 minutes of waking.[2] Serum T decreases with age and has shown to have an association with diabetes, bone density loss, infertility, and other health disorders.[3–5] Based on the most recent American Urologic Association (AUA) guidelines, clinicians should use a total T level of less than 300 ng/dL, or a free T below the normal range, as a reasonable cut-off in support of the diagnosis of low T.[6] Further evaluation is often needed to determine the etiology of the hypogonadism. The

[a] Johns Hopkins School of Medicine Brady Urological Institute, 600 North Wolfe Street Park 2, Baltimore, MD 21287, USA; [b] Johns Hopkins School of Medicine Brady Urological Institute, 600 North Wolfe Street, Marburg 407, Baltimore, MD 21287, USA; [c] Johns Hopkins Clinical Research Network, 1830 Monument Street, Suite 328, Baltimore, MD 21205, USA
* Corresponding author.
E-mail address: adobs@jhmi.edu

Endocrinol Metab Clin N Am 51 (2022) 123–131
https://doi.org/10.1016/j.ecl.2021.11.011
0889-8529/22/© 2021 Elsevier Inc. All rights reserved.

endo.theclinics.com

intent of this article is to understand the effects T may have in the development and alteration of normal prostatic physiology and how it influences clinical applications in the hypogonadotropic male.

TESTOSTERONE AND THE PROSTATE
The Prostate

The normal prostate gland develops from the urogenital sinus where circulating androgens produced by fetal testes play a critical role in its development. It is ovoid in shape and measures 3 cm in length, 4 cm in width, and 2 cm in depth with an estimated weight of 18 to 20 g. The base is situated at the bladder–prostate junction with the narrowed apex the most inferior portion of the prostate gland. It is divided into 3 distinct zones: the peripheral zone (the largest zone approximately 70% of tissue) and most susceptible to carcinoma, the transitional zone in which benign prostatic hyperplasia and ultimately obstruction may occur, and finally the central zone. The prostate is composed of both glandular elements (70%) as well as fibromuscular stroma (30%).[7]

The prostate depends on hormonal stimulation to develop, and previous studies have demonstrated that a lack of T has resulted in inability of the prostate to develop normally.[8] T is converted to dihydrotestosterone via the enzyme 5-alpha reductase. Inhibiting this enzyme with pharmaceuticals such as finasteride and dutasteride decreases the amount of dihydrotestosterone available to the prostate and subsequently may result in not only cessation of growth, but also a shrinking of the gland as well. Exogenous T effects on the prostate remain controversial. Total prostate volume as well as transitional zone growth, as measured by ultrasound examination, were not significantly changed in patients undergoing T therapy. Numerous studies evaluating prostate-specific antigen (PSA) have demonstrated varying results as to whether PSA levels increase in T-deficient men.[9] Kang and colleagues[10] reviewed 15 studies with a total of 739 patients receiving T compared with 385 controls that demonstrated T therapy does not increase PSA levels in men being treated for hypogonadism, except when it is given by the intramuscular route, and even the increase with intramuscular administration is minimal.

Benign Prostatic Hyperplasia and Testosterone

Lower urinary tract symptoms (LUTS), which include frequency, urgency, incomplete voiding, and slow stream, are common in both men and women with advancing age. The most common cause of LUTS in men is prostate enlargement and progression of BPH. Although there remains conflicting evidence about the benefits of T therapy in men with BPH and LUTS, the current body of literature demonstrates the safety of using T in men with BPH and LUTS.[11] In regard to treating LUTS, numerous animal and human studies have been conducted to determine the effect of T on LUTS. T is hypothesized to improve LUTS via regulation of the expression of alpha-1 adrenergic receptors, phosphodiesterase type 5 activity, Rho-kinase activation, endothelin activity, and neuronal nitric oxide synthase.[12,13] The effects of T on LUTS are not limited to overall effects on the prostate. In fact, in a rat model T has been shown to improve bladder function via increasing bladder capacity and compliance by decreasing detrusor pressure.[14] Similarly, Celayir[15] measured baseline urodynamics and T levels in both control patients and those undergoing orchiectomy followed by treatment with or without T. Bladder capacity and compliance were increased on days 5 and 10 with T treatment, but decreased thereafter and returned to baseline levels on day 30, suggesting that T modulates bladder capacity and compliance.[15]

The aforementioned thought of T's effects on LUTS transitioned similarly from animal models to human studies. T therapy has been reported to improve lower urinary tract function by increasing bladder capacity and compliance by decreasing detrusor pressure at maximal flow in men with T deficiency. Two separate studies, one with 30 men enrolled and another with 25 demonstrated statistically significant improvements in the International Prostate Symptom Score (IPSS) in addition to decreased mean detrusor pressure.[16,17] Sixty Japanese men were recently enrolled in a clinical trial investigating the effects of T on various parameters. No statistical differences were observed regarding body mass index, postvoid residual urine volume, or prostate volume. However, similar to previous studies IPSS and International Index of Erectile Function scores improved significantly. Subgroup analysis demonstrated significant improvements in storage symptoms scores but not voiding symptoms scores.[18]

Last, the 2 largest studies to date involving 428 men with follow-up at 8 years and 999 men with follow-up at 3 years demonstrated conflicting results. Permpongkosol[19] studied 428 men with late-onset hypogonadism, 120 of whom had 5 to 8 years of continuous T therapy. The study demonstrated a statistically significant improvement in the IPSS from a baseline of 8.54 ± 6.6 to 6.78 ± 5.44 and also statistically significantly increased the median PSA (0.96 μg/L).[19] Conversely, the latter study by Debruyne and colleagues[20] demonstrated mean baseline unadjusted PSA levels slightly higher for untreated men 2.2 ± 9.1 ng/mL versus 1.1 ± 1.7 ng/mL with treated men. Similarly, untreated men showed a slight increase in adjusted total IPSS over time, although little change was seen overall at baseline 5.13 on T therapy compared with 4.36 not on T therapy.[20] **Table 1** demonstrates a summary of T therapy on LUTS.

A recent meta-analysis by Rastrelli and associates[21] helped to reiterate previous findings that T "is not detrimental for the prostate, and treating hypogonadism could even produce relief from LUTS and limit prostatic inflammation, which generates and maintains the process leading to BPH." Because of the significant number of studies regarding the effect of T and BPH, the most recent guidelines from the European Association of Urology state there are no grounds to discourage T therapy in hypogonadal patients with BPH/LUTS and there is evidence of limited benefit from androgen administration.[22]

Testosterone and Prostate Cancer

Prostate cancer (PCa) is the most commonly diagnosed cancer in men, with approximately 1 in 7 who will ultimately be diagnosed. In the United States, 170,000 men are

Table 1 The effects of T therapy on lower urinary tract symptoms	
Bladder capacity	Increased
Compliance	Increased
Detrusor pressure	Decreased
Storage symptoms	Improved
Voiding symptoms	Unchanged
Postvoid residual	Unchanged
PSA	Increased or decreased (varying evidence)
IPSS (varying evidence)	Decreased or unchanged (varying evidence)

diagnosed with PCa each year with a lifetime risk of death from PCa approximating nearly 2.8%. This totaled an estimated 31,620 PCa-related deaths in 2019. The pathogenesis of PCa is hormone dependent, and it is thus important to assess the potential risks and benefits that exogenous T may have before a diagnosis of cancer and the role for T therapy after a cancer diagnosis.[23–25]

In 2017, Lopez and colleagues[26] identified studies investigating the association of endogenous total T and use of T therapy with PCa events, ranging from 1990 to 2016. Most studies identified included observational studies as well as randomized controlled trials. The meta-analysis was subdivided into 3 parts. The first part demonstrated the association of endogenous total T with PCa in 31 observational studies (20 prospective and 11 prospective/retrospective). None of the 20 prospective studies demonstrated a relationship with PCa and 2 of 11 prospective/retrospective demonstrated an increased risk of PCa, whereas 2 demonstrated a decreased risk. Second, the relationship of categorical high versus low endogenous T was examined in 25 studies, 8 of which reported an increased risk of PCa in men with high T compared with low, but only 4 of these 8 were statistically significant. The remaining 17 studies showed a decreased risk of PCa after comparing high versus low, 11 of which were statistically significant. Finally, and perhaps most importantly in regards to T therapy were 2 meta-analyses of the randomized controlled trials (n = 8 and n = 11) involving associations with T therapy and PCa. These trials demonstrated a nonsignificant decreased risk of PCa.[26] A more recent meta-analysis of 27 randomized controlled trials found no evidence of increased PSA levels after T therapy for 1 year. Included in the meta-analysis were 11 studies that found no evidence of increased risk of PCa.[27]

In conjunction with one another, both the AUA and European Association of Urology concluded that the current literature demonstrates an absence of evidence linking T to the development of PCa.

Testosterone Replacement in Men with a Prior Diagnosis of Prostate Cancer

T therapy can be considered in those men who have undergone radical prostatectomy with favorable pathology (ie, negative margins, negative seminal vesicles, negative lymph nodes), and who have undetectable PSA postoperatively. Three separate studies in patients undergoing T therapy demonstrated that patients who had undergone radical prostatectomy and had undetectable PSAs postoperatively demonstrated no cancer recurrence and maintained undetectable PSAs. The first study in 2004 included 7 hypogonadal men who underwent treatment with T therapy after undergoing radical prostatectomy, none of whom demonstrated recurrence. The next study in 2005 demonstrated similar results in 10 hypogonadal patients previously treated with radical prostatectomy and who had a median follow-up of 19 months after starting T therapy. Finally, the largest study in 2005 compared 103 hypogonadal men with PCa treated with radical prostatectomy and T therapy compared with 49 after radical prostatectomy in the reference group. Overall, 4 and 8 cases of recurrence were observed in the treatment group and reference groups, respectively.[28–30]

There remains a paucity of literature in patients treated with T therapy who were diagnosed with PCa previously and received radiation therapy as definitive treatment. Although scarce, retrospective studies of patients undergoing T therapy have been reported. In 2007, Sarosdy[31] reported on 31 patients who had previously undergone brachytherapy for treatment of their PCa. T was started at a median of 4.5 years from brachytherapy treatment and, most notably, no patients stopped T therapy because of cancer recurrence or documented cancer progression, although 1 patient had transient increases in PSA.[31] A similar retrospective study was published in 2014 with 20 patients who had previously undergone brachytherapy treatment for PCa.

Similarly, none of these patients had PCa progression or recurrence and no patient had an increasing serum PSA. They were also shown to have clinically significant benefits in both increase in T as well as improvements on the Sexual Health Inventory for Men questionnaire.[32] A small case series of 5 patients who had previously been treated with external beam radiation after PSA nadir demonstrated marked clinical response to T therapy; however, 1 patient did have a transitory increase in the PSA.[33]

The final patient cohort that should be considered are those individuals who have been diagnosed previously with PCa but remain on an active surveillance protocol. The greatest concern patients and providers have regarding those individuals on active surveillance begs the question "will starting T therapy cause progression of previously diagnosed PCa?" In 2003, Rhoden and Morgentaler[34] published a retrospective study of 75 patients previously diagnosed with prostatic intraepithelial neoplasia, but not PCa. They concluded at 1 year after treatment with T therapy that men with prostatic intraepithelial neoplasia do not have a greater increase in PSA or a significantly increased risk of cancer than men without prostatic intraepithelial neoplasia.[34] In 2011, Morgentaler and colleagues[35] retrospectively reviewed 13 men with untreated PCa and T deficiency who had received T therapy. They concluded that T therapy in men with untreated, low-volume, low to moderate grade PCa was not associated with progression in the short to medium term.[35] More recently, a systematic review for T therapy in men with untreated PCa implied that T therapy might be harmful in men with advanced disease who undergo active surveillance.[36]

In practice, many men who have been diagnosed with and treated for PCa, may have sufficiently low serum T levels and symptoms that may warrant T therapy. This may be particularly true in men who in the past were treated with androgen deprivation therapy and never fully regained activity of their hypothalamic–pituitary–gonadal axis. In this population, the resulting reduction in bone density, sexual function, and muscle mass may be particularly detrimental. Patients with T deficiency and a history of PCa should be informed that there is inadequate evidence to quantify the risk–benefit ratio of T therapy.[6]

Clinical Evaluation and Initiation of Testosterone Replacement

Patients undergoing any type of hormone replacement therapy should undergo a comprehensive medical, surgical, and social history, as well as a physical examination. Obesity is strongly associated with hypogonadism, so body mass index as well as measurement of waist circumference are strongly recommended. When reviewing a patient's LUTS, validated questionnaires such as the IPSS or AUA Symptom Index help not only to determine how bothersome an individual's symptoms are, but also how they are responding to treatment. Similar questionnaires are used to assess patients with erectile dysfunction, such as the International Index of Erectile Function questionnaire, which helps to discern erectile dysfunction severity and also can be helpful in assessing future improvements. In regards to a physical examination, components should include testicular size in addition to secondary sexual characteristics regarding overall androgen status. Finally, a digital rectal examination (DRE) should be performed to exclude any prostate abnormalities.[22]

PSA should be measured in men over 40 years of age before the commencement of T therapy to exclude a PCa diagnosis. In patients who have an elevated PSA at baseline, a second PSA test is recommended to rule out a spurious elevation. In patients who have 2 PSA levels at baseline that raise suspicion for the presence of PCa, a more formal evaluation should be conducted.[6] Once a baseline PSA is established with no concern to pursue further testing for PCa, T supplementation may be started. Once patients who are started on T are maintained in the normal range, PSA testing should revert back to the AUA for PCa screening. Men aged 55 to 69 years undergo PSA screening via a shared decision-making process between the patient and their physician. Decisions in screening of men aged 40 to 54 years at higher risk for PCa should be individualized. The AUA defines men who may be at higher risk for PCa to include men of African American race, those with a family history of metastatic or lethal adenocarcinomas (ie, PCa, breast, ovarian, and pancreatic cancers), those affecting multiple first-degree relatives, and PCa that developed at younger ages.[37]

Although PSA remains the gold standard serum marker for diagnosis of PCa and DRE remains the gold standard physical examination, the amount of PCa missed in patients who have normal PSAs should be considered. Thompson and colleagues[38] enrolled more than 18,000 men in a prevention trial and, among these, a cohort of 2950 men underwent prostate biopsy though they never had a PSA that was abnormal (>4.0 ng/mL) and never had an abnormal DRE. Of the 2950 men in the normal PSA/DRE cohort, 449 (15.2%) had PCa and 449 (14.9%) had a clinically significant PCa (Gleason grade 7 or higher).[38] The DRE remains a common physical examination tool to help identify abnormalities in the prostate, which may prompt prostate biopsy owing to concerns for cancer. A further subanalysis of 35,350 men who underwent DRE from the Prostate, Lung, Colorectal, and Ovarian Cancer Screening trial (PLCO) by Halpern and colleagues[39] demonstrated that DRE has prognostic usefulness when the PSA was greater than 3 ng/mL, limited usefulness at less than 2 ng/mL, and marginal usefulness for 2 to 3 ng/mL.[39] Although new technologies (such as prostate MRI) and biomarkers are being used in practice more often, PSA and DRE remain the gold standard for PCa screening.

In the aforementioned study by Morgentaler and colleagues from 2011, patients who were treated with T therapy and had a previous diagnosis of PCa on active surveillance underwent PSA and DRE every 3 months with annual prostate biopsy. Furthermore, patients with high-risk or advanced PCa should not be candidates for T therapy. The authors remain in agreement with the following AUA guideline recommendations. For patients undergoing T therapy, T levels should be measured every 6 to 12 months. Finally, clinicians should discuss the cessation of T therapy 3 to 6 months after commencement of treatment in patients who experience normalization of total T levels but fail to achieve symptom or sign improvement.[6]

SUMMARY

The signs and symptoms of hypogonadism are becoming increasingly recognized and there is an increasing desire for both patients and providers to initiate T therapy to help mitigate issues with low libido, erectile function, anemia, bone mineral density, lean body mass, and even depressive symptoms. The benefit of T therapy remains a subject for debate, but the risk for adverse events on prostate health is likely minimal. As clinicians, it is important to weigh the benefits of prescribing any type of medication or hormone replacement therapy as well as understanding the risks associated with such. A substantial amount of literature regarding T therapy and its relation to both benign and malignant etiologies involving the prostate currently exists. However, most of this literature is not definitive and in fact many studies contradict one another. Based on the currently available literature and in conjunction with current guidelines, T therapy should not be discouraged and may be of limited benefit in patients with BPH/LUTS. Moreover, in relation to prostate malignancy, there is an absence of literature linking exogenous T to the development of PCa. Finally, in patients with a history of PCa, there remains inadequate evidence to quantify the risk–benefit ratio of exogenous T.

CLINICS CARE POINTS

- Clinicians should obtain 2 separate morning total T levels drawn in the morning (approximately 8 AM) with values of less than 300 ng/dL as a reasonable cut-off to establish the diagnosis of low T. Further evaluations should be done to determine its underlying etiology.

- Candidates for T therapy should undergo a through history and physical examination, including using various questionnaires to objectively define BPH/LUTS, erectile dysfunction (IPSS, AUA Symptom Index, Index of Erectile Function), and establishing risk factors that may predispose a patient to PCa. A full physical examination should include palpation of testicular size and a DRE.

- In addition to serum morning sex hormone measures, any male over the age of 40 should have a PSA drawn to establish a baseline. Afterward, standard AUA guidelines can be applied.

- Although the risks seem to be minimal, future studies are needed to affirm the benefits of T therapy in men with BPH/LUTS, rule out any association with PCa, and help to establish better risk–benefit profiles of men who have a previous diagnosis of PCa.

DISCLOSURE

The authors have nothing to disclose.

REFERENCES

1. Matsumoto AM, Bremner WJ. Testicular disorders. In: Melmed S, Polansky KS, Larsen PR, Kronenberg HM, editors. Williams textbook of endocrinology. 13th edition. New York (NY): Elsevier; 2016. p. 688–777.
2. Plymate SR, Tenover JS, Bremner WJ. Circadian variation in testosterone, sex hormone-binding globulin, and calculated nonsex hormone-binding globulin bound testosterone in healthy young and elderly men. J Androl 1989;10:366.
3. Harman SM, Metter EJ, Tobin JD, et al. Longitudinal effects of aging on serum total and free testosterone levels in healthy men. J Clin Endocrinol Metab 2001;86:724–31.
4. Garvey WT, Mechanick JI, Brett EM, et al. American Association of Clinical Endocrinologists and American College of Endocrinology comprehensive clinical practice guidelines for medical care of patients with obesity. Endocr Pract 2016;22(Suppl 3):1.
5. Sussman EM, Chudnovsky A, Niederberger CS. Hormonal evaluation of the infertile male: has it evolved? Urol Clin North Am 2008;35:147.
6. Mulhall JP, Trost LW, Brannigan RE, et al. Evaluation and management of testosterone deficiency: AUA guideline. J Urol 2018;200:423.
7. Wein AJ, Kavoussi LR, Campbell MF. Campbell-Walsh urology. 11th edition. Philadelphia (PA): Elsevier Saunders; 2016.
8. Wu CP, Gu FL. The prostate in eunuchs. Prog Clin Biol Res 1991;370:249–55.
9. Marks LS, Mazer NA, Mostaghel E, et al. Effect of testosterone replacement therapy on prostate tissue in men with late-onset hypogonadism: a randomized controlled trial. JAMA 2006;296(19):2351–61.
10. Kang DY, Li HJ. The effect of testosterone replacement therapy on prostate-specific antigen (PSA) levels in men being treated for hypogonadism: a systematic review and meta-analysis. Medicine (Baltimore) 2015;94(3):e410.
11. Traish AM, Johansen V. Impact of Testosterone Deficiency and Testosterone Therapy on Lower Urinary Tract Symptoms in Men with Metabolic Syndrome. World J Mens Health 2018;36(3):199–222.

12. Koritsiadis G, Stravodimos K, Mitropoulos D, et al. Androgens and bladder outlet obstruction: a correlation with pressure-flow variables in a preliminary study. CBJU Int 2008;101(12):1542–6.

13. Traish AM, Park K, Dhir V, et al. Effects of castration and androgen replacement on erectile function in a rabbit model. Endocrinology 1999;140(4):1861–8.

14. Tek M, Balli E, Cimen B, et al. The effect of testosterone replacement therapy on bladder functions and histology in orchiectomized mature male rats. Urology 2010;75(4):886–90.

15. Celayir S. Effects of different sex hormones on male rabbit urodynamics: an experimental study. Horm Res 2003;60(5):215–20.

16. Kalinchenko S, Vishnevskiy EL, Koval AN, et al. Saad F Beneficial effects of testosterone administration on symptoms of the lower urinary tract in men with late-onset hypogonadism: a pilot study. Aging Male 2008;11(2):57–61.

17. Karazindiyanoğlu S. Cayan S The effect of testosterone therapy on lower urinary tract symptoms/bladder and sexual functions in men with symptomatic late-onset hypogonadism. Aging Male 2008;11(3):146–9.

18. Okada K. Improved Lower Urinary Tract Symptoms Associated With Testosterone Replacement Therapy in Japanese Men With Late-Onset Hypogonadism. Am J Mens Health 2018;12(5):1403–8.

19. Permpongkosol S. Effects of 8-year treatment of long-acting testosterone undecanoate on metabolic parameters, urinary symptoms, bone mineral density, and sexual function in men with late-onset hypogonadism. J Sex Med 2016; 13(8):1199–211.

20. Debruyne FM, Behre HM, Roehrborn CG, et al. Testosterone treatment is not associated with increased risk of prostate cancer or worsening of lower urinary tract symptoms: prostate health outcomes in the Registry of Hypogonadism in Men. BJU Int 2017;119(2):216–24. https://doi.org/10.1111/bju.13578.

21. Rastrelli G, Vignozzi L, Corona G, et al. Testosterone and benign prostatic hyperplasia. Sex Med Rev 2019;7(2):259–71.

22. Salonia A, Bettocchi C, Carvalho J, et. al. EAU guidelines on sexual and reproductive health. Publisher: EAU Guidelines office. Place published: Arnhem (The Netherlands).

23. American Cancer Society.

24. Siegel RL, Miller KD, Jemal A. Cancer statistics, 2019. CA Cancer J Clin 2019; 69(1):7–34.

25. Leyh-Bannurah SR, Karakiewicz PI, Pompe RS, et al. 'Inverse stage migration patterns in North American patients undergoing local prostate cancer treatment: a contemporary population-based update in light of the 2012 USPSTF recommendations'. World J Urol 2019;37:469–79.

26. Lopez DS, Advani S, Tsilidis KK, et al. Endogenous and exogenous testosterone and prostate cancer: decreased-, increased- or null-risk? Transl Androl Urol 2017;6(3):566–79.

27. Boyle P, Koechlin A, Bota M, et al. Endogenous and exogenous testosterone and the risk of prostate cancer and increased prostate-specific antigen (PSA) level: a meta-analysis. BJU Int 2016;118:731.

28. Kaufman JM, Graydon RJ. Androgen replacement after curative radical prostatectomy for prostate cancer in hypogonadal men. J Urol 2004;172:920.

29. Agarwal PK, Oefelein MG. Testosterone replacement therapy after primary treatment for prostate cancer. J Urol 2005;173:533.

30. Khera M, Grober ED, Najari B, et al. Testosterone replacement therapy following radical prostatectomy. J Sex Med 2009;6:1165.

31. Sarosdy MF. Testosterone replacement for hypogonadism after treatment of early prostate cancer with brachytherapy. Cancer 2007;109:536.

32. Balbontin FG, Moreno SA, Bley E, et al. Long-acting testosterone injections for treatment of testosterone deficiency after brachytherapy for prostate cancer. BJU Int 2014;114:125.

33. Morales A, Black AM, Emerson LE. Testosterone administration to men with testosterone deficiency syndrome after external beam radiotherapy for localized prostate cancer: preliminary observations. BJU Int 2009;103:62.

34. Rhoden EL, Morgentaler A. Testosterone replacement therapy in hypogonadal men at high risk for prostate cancer: results of 1 year of treatment in men with prostatic intraepithelial neoplasia. J Urol 2003;170:2348.

35. Morgentaler A, Lipshultz LI, Bennett R, et al. Testosterone therapy in men with untreated prostate cancer. J Urol 2011;185:1256.

36. Kim M, Byun SS, Hong SK. Testosterone replacement therapy in men with untreated or treated prostate cancer: do we have enough evidences? World J Mens Health 2021;39(4):705–23.

37. Carter HB, Albertsen PC, Barry MJ, et al. Early detection of prostate cancer: AUA guideline. J Urol 2013;190:419.

38. Thompson IM, Pauler DK, Goodman PJ, et al. Prevalence of prostate cancer among men with a prostate-specific antigen level < or =4.0 ng per milliliter. N Engl J Med 2004;350(22):2239–46 [Erratum appears in N Engl J Med 2004; 351(14):1470].

39. Halpern JA, Oromendia C, Shoag JE, et al. Use of digital rectal examination as an adjunct to prostate specific antigen in the detection of clinically significant prostate cancer. J Urol 2018;199(4):947–53.

Fertility Considerations in Hypogonadal Men

Nikoleta Papanikolaou, MBBS, MRCP, Rong Luo, MBBS,
Channa N. Jayasena, MA, PhD, MRCP, FRCPath*

KEYWORDS

- Hypogonadism • Hypogonadal men • Male infertility • Hormone stimulation
- Gonadotropins • GnRH • SERM • Aromatase inhibitors

KEY POINTS

- Hypogonadism may affect up to 40% of men who present with couple infertility; therefore, it is important to investigate for underlying hypogonadism.
- The clinical impact of hypogonadism on fertility potential depends on the timing of its onset (fetal, prepubertal, or postpubertal) and effect on semen parameters.
- Testosterone replacement therapy is routinely used in men with hypogonadism to induce virilization, bolster desirable secondary sexual characteristics as well as to improve libido and bone density, but it has no effect on inducing fertility.
- Hypogonadotropic hypogonadism is one of the few medically treatable causes of male infertility. Hormone stimulation with gonadotropins or pulsatile gonadotrophin-releasing hormone is highly effective, although a prolonged course is required.
- Assisted reproductive technologies, and especially intracytoplasmic sperm injection, have enhanced fertility potential of men with primary hypogonadism. Some centers use hormone stimulation in this cohort of patients before sperm harvesting; results are scant, and therefore, the American Society for Reproductive Medicine does not support endocrine stimulation as standard clinical practice.

INTRODUCTION

Male factors are increasingly recognized to be a causative or contributory factor in approximately 50% of infertile couples.[1,2] Hypogonadism may be present in up to 40% of men who present with couple infertility.[3] Testosterone is the major androgen-regulating spermatogenesis in men; as a result, men with either primary or secondary hypogonadism may be subfertile because of impaired spermatogenesis. The clinical impact of hypogonadism on fertility potential depends on the timing of its onset (fetal, prepubertal, or postpubertal) and effect on semen parameters. Secondary hypogonadism is one of the few medically treatable causes of male infertility.

N. Papanikolaou and R. Luo have contributed equally to the preparation of this article.
Section of Investigative Medicine Imperial College London, Hammersmith Hospital, 6th Floor, Commonwealth Building, 150 Du Cane Road, London W12 0NN, UK
* Corresponding author.
E-mail address: c.jayasena@imperial.ac.uk

Hormonal treatment with gonadotropins, pulsatile gonadotrophin-releasing hormone (GnRH) as well as off-label medications, such as selective estrogen receptor modulators (SERMs) and aromatase inhibitors (AI), has been trialed in men with hypogonadism with various results. Treatment pathways and success rates differ according to the cause of hypogonadism and the time of its onset. Assisted reproductive technologies account for another treatment pathway that has further improved fertility potential of hypogonadal men.

BACKGROUND PHYSIOLOGY

Boys have a surge of GnRH during the first 3 months of life, leading to pulsatile follicle-stimulating hormone (FSH) and luteinizing hormone (LH) secretion known as "mini-puberty."[4] The increase in serum LH stimulates the Leydig cells to synthesize testosterone, leading to increase in penile length and testicular volume.[5] Crucially for fertility, the surge in FSH induces proliferation of immature Sertoli cells (SC) by 5-fold from approximately 260×10^6 at birth to 1500×10^6 by 3 months of age.[6] These SC begin to express androgen receptors at around 12 months of age in humans.[7,8] After 6 months of age, the hypothalamic-pituitary-gonadal (HPG) axis is quiescent, and testosterone levels remain low until puberty.[4,6] Reactivation of the HPG axis during puberty stimulates a second wave of SC proliferation, doubling the number of SC to approximately 2900 million.[6] By now, the vast majority (87%–95%) of SC express androgen receptors.[7] In healthy men, LH pulses stimulated by GnRH pulsatility are generated every 1.5 to 2 hours,[9] but this pattern is largely lost in hypogonadotropic hypogonadism (HH).

Testosterone is the major androgen-regulating spermatogenesis in men. It is synthesized by Leydig cells in response to LH and binds to androgen receptors expressed on SC to support spermatogenesis.[10,11] The classical testosterone signaling pathway takes 30 to 45 minutes for cellular response.[12] Testosterone first diffuses across the plasma membrane to bind with intracellular androgen receptors that are sequestrated by heat shock proteins in the cytoplasm. Binding of testosterone to androgen receptors induces phosphorylation and subsequent homodimerization, and a conformational change in the receptor structure allows recruitment of co-regulators and its nuclear translocation and upregulation and downregulation of target genes transcription.[13] The nonclassical pathways of testosterone signaling are much more rapid, occurring within seconds to minutes.[14] One pathway involves activation of Src tyrosine kinases, resulting in phosphorylation of epidermal growth factor receptor and consequent activation of the MAP kinase cascade (Raf, MEK, ERK).[15] This pathway has been shown to facilitate Sertoli-germ cell attachment and release of mature sperm.[15,16]

Because of localized production of testosterone within the testes, intratesticular concentrations of testosterone are reported to be 200-fold higher than serum level samples from peripheral venous blood.[17,18] Below a critical concentration of testosterone, spermatogenesis becomes impaired.[19]

Testosterone replacement therapy (TRT) in men with hypogonadism is often used to induce virilization and bolster secondary sexual characteristics as well as to improve libido, bone composition, and bone mineral density.[20,21] TRT may be administered enterally, parenterally, and transdermally. TRT does not support spermatogenesis because of its negative feedback on the GnRH and gonadotrophin secretion. In one study, regular administration of exogenous testosterone in 271 healthy fertile men induced azoospermia after a mean of 4 months, whereas restoration of spermatogenesis after cessation of testosterone therapy took 6 months.[22] Therefore, testosterone therapy is not recommended in men with hypogonadism who desire fertility in the next

6 to 12 months.[23] In addition, there have been concerns regarding persistent suppression of spermatogenesis following discontinuation of TRT.[23] A meta-analysis by Rastrelli and colleagues[24] reported that previous TRT in men with HH did not have a negative effect on treatment outcomes with gonadotrophins/GnRH fertility induction. Appropriate fertility counseling of men who are being considered for TRT should take place.

SECONDARY HYPOGONADISM OR HYPOGONADOTROPIC HYPOGONADISM

HH is one of the few medically reversible causes of male infertility (**Table 1**). It is characterized by low or inappropriately normal FSH and or LH; hence, treatment with gonadotrophins or pulsatile GnRH to stimulate gonadotrophins represents a logic approach. Men with congenital hypogonadotropic hypogonadism (CHH) typically present in their adolescence with either partial (25%) or complete absence of puberty (75%).[25] Pitteloud and colleagues[26] studied 78 men with HH and found that 80% had apulsatile LH activity resulting in absent puberty, whereas 20% had discernible LH pulses, which were either low in frequency or amplitude or both, resulting in partial puberty. There were significantly higher rates of cryptorchidism, microphallus, and severely reduced testicular volume in men with complete compared with partial HH.[26] If HH has a postpubertal onset, secondary sexual characteristics and testicular development are normal. Men with HH usually present with reduced libido, fewer nighttime and spontaneous erections, decreased sexual activity, and reduced or absent sperm in ejaculate.

Table 1
Treatment strategies for treatment of men with hypogonadotropic hypogonadism

Hormone Regimen	Doses	Rationale	Considerations/ Outcomes
hCG monotherapy	Initial dose 500 IU S/C twice weekly and increased up to 5000 IU weekly[a]	hCG exert similar effects of LH on Leydig cells	• More likely to be effective in men with postpubertal onset of HH • Inferior to combination therapy (hCG + FSH) in CHH • Injectable
hCG + FSH combination therapy	rFSH dose 75–150 IU S/C 3 times weekly[a]	FSH is added after 3–6 months of hCG monotherapy	• Superior to hCG monotherapy (especially in CHH cases) • More costly than hCG monotherapy • Injectable
Pulsatile GnRH	SC pump: 25 ng/kg per pulse every 2 h, up to 600 ng/kg per pulse[a]	Mimics physiologic GnRH pulses	• Effective when normal pituitary • Requires pump use • Limited use in clinical practice by cost, availability, & complexity

(continued on next page)

Table 1
(continued)

Hormone Regimen	Doses	Rationale	Considerations/Outcomes
SERMS, for example, clomiphene citrate, tamoxifen (off label)	Clomiphene: 25 mg every other day, up to 50 mg daily[b] Tamoxifen: 20–30 mg daily[b]	Inhibits negative feedback of estrogen to hypothalamus/pituitary	• Requires intact hypothalamic-pituitary-gonadal axis • Less evidence base compared with gonadotropins/pulsatile GnRH • Some effect in LOH • Oral route of administration • Inconsistent fertility outcomes
Aromatase inhibitors, for example, anastrozole (off label)	Anastrozole 1 mg, 3 times per week, up to 1 mg daily[c]	Inhibits negative feedback of estrogen to hypothalamus/pituitary Improves T/E2 ratio	• Some effect in special HH groups, that is, obesity driven • Oral route of administration • Safety risk for skeletal bone loss with long-term usage • Less evidence base compared with gonadotropins/pulsatile GnRH

Abbreviations: LOH, late onset hypogonadism; S/C, subcutaneous.

[a] Young J, Xu C, Papadakis GE, et al. Clinical management of congenital hypogonadism. Endocr Rev 2019;40(2). https://doi.org/10.1210/er.2018-00116.

[b] Ide V, Vanderscchueren D, Antonio L. Treatment of men with central hypogonadism: alternatives to testosterone replacement therapy. Int J Mol Sci. 2021:22(1). https://doi.org/10.3390/ijms22010021.

[c] Leder BZ, Rohrer JL, Rubin SD, et al. Effects of aromatase inhibition in elderly man with low or boderline-low serum testosterone levels. J Clin Endocrinol Metab. 2004:8. https://doi.org/10.1210/jc.2003-031467.

Gonadotropins

Human chorionic gonadotropin (hCG) hormone exerts similar actions to LH on Leydig cells. Several studies have shown that hCG can increase the intratesticular testosterone in a dose-dependent manner[27,28] and induce spermatogenesis.[29] However, hCG monotherapy appears to have inferior results to the combination therapy with FSH in cases where there has been lack of pubertal development and/or history of cryptorchidism. Men with postpubertal onset of HH or some degree of gonadal development are more likely to respond to hCG alone.[30] A study by Depenbusch and colleagues[31] observed that LH monotherapy could sustain sufficient spermatogenesis for extended periods following initial treatment with either a combination of gonadotrophins or GnRH in a small cohort of 13 patients with idiopathic HH (IHH). A European consensus statement on the treatment of CHH recommends that hCG should be the first-line therapy for patients with some gonadal development (testicular volume >4 mL) and no history of undescended testes and that duration of treatment should be at least for 3 to 6 months before adding FSH.[30]

FSH induces proliferation and maturation of SC, which support the spermatogenesis process within the testis. In clinical practice, either urine-derived FSH (human menopausal gonadotrophin) or recombinant FSH (rFSH) is commonly used. The safety and efficacy of rFSH have been demonstrated in many studies.[32,33] Furthermore, by modifying the glycosylation sites of the rFSG, long-acting FSH analogues have been developed; these long-acting FSH analogues have been shown to be safe and efficacious in women seeking infertility care. Corifollitropin alfa has the same pharmacodynamic profile as the rFSH, but it has a longer half-life,[34] reducing the frequency of multiple injections. A small number of studies of long-acting rFSH in men with HH[35,36] have shown these preparations to be safe and able to induce greater than 1 million sperm in more than 75% of men with HH, but further studies are warranted before they are established in clinical practice.

Combination FSH with hCG hormone stimulation has yielded improved results in producing sperm and promoting fertility compared with hCG alone. Approximately 50% of those remaining azoospermic with LH monotherapy produced greater than 1×10^6 sperm when FSH was added.[33] FSH is usually added after 3 to 6 months of LH hormone stimulation if LH alone has failed to induce spermatogenesis. Baseline testicular volume and sexual development are important prognostic factors for response to combination gonadotropins therapy.[37,38] In addition, body mass index (BMI) has been recognized as a prognostic marker of inducing spermatogenesis with gonadotrophins therapy, with lower BMI being associated with a better response.[39] Given the improved outcomes with combination gonadotropins therapy, FSH was evaluated as an adjunct to standard testosterone therapy in an early study aiming to assess spermatogenesis induction and maintenance in HH men without cryptorchidism. Following 24 months of cotreatment, combined treatment with testosterone and FSH failed to show sperm induction; instead, the sperm count decreased even further.[40]

A meta-analysis of 49 studies by Rastrelli and colleagues[24] reported an overall success rate of 75% in achieving at least 1 spermatozoa in the semen from baseline of azoospermia and a mean sperm concentration of 5.92 million/mL after gonadotrophin therapy. Prior therapy with TRT did not affect the outcome of gonadotrophin therapy. Higher success rates were observed with combination therapy of hCG and FSH than with hCG alone; poorer outcomes were noted in men with prepubertal onset of HH.[24]

Gonadotropin therapy is in general effective in inducing spermatogenesis in men with HH. Several different gonadotropin therapy protocols exist, but insufficient data exist on the relative efficacy of various regimens. The treatment regimens typically include hCG at a dose from 500 to 2500 IU twice or thrice weekly and FSH at a dose from 75 to 150 IU 2 to 3 times weekly.[25,41] To date, no randomized prospective trials exist to confirm the best treatment regimen, and these protocols are based on expert opinions.[42,43]

When gonadotropin therapy fails to induce enough sperm for a couple to conceive naturally, assistive reproductive technologies (ART) can enhance paternity potential in men with HH. A meta-analysis of 709 patients with CHH showed that the rates of fertilization, implantation, and live births (72%, 36%, and 40%) did not differ in men with CHH compared with men with other causes of infertility.[44] Thus, ART is a rational next step in the management of infertility in men with HH who fail to respond to gonadotrophin treatment.

Pulsatile Gonadotrophin-Releasing Hormone

Pulsatile GnRH represents another approach for managing infertility in men with CHH. Several studies have investigated the efficacy of GnRH treatment, and some studies have compared GnRH treatment with combined gonadotropins treatment.[25] However, no head-to-head trials have compared GnRH treatment with combined gonadotropin treatment. GnRH pumps are not widely available, and in many countries, these pumps are available only in research settings. A meta-analysis of 8 studies reported that treatment with GnRH resulted in earlier onset of spermatogenesis compared with gonadotropins treatment in men with CHH, but there were no differences in sperm concentration and pregnancy rate.[45] To mimic the pulsatile pattern of release in normal physiology, GnRH is given either intravenously or subcutaneously via a pump. Standard commencement dose is 25 ng/kg per pulse every 2 hours, and the dose is titrated to achieve serum testosterone levels in the normal reference range.[25] Duration of GnRH pump therapy normally exceeds 12 months in men with HH. Response to treatment varies according to degree of GnRH deficiency, baseline inhibin B level, and presence of cryptorchidism.[46]

Another therapeutic regimen that has been evaluated is pulsatile GnRH with rFSH pretreatment.[47] This small, open-label study showed that 24 months of GnRH therapy with preceding 6-month rFSH administration had a possible favorable effect on gonadal development, attaining testicular growth, normalizing levels of inhibin B levels, and promoting fertility in patients with CHH compared with 24 months of GnRH therapy alone; however, the 2 regimens did not differ significantly in the final testicular volume, sperm count, time to sperm appearance in the ejaculate, and fertility outcomes.[47] The study had a small number of participants (n = 13), and it was not powered to prove superiority of FSH/GnRH group in either sperm count or fertility outcomes.

Pulsatile GnRH is effective in cases with intact pituitary. GnRH appears to have less estrogenic derived side effects, but it has not been found to expedite testicular growth or the presence of sperm in the ejaculate compared with FSH/hCG treatment.[48] A mean sperm concentration of 4.27 million/mL was reported following hormonal stimulation with GnRH treatment in men with HH.[24] Although these values decreased well below the lower reference limit according to World Health Organization 2010 classification,[49] they were sufficient to obtain a pregnancy in 30% to 50% of cases of those who wanted to achieve paternity through both natural conception and assisted reproduction. This is further supported by a previous study that demonstrated that 16% of pregnancies occurred when the mean sperm concentration was less than 1×10^6 million/mL and 71% of pregnancies occurred when the mean sperm concentration was less than 20×10^6 million/mL.[50]

Selective Estrogen Receptor Modulators

SERMs have been used off label to treat men with low testosterone. Clomiphene citrate (CC) and tamoxifen are the most commonly used SERM agents. SERMs provide a potential advantage over TRT because they work by inhibiting the negative feedback of estrogen to the hypothalamus/pituitary, resulting in increased gonadotrophin secretion and subsequent testosterone secretion. Many studies have shown an improvement in endogenous testosterone levels in hypogonadal men[51–53]; however, the improvement in hypogonadal symptoms with SERM treatment has been inconsistent in published studies.[51,54,55] Furthermore, these studies included predominantly men with late-onset hypogonadism. The men with congenital or acquired HH secondary to pituitary tumor did not respond to high doses or prolonged course of clomiphene (50 mg twice daily).[56] Similarly, Kulin and colleagues[57] observed that prepubertal boys, before the maturation of their hypothalamic-pituitary axis, did not respond to CC. Thus, an intact and functioning HPG axis is necessary for the mechanism of action of SERM to activate testicular function.

Common adverse effects of SERMs include headache, visual changes, nausea and vomiting, and mood swings. Clomiphene has been reported to cause gynecomastia, and there have been rare reports showing induced azoospermia.[58] Only a few studies have addressed possible side effects after long-term use of clomiphene (>3 years); the long-term side effects appear to be similar to those with short-term use. Given the antiestrogenic effects, there had been concern regarding bone density. Three years of CC usage resulted in improvement of bone mass across all 29 patients who had either normal or reduced bone mineral density at baseline.[53] This is explained by the estrogenic agonistic effect on bones. However, this could not be extrapolated for all class drugs, and tamoxifen's effect on bone density remains questionable.[59,60]

Aromatase Inhibitors

AI, such as anastrozole, also have been used off label in hypogonadal men to increase testosterone production. A randomized control trial with 26 hypogonadal men suggested that anastrozole resulted in a significantly larger increase in T/E_2 ratio than CC.[61] A low T/E_2 ratio has been suggested as a separate endocrine parameter of male infertility.[62] A few studies observed that treatment of hypogonadal men with low T/E_2 ratio with anastrozole resulted in improvement of this ratio, and this correlated with a 3-fold improvement in sperm concentration.[63,64] These findings instigated the design of following studies where both anastrozole and CC were administered aiming to tackle the hyperestrogenemia derived from the latter. A retrospective study investigating the efficacy and safety of combination therapy in 51 men with low testosterone concluded that therapy was safe and effective in raising testosterone levels and normalizing estrogen levels and T/E2 ratio.[65] However, effect on semen parameters was not reported.

AI's commonest side effects include headache, gastrointestinal disturbances, hot flushes, and bone pains. In addition, the long-term skeletal safety remains an issue of concern with anastrozole, which has been associated with accelerated bone loss in postmenopausal women with breast cancer.[66] Therefore, anastrozole in not routinely used. Last, AI and SERMs have been associated with increased risk of thromboembolic events[67]; it is unclear if thrombosis risk is higher in comparison to TRT or to baseline risk in an age-matched population.

PRIMARY HYPOGONADISM

The men with primary hypogonadism may be azoospermic (nonobstructive azoospermia [NOA]) or have reduced semen quality. The histopathological finding can vary from absence of germ cells (SC only) to maturation arrest and hypospermatogenesis and is directly linked to the cause of the testicular failure. Historically, the only viable options to paternity in men with azoospermia were sperm donation or adoption. Recent advances in surgical extraction of sperm in some men with NOA along with ART have enabled many men with primary testicular failure to father their own biological children.

There are different surgical methods to retrieve sperm in men with NOA. Conventional testicular sperm extraction (cTESE) involves exposure of the testis through a small incision and the acquisition of multiple biopsies blindly as a means to isolate sperm. Microdissection testicular sperm extraction (mTESE) is performed with the aid of a surgical microscope to identify engorged seminiferous tubules (containing sperm, it is hoped) in situ and to take out a small amount of testicular tissue for sperm extraction[68] (**Fig. 1**). Although mTESE is now considered the gold-standard method for sperm retrieval, a meta-analysis did not show superiority of mTESE over cTESE with regards to sperm recovery.[69] TESA (testicular sperm aspiration), which is performed by introducing a needle into the testis and aspirating fluid and tissue, has been shown to be inferior to testicular sperm extraction (TESE).[70]

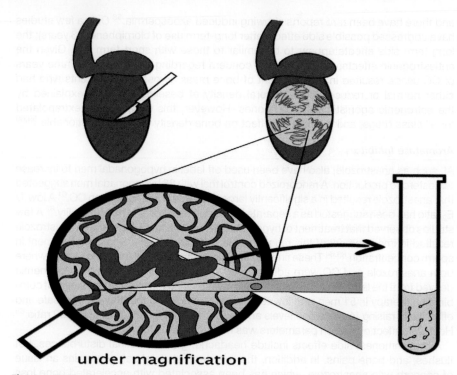

under magnification

Fig. 1. mTESE. Microdissection of seminiferous tubules is done under ×20 to 40 magnification. Isolated sperm are used during ICSI of eggs from the female partner but may be cryopreserved beforehand.

Endocrine stimulation is an emerging area with a potential role in the treatment of men with NOA undergoing surgical sperm retrieval (SSR). Although at a first glance it seems counterintuitive to use medications that increase gonadotrophins, there are pathophysiological arguments to support this approach: maximization of intratesticular testosterone, SC desensitization theory.[71–73] Low testosterone and T/E_2 appear to be implicated in the pathophysiology of NOA.[62] Also, it has been observed that HCG therapy can increase testosterone production in men with hypergonadotropic hypogonadism.[74] SC desensitization theory has emanated from animal studies; SC appear to be less sensitive when chronic stimulation of FSH occurs, resulting in downregulation of testicular gonadotropin receptor binding sites.[75] Foresta and colleagues[72] demonstrated that in their population of men with high baseline FSH and oligozoospermia, improved SC function was observed in response to FSH therapy following a 4-month period of temporary GnRH blockage. This postulates that SC desensitization can be reversed.[72] However, hormonal stimulation as a means to optimize intratesticular testosterone before SSR has only been insufficiently reviewed in small-scale studies, and there is conflicting evidence of whether it increases SSR rates in men with primary testicular failure.[73,76,77] Moreover, there is no clear evidence base for drug selection. SERMs and AI are commonly preferred given their oral route of administration and relatively low cost compared with gonadotropins/GnRH therapy. Although some centers use endocrine stimulation to optimize testosterone levels before SSR owing to some reports that showed favorable outcomes,[62,74,78,79] because of insufficient data, the practice committee of the American Society for Reproductive Medicine does not support the endocrine stimulation as standard clinical practice.[80]

Klinefelter syndrome (KS) is a chromosomal disorder typically associated with 47,XXY karyotype or mosaicism (47,XXY/46,XY) and primary testicular failure. Classical KS is characterized by tall stature, eunuchoid body proportions, gynecomastia, small testes, and NOA. Only a minority of men with nonmosaic KS (7%–8%) has been reported to produce few spermatozoa in ejaculate.[81,82] Most men with KS (XXY, karyotype) are azoospermic[83] and require surgical sperm extraction to achieve fatherhood. A successful rate of SSR using cTESE or mTESE in KS is estimated at 44% to 61%[69,84,85]; however, the likelihood of live childbirth decreases to approximately 16%.[86]

It is worth noting that KS is a cause of primary testicular failure, yet with a progressive course. Men with KS are born with spermatogonia, but during puberty there is an accelerated reduction in germ cells. Sperm have been identified in 70% of ejaculated semen specimens in adolescents with KS aged 12 to 20 years.[85] Moreover, adolescents with KS are known to have normal or low normal testosterone levels, whereas exogenous testosterone might further complicate their fertility potential in their adulthood. For those reasons, there is an ongoing discussion about the appropriate time of sperm harvesting and sperm cryopreservation. Isolation of good-quality sperm in the ejaculate and cryopreservation would mitigate the need to undergo invasive TESE in the future. However, sperm cryopreservation at a young age raises issues of emotional immaturity to make such a decision and financial burden for health service or family. Recent studies have not shown improved SSR rates in adolescents versus adults, and a 2017 meta-analysis did not show improved live birth and pregnancy outcomes with frozen versus fresh sperm in 1248 KS patients.[86]

ASSISTIVE REPRODUCTIVE TECHNOLOGIES/INTRACYTOPLASMIC SPERM INJECTION RISKS

ART have revolutionized the field of couple infertility with more than 7 million children born worldwide with these methods. Intracytoplasmic sperm injection (ICSI), in particular, has overcome to an extent the problem of fertilization in cases with severe oligospermia or azoospermia. ICSI involves the injection of a single sperm directly into a mature oocyte (**Fig. 2**). However, ART treatments do not come without risks. Although the risks are considered modest, there are a few key factors that may contribute to this relatively higher risk compared with naturally conceived pregnancies: infertility itself, risks associated with culture of embryos and gametes, type of ART, and epigenetic imprinting. A recent study using data from the Society for Assisted Reproductive Technology Clinic Outcome Reporting System registry concluded that ART is associated with increased risks of a major nonchromosomal birth defect, cardiovascular defect, and any defect in singleton children, and chromosomal defects in twins.[87] In

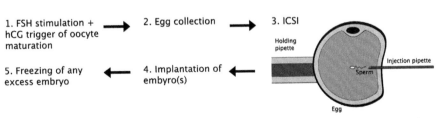

Fig. 2. ICSI. Following superovulation using FSH and hCG injections, eggs are retrieved under ultrasonographic guidance. Eggs are stripped and then injected with a single sperm. Following 3 to 5 days' incubation, 1 to 2 embryos are transferred to the uterine cavity. Remaining embryos may be stored for a later frozen embryo transfer.

addition, the use of ICSI further increases this risk, and particularly when male factor infertility is implicated.[87] It remains unclear though if one of the aforementioned key factors contributes more to this relative increased risk. There is not enough evidence to consolidate the long-term health risks of ART. Limited data suggest that altered blood pressure and cardiovascular function are more commonly encountered in ART children compared with children born from natural conception. It has also been described as a plausible association between cerebral palsy and ART. To date, no evidence to support increased risks of malignancies exists.[88]

SUMMARY

Fertility potential of hypogonadal men has been enhanced over the past 40 years. It is of utmost importance that fertility care is delivered by an experienced multidisciplinary team to ensure appropriate investigation, counseling, pharmacologic therapy, and follow-up as well as a timely referral for ART should it be required.

HH represents one of the few medically treatable causes of male infertility. Treatment pathways and success rates differ according to the cause of hypogonadism and the time of onset. Puberty, a crucial milestone in a man's life, informs the definitive management and response to treatment.[89,90] Postpubertal onset, early arrest of puberty, and complete failure of puberty have different fertility induction outcomes listed from more to least favorable. Hormonal treatment with gonadotropins and pulsatile GnRH has a much stronger evidence base in men with HH than SERMs or AI. In addition, hCG with or without FSH and pulsatile GnRH have been shown to be consistently effective in HH, but pulsatile GnRH is less favored in clinical practice mainly because of cumbersomeness and cost. The role for hormonal stimulation in cases with primary hypogonadism remains equivocal: ART with ICSI represents the gold standard of treatment. Modest risks have been reported with ART/ICSI.

CLINICS CARE POINTS

- Testosterone replacement therapy in men with hypogonadism is useful for virilization and bolstering of desirable secondary sexual characteristics but does not support spermatogenesis because of negative feedback on the hypothalamic-pituitary-gonadal axis.

- Human chorionic gonadotropin represents the first-line therapy for patients with secondary hypogonadism and some gonadal development (testicular volume >4 mL) with no history of undescended testes. Duration of treatment should be at least 3 to 6 months before adding follicle-stimulating hormone.

- Poorer outcomes to gonadotropins therapy were noted in men with prepubertal onset of hypogonadotropic hypogonadism.

- Medications that increase endogenous testosterone have been implicated with deep vein thrombosis (DVT) risk.

DISCLOSURE

The Section of Endocrinology and Investigative Medicine is funded by grants from the MRC and NIHR and is supported by the NIHR Imperial Biomedical Research Centre (BRC) Funding Scheme. C.N. Jayasena is funded by an NIHR Post-Doctoral Fellowship. The views expressed are those of the authors and not necessarily those of the above-mentioned funders, the NHS, the NIHR, or the Department of Health.

REFERENCES

1. Anderson JE, Farr SL, Jamieson DJ, et al. Infertility services reported by men in the United States: national survey data. Fertil Steril 2009;91(6):2466–70.
2. Thonneau P, Marchand S, Tallec A, et al. Incidence and main causes of infertility in a resident population (1,850,000) of three French regions (1988-1989). Hum Reprod 1991;6(6):811–6.
3. Ahmad AE, Lao M, Mechlin CW, et al. Prevalence of male hypogonadism in couples presenting to a reproductive endocrinology infertility clinic. Fertil Steril 2013; 100(3):S211.
4. Andersson A-M, Toppari J, Haavisto A-M, et al. Longitudinal reproductive hormone profiles in infants: peak of inhibin B levels in infant boys exceeds levels in adult men. J Clin Endocrinol Metab 1998;83(2):675–81.
5. Kuiri-Hänninen T, Sankilampi U, Dunkel L. Activation of the hypothalamic-pituitary-gonadal axis in infancy: minipuberty. Horm Res Paediatr 2014;82(2): 73–80.
6. Cortes D, Müller J, Skakkebæk NE. Proliferation of Sertoli cells during development of the human testis assessed by stereological methods. Int J Androl 1987;10(4):589–96.
7. Chemes HE, Rey RA, Nistal M, et al. Physiological androgen insensitivity of the fetal, neonatal, and early infantile testis is explained by the ontogeny of the androgen receptor expression in Sertoli cells. J Clin Endocrinol Metab 2008; 93(11):4408–12.
8. Rey RA, Musse M, Venara M, et al. Ontogeny of the androgen receptor expression in the fetal and postnatal testis: its relevance on Sertoli cell maturation and the onset of adult spermatogenesis. Microsc Res Tech 2009;72(11):787–95.
9. Spratt DI, O'Dea StLL, Schoenfeld D, et al. Neuroendocrine-gonadal axis in men: frequent sampling of LH, FSH, and testosterone. Am J Physiol Endocrinol Metab 1988;254(5). https://doi.org/10.1152/ajpendo.1988.254.5.e658.
10. Griswold MD. The central role of Sertoli cells in spermatogenesis. Semin Cell Dev Biol 1998;9(4):411–6.
11. Zhou Q, Nie R, Prins GS, et al. Localization of androgen and estrogen receptors in adult male mouse reproductive tract. J Androl 2002;23(6):870–81.
12. Shang Y, Myers M, Brown M. Formation of the androgen receptor transcription complex. Mol Cell 2002;9(3):601–10.
13. Li J, Al-Azzawi F. Mechanism of androgen receptor action. Maturitas 2009;63(2): 142–8.
14. Fix C, Jordan C, Cano P, et al. Testosterone activates mitogen-activated protein kinase and the cAMP response element binding protein transcription factor in Sertoli cells. Proc Natl Acad Sci U S A 2004;101(30):10919–24.
15. Cheng J, Watkins SC, Walker WH. Testosterone activates mitogen-activated protein kinase via Src kinase and the epidermal growth factor receptor in Sertoli cells. Endocrinology 2007;148(5):2066–74.
16. Walker WH. Testosterone signaling and the regulation of spermatogenesis. Spermatogenesis 2011;1(2):116–20.
17. Maddocks S, Hargreave TB, Reddie K, et al. Intratesticular hormone levels and the route of secretion of hormones from the testis of the rat, guinea pig, monkey and human. Int J Androl 1993;16(4):272–8.
18. Jarow JP, Chen H, Rosner W, et al. Assessment of the androgen environment within the human testis: minimally invasive method to obtain intratesticular fluid. J Androl 2001;22(4):640–5.

19. Zirkin BR, Santulli R, Awoniyi CA, et al. Maintenance of advanced spermatogenic cells in the adult rat testis: quantitative relationship to testosterone concentration within the testis. Endocrinology 1989;124(6):3043–9.

20. Rodriguez-Tolrà J, Torremadé J, di Gregorio S, et al. Effects of testosterone treatment on bone mineral density in men with testosterone deficiency syndrome. Andrology 2013;1(4):570–5.

21. Traish AM, Haider A, Doros G, et al. Long-term testosterone therapy in hypogonadal men ameliorates elements of the metabolic syndrome: an observational, long-term registry study. Int J Clin Pract 2014;68(3):314–29.

22. Griffin PD, Aribarg A, Gui-yuan Z, et al. Contraceptive efficacy of testosterone-induced azoospermia and oligozoospermia in normal men. Fertil Steril 1996; 65(4):821–9.

23. Bhasin S, Brito JP, Cunningham GR, et al. Testosterone therapy in men with hypogonadism: an Endocrine Society Clinical Practice Guideline. J Clin Endocrinol Metab 2018;103(5):1715–44.

24. Rastrelli G, Corona G, Mannucci E, et al. Factors affecting spermatogenesis upon gonadotropin-replacement therapy: a meta-analytic study. Andrology 2014;2(6): 794–808.

25. Young J, Xu C, Papadakis GE, et al. Clinical management of congenital hypogonadotropic hypogonadism. Endocr Rev 2019;40(2):669–710.

26. Pitteloud N, Hayes FJ, Boepple PA, et al. The role of prior pubertal development, biochemical markers of testicular maturation, and genetics in elucidating the phenotypic heterogeneity of idiopathic hypogonadotropic hypogonadism. J Clin Endocrinol Metab 2002;87(1):152–60.

27. Coviello AD, Matsumoto AM, Bremner WJ, et al. Low-dose human chorionic gonadotropin maintains intratesticular testosterone in normal men with testosterone-induced gonadotropin suppression. J Clin Endocrinol Metab 2005; 90(5):2595–602.

28. Roth MY, Page ST, Lin K, et al. Dose-dependent increase in intratesticular testosterone by very low-dose human chorionic gonadotropin in normal men with experimental gonadotropin deficiency. J Clin Endocrinol Metab 2010;95(8): 3806–13.

29. Vicari E, Mongioì A, Calogero AE, et al. Therapy with human chorionic gonadotrophin alone induces spermatogenesis in men with isolated hypogonadotrophic hypogonadism—long-term follow-up. Int J Androl 1992;15(4):320–9.

30. Pasteur I, Boehm U, Bouloux P-M, et al. Expert consensus document: European Consensus Statement on congenitaln hypogonadotropic hypogonadism—pathogenesis, diagnosis and treatment. Nat Publ Gr 2015;11:547–64.

31. Depenbusch M, Von Eckardstein S, Simoni M, et al. Maintenance of spermatogenesis in hypogonadotropic hypogonadal men with human chorionic gonadotropin alone. Vol 147. Available at: www.eje.org. Accessed March 26, 2021.

32. Loumaye E, Dreano M, Galazka A, et al. Recombinant follicle stimulating hormone: development of the first biotechnology product for the treatment of infertility. Hum Reprod Update 1998;4(6):862–81.

33. Bouloux PMG, Nieschlag E, Burger HG, et al. Induction of spermatogenesis by recombinant follicle-stimulating hormone (Puregon) in hypogonadotropic azoospermic men who failed to respond to human chorionic gonadotropin alone. J Androl 2003;24(4):604–11.

34. Fauser BCJM, Mannaerts MJL, Devroey P, et al. Advances in recombinant DNA technology: corifollitropin alfa, a hybrid molecule with sustained follicle-

stimulating activity and reduced injection frequency. Hum Reprod Update 2009; 15(3):309–21.

35. Bouloux PMG, Handelsman DJ, Jockenhövel F, et al. First human exposure to FSH-CTP in hypogonadotrophic hypogonadal males. Hum Reprod 2001;16: 1592–7.

36. Nieschlag E, Bouloux PMG, Stegmann BJ, et al. An open-label clinical trial to investigate the efficacy and safety of corifollitropin alfa combined with hCG in adult men with hypogonadotropic hypogonadism. Reprod Biol Endocrinol 2017;15(1). https://doi.org/10.1186/s12958-017-0232-y.

37. Miyagawa Y, Tsujimura A, Matsumiya K, et al. Outcome of gonadotropin therapy for male hypogonadotropic hypogonadism at university affiliated male infertility centers: a 30-year retrospective study. J Urol 2005;173(6):2072–5.

38. Liu PY, Baker HWG, Jayadev V, et al. Induction of spermatogenesis and fertility during gonadotropin treatment of gonadotropin-deficient infertile men: predictors of fertility outcome. J Clin Endocrinol Metab 2009;94(3):801–8.

39. Warne DW, Decosterd G, Okada H, et al. A combined analysis of data to identify predictive factors for spermatogenesis in men with hypogonadotropic hypogo-nadism treated with recombinant human follicle-stimulating hormone and human chorionic gonadotropin. Fertil Steril 2009;92(2):594–604.

40. Schaison G, Young J, Pholsena M, et al. Failure of combined follicle-stimulating hormone-testosterone administration to initiate and/or maintain spermatogenesis in men with hypogonadotropic hypogonadism. J Clin Endocrinol Metab 1993; 77(6):1545–9.

41. Lee JA, Ramasamy R. Indications for the use of human chorionic gonadotropic hormone for the management of infertility in hypogonadal men. Transl Androl Urol 2018;7(Suppl 3):S348–52.

42. Rastrelli G, Vignozzi L, Maggi M. Different medications for hypogonadotropic hypogonadism. Endocr Dev 2016;30:60–78.

43. Behre HM. Clinical use of FSH in male infertility. Front Endocrinol (Lausanne) 2019;10. https://doi.org/10.3389/fendo.2019.00322.

44. Gao Y, Yu B, Mao J, et al. Assisted reproductive techniques with congenital hypogonadotropic hypogonadism patients: a systematic review and meta-analysis. BMC Endocr Disord 2018;18(1). https://doi.org/10.1186/s12902-018-0313-8.

45. Wei C, Long G, Zhang Y, et al. Spermatogenesis of male patients with congenital hypogonadotropic hypogonadism receiving pulsatile gonadotropin-releasing hormone therapy versus gonadotropin therapy: a systematic review and meta-analysis. World J Mens Health 2020. https://doi.org/10.5534/wjmh.200043.

46. Pitteloud N, Hayes FJ, Dwyer A, et al. Predictors of outcome of long-term GnRH therapy in men with idiopathic hypogonadotropic hypogonadism. J Clin Endocrinol Metab 2002;87(9):4128–36.

47. Dwyer AA, Sykiotis GP, Hayes FJ, et al. Trial of recombinant follicle-stimulating hormone pretreatment for GnRH-induced fertility in patients with congenital hypogonadotropic hypogonadism). E1790 jcem.endojournals.org. J Clin Endocrinol Metab 2013;98(11):1790–5.

48. Liu L, Banks SM, Barnes KM, et al. Two-year comparison of testicular responses to pulsatile gonadotropin-releasing hormone and exogenous gonadotropins from the inception of therapy in men with isolated hypogonadotropic hypogonadism. J Clin Endocrinol Metab 1988;67(6):1140–5.

49. WHO laboratory manual for the examination and processing of human semen. Available at: https://www.who.int/publications/i/item/9789241547789. Accessed April 28, 2021.

50. Burris AS, Clark RV, Vantman DJ, et al. A low sperm concentration does not preclude fertility in men with isolated hypogonadotropic hypogonadism after gonadotropin therapy. Fertil Steril 1988;50(2):343–7.
51. Habous M, Giona S, Tealab A, et al. Clomiphene citrate and human chorionic gonadotropin are both effective in restoring testosterone in hypogonadism: a short-course randomized study. BJU Int 2018;122(5):889–97.
52. Whitten SJ, Nangia AK, Kolettis PN. Select patients with hypogonadotropic hypogonadism may respond to treatment with clomiphene citrate. Fertil Steril 2006; 86(6):1664–8.
53. Moskovic DJ, Katz DJ, Akhavan A, et al. Clomiphene citrate is safe and effective for long-term management of hypogonadism. BJU Int 2012;110(10):1524–8.
54. Soares AH, Horie NC, Chiang LAP, et al. Effects of clomiphene citrate on male obesity-associated hypogonadism: a randomized, double-blind, placebo-controlled study. Int J Obes 2018;42(5):953–63.
55. Guay AT, Jacobson J, Perez JB, et al. Clomiphene increases free testosterone levels in men with both secondary hypogonadism and erectile dysfunction: who does and does not benefit? Int J Impot Res 2003;15(3):156–65.
56. Santen RJ, Leonard JM, Sherins RJ, et al. Short- and long-term effects of clomiphene citrate on the pituitary-testicular axis. J Clin Endocrinol Metab 1971;33(6): 970–9.
57. Kulin HE, Grumbach MM, Kaplan SL. Changing sensitivity of the pubertal gonadal hypothalamic feedback mechanism in man. Science 1969;166(3908): 1012–3.
58. Pasqualotto FF, Fonseca GP, Pasqualotto EB. Azoospermia after treatment with clomiphene citrate in patients with oligospermia. Fertil Steril 2008;90(5): 2014.e11-2.
59. Riggs BL, Hartmann LC. Selective estrogen-receptor modulators—mechanisms of action and application to clinical practice. N Engl J Med 2003;348(7):618–29.
60. Lee J, Alqudaihi HM, Kang MS, et al. Effect of tamoxifen on the risk of osteoporosis and osteoporotic fracture in younger breast cancer survivors: a nationwide study. Front Oncol 2020;10:366.
61. Helo S, Ellen J, Mechlin C, et al. A randomized prospective double-blind comparison trial of clomiphene citrate and anastrozole in raising testosterone in hypogonadal infertile men. J Sex Med 2015;12(8):1761–9.
62. Pavlovich CP, King P, Goldstein M, et al. Evidence of a treatable endocrinopathy in infertile men. J Urol 2001;165(3):837–41.
63. Raman JD, Schlegel PN. Aromatase inhibitors for male infertility. J Urol 2002; 167(2 Pt 1):624–9.
64. Shoshany O, Abhyankar N, Mufarreh N, et al. Outcomes of anastrozole in oligozoospermic hypoandrogenic subfertile men. Fertil Steril 2017;107(3):589–94.
65. Alder NJ, Keihani S, Stoddard GJ, et al. Combination therapy with clomiphene citrate and anastrozole is a safe and effective alternative for hypoandrogenic subfertile men. BJU Int 2018;122(4):688–94.
66. Eastell R, Adams JE, Coleman RE, et al. Effect of anastrozole on bone mineral density: 5-year results from the anastrozole, tamoxifen, alone or in combination trial 18233230. J Clin Oncol 2008;26(7):1051–8.
67. Anastrozole 1 mg film-coated tablets - summary of product characteristics (SmPC) - (EMC). Available at: https://www.medicines.org.uk/emc/product/2749/smpc. Accessed April 28, 2021.
68. Schlegel PN. Testicular sperm extraction: microdissection improves sperm yield with minimal tissue excision. Hum Reprod 1999;14(1):131–5.

69. Corona G, Minhas S, Giwercman A, et al. Sperm recovery and ICSI outcomes in men with non-obstructive azoospermia: a systematic review and meta-analysis. Hum Reprod Update 2019;25(6):733–57.

70. Hauser R, Yogev L, Paz G, et al. Comparison of efficacy of two techniques for testicular sperm retrieval in nonobstructive azoospermia: multifocal testicular sperm extraction versus multifocal testicular sperm aspiration. J Androl 2006; 27(1):28–33.

71. Tharakan T, Salonia A, Corona G, et al. The role of hormone stimulation in men with nonobstructive azoospermia undergoing surgical sperm retrieval. J Clin Endocrinol Metab 2020;105(12). https://doi.org/10.1210/clinem/dgaa556.

72. Foresta C, Bettella A, Spolaore D, et al. Suppression of the high endogenous levels of plasma FSH in infertile men are associated with improved Sertoli cell function as reflected by elevated levels of plasma inhibin B. Hum Reprod 2004; 19(6):1431–7.

73. Shinjo E, Shiraishi K, Matsuyama H. The effect of human chorionic gonadotropin-based hormonal therapy on intratesticular testosterone levels and spermatogonial DNA synthesis in men with non-obstructive azoospermia. Andrology 2013; 1(6):929–35.

74. Shiraishi K, Ohmi C, Shimabukuro T, et al. Human chorionic gonadotrophin treatment prior to microdissection testicular sperm extraction in non-obstructive azoospermia. Hum Reprod 2012;27(2):331–9.

75. Gnanaprakasam MS, Chen CJH, Sutherland JG, et al. Receptor depletion and replenishment processes: in vivo regulation of gonadotropin receptors by luteinizing hormone, follicle stimulating hormone and ethanol in rat testis. Biol Reprod 1979;20(5):991–1000.

76. Reifsnyder JE, Ramasamy R, Husseini J, et al. Role of optimizing testosterone before microdissection testicular sperm extraction in men with nonobstructive azoospermia. J Urol 2012;188(2):532–7.

77. Amer MK, Ahmed AR, Abdel Hamid AA, et al. Can spermatozoa be retrieved in non-obstructive azoospermic patients with high FSH level?: a retrospective cohort study. Andrologia 2019;51(2):e13176.

78. Foresta C, Selice R, Moretti A, et al. Gonadotropin administration after gonadotropin-releasing-hormone agonist: a therapeutic option in severe testiculopathies. Fertil Steril 2009;92(4):1326–32.

79. Hussein A, Ozgok Y, Ross L, et al. Optimization of spermatogenesis-regulating hormones in patients with non-obstructive azoospermia and its impact on sperm retrieval: a multicentre study. BJU Int 2013;111(3b):E110–4.

80. Practice Committee of the American Society for Reproductive Medicine. Management of nonobstructive azoospermia: a committee opinion. Fertil Steril 2018; 110(7):1239–45.

81. Kitamura M, Matsumiya K, Koga M, et al. Ejaculated spermatozoa in patients with non-mosaic Klinefelter's syndrome. Int J Urol 2000;7(3):88–92.

82. Lanfranco F, Kamischke A, Zitzmann M, et al. Klinefelter's syndrome. Lancet 2004;364(9430):273–83.

83. Smyth CM, Bremner WJ. Klinefelter syndrome. Arch Intern Med 1998;158(12): 1309–14.

84. Fullerton G, Hamilton M, Maheshwari A. Should non-mosaic Klinefelter syndrome men be labelled as infertile in 2009? Hum Reprod 2010;25(3):588–97.

85. Mehta A, Paduch DA. Klinefelter syndrome: an argument for early aggressive hormonal and fertility management. Fertil Steril 2012;98(2):274–83.

86. Corona G, Pizzocaro A, Lanfranco F, et al. Sperm recovery and ICSI outcomes in Klinefelter syndrome: a systematic review and meta-analysis. Hum Reprod Update 2017;23(3):265–75.

87. Luke B, Brown MB, Wantman E, et al. The risk of birth defects with conception by ART. Hum Reprod 2021;36(1):116–29.

88. Berntsen S, Söderström-Anttila V, Wennerholm U-B, et al. The health of children conceived by ART: "the chicken or the egg? Hum Reprod Update 2019;25(2): 137–58.

89. McLachlan RI. The endocrine control of spermatogenesis. Best Pract Res Clin Endocrinol Metab 2000;14(3):345–62.

90. Rohayem J, Sinthofen N, Nieschlag E, et al. Causes of hypogonadotropic hypogonadism predict response to gonadotropin substitution in adults. Andrology 2016;4(1):87–94.

The Benefits and Risks of Testosterone Treatment in Older Hypogonadal Men

Peter J. Snyder, MD

KEYWORDS

- Testosterone • Hypogonadal • Sexual function • Walking • Mood • Hemoglobin
- Bone mineral density

KEY POINTS

- The serum testosterone concenmtration decreases very little with increasing age, but the free testosterone concentration decreases more
- Testosterone treatment of older hypogonadal men improves their sexual function, walking, hemoglobin and bone mineral density and strength, but no vitality or cognition.
- The possibility has been raised that testosterone treatment of older hypogonadal men would increase the risk of benign prostatic hyperplasia, prostate cancer or heart disesase, but no trial has yet been large enough or long enough to evaluate this possibility.

As men age, their serum testosterone concentrations decrease. Also as men age, other changes occur that are similar to changes in men who become hypogonadal owing to pituitary and testicular disease, suggesting that the decrease in testosterone may be a cause of the other changes. Recent studies have been completed to determine if treating older men with testosterone will reverse these changes.

TESTOSTERONE DECREASES WITH ADVANCING AGE

Testosterone concentrations in men decrease with age throughout adulthood, as demonstrated in both cross-sectional and longitudinal studies. In a cross-sectional study, the mean ± standard deviation testosterone concentration in men 20 to 39 years old was 683 ± 289 ng/dL and in men 70 to 79 year old was 428 ± 128 ng/dL.[1] The relative decrease in calculated free testosterone concentration was even greater, from 10.7 ± 3.4 ng/dL in the younger men to 5.8 ± 2.5 ng/dL in the older men. In the cross-sectional European Male Aging Study of 3220 men aged 40 to 79 years, the serum total testosterone decreased only 0.04% per year, but the decrease in free testosterone was greater, at 1.3% per year.[2]

Perelman School of Medicine, University of Pennsylvania, 12-135 Smilow Center for Clinical Research, 3400 Civic Center Boulevard, Philadelphia, PA 19104, USA
E-mail address: pjs@pennmedicine.upenn.edu

Endocrinol Metab Clin N Am 51 (2022) 149–156
https://doi.org/10.1016/j.ecl.2021.11.003
0889-8529/22/© 2021 Elsevier Inc. All rights reserved.

Longitudinal studies show a somewhat greater decrease in serum total testosterone concentrations. In the Baltimore Longitudinal Study on Aging, 890 men experienced a decrease in serum total testosterone concentration of from approximately 519 ng/dL at age 30 to 346 ng/dL at age 80.[3] In the Massachusetts Male Aging Study, 1709 men were evaluated initially, 1156 were evaluated a second time—an average of 8 years later—and 853 were evaluated a third time, at an average of 7 years after the second time.[4] By regression modeling, the total serum testosterone concentration decreased 14.5% per decade.

In sum, studies show a modest decrease in testosterone with increasing age in men, best shown in longitudinal studies and more apparent by measurement of free testosterone.

BENEFITS OF TESTOSTERONE TREATMENT OF OLDER HYPOGONADAL MEN

Similarities between the consequences of frank hypogonadism and the consequences of aging, such as a decline in sexual function, decrease in muscle mass and strength, decrease in bone mineral density, and lower hemoglobin, suggest the possibility that the decreasing testosterone in older men might contribute to these consequences of aging. To test this possibility, The Testosterone Trials, a group of 7 coordinated trials, were conducted to determine if increasing the serum testosterone levels of older men to normal for young men would have any benefit.[5] The results were reported from 2010 to 2020. Results of a few other studies were reported during the same period.

The Testosterone Trials enrolled 790 men, with a mean age of 72 years, whose median serum testosterone concentration at baseline was 234 ng/dL.[6] They were allocated to receive testosterone or placebo gel for 1 year. Men who received testosterone experienced an increase in serum testosterone to the mid-500s during treatment. They were assessed for the beneficial and deleterious effects of testosterone during the 1 year of treatment. Testosterone had beneficial effects on sexual function, walking, mood, bone density and strength, and hemoglobin.

Sexual Function

Testosterone treatment, compared with placebo, increased all aspects of sexual function, especially sexual activity (**Fig. 1**) and libido and, to a lesser degree, erectile function.[6,7] The effects on sexual function and libido were associated with increases in total and free testosterone and estradiol. Testosterone also increased sexual function in another trial of 751 men, 18 years or older, with low testosterone level and one or more symptoms of testosterone deficiency.[8]

Physical Function

Testosterone treatment increased the distance walked in 6 minutes to a small degree in all men in The Testosterone Trials and also improved their perception that their walking was better.[6,9] The increase in walking was associated with increases in total and free testosterone and hemoglobin. In 2 smaller trials, testosterone treatment did not improve walking, although it did improve strength.[10,11]

Mood and Depressive Symptoms

Testosterone treatment improved mood to a small but statistically significant degree, both increasing positive mood and decreasing negative mood.[6] Testosterone also decreased depressive symptoms.

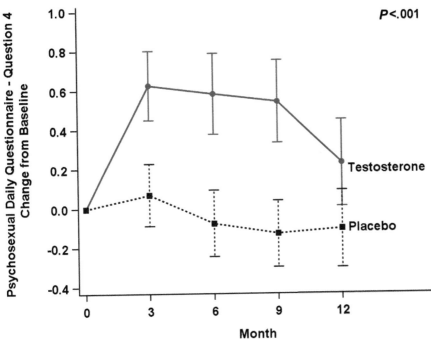

Fig. 1. The effect of testosterone treatment for 1 year on sexual function in older, hypogonadal men. (*From* Snyder PJ, Bhasin S, Cunningham GR, Matsumoto AM, Stephens-Shields AJ, Cauley JA, Gill TM, Barrett-Connor E, Swerdloff RS, Wang C, Ensrud KE, Lewis CE, Farrar JT, Cella D, Rosen RC, Pahor M, Crandall JP, Molitch ME, Cifelli D, Dougar D, Fluharty L, Resnick SM, Storer TW, Anton S, Basaria S, Diem SJ, Hou X, Mohler ER 3rd, Parsons JK, Wenger NK, Zeldow B, Landis JR, Ellenberg SS; Testosterone Trials Investigators. Effects of Testosterone Treatment in Older Men. N Engl J Med. 2016 Feb 18;374(7):611-24.)

Bone

A subset of 211 men in The Testosterone Trials were assessed for volumetric bone mineral density and estimated bone strength by quantitative computerized tomography at baseline and month 12 (**Fig. 2**).[12] Testosterone treatment increased the volumetric bone mineral density of the trabecular spine by 6.8% more than placebo and increased estimated bone strength similarly. The improvements in the hip were less but also significant.

Erythropoiesis

One hundred twenty-six men in The Testosterone Trials were anemic at baseline, about one-half owing to known causes, such as iron deficiency, and one-half whose anemia was unexplained.[13] Testosterone treatment increased hemoglobin in men with unexplained anemia, but also in men with anemia of known cause, by approximately 1.0 g/dL in both, correcting the anemia in more than 50% of the men (**Fig. 3**).

OUTCOME MEASURES THAT DID NOT IMPROVE WITH TESTOSTERONE TREATMENT IN OLDER MEN WITH HYPOGONADISM

Testosterone had been postulated to have beneficial effects on vitality, cognitive function and lipids and glucose, but in The Testosterone Trials, testosterone either had no effect or had an effect so small as to be of uncertain clinical meaning.

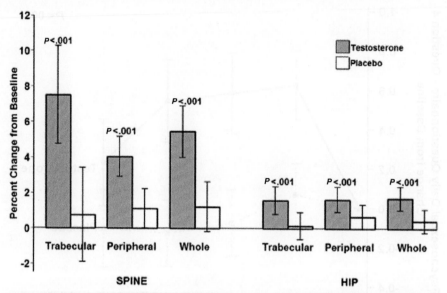

Fig. 2. The effect of testosterone treatment for 1 year on trabecular volumetric bone mineral density of the lumbar spine in older, hypogonadal men. (*From* Snyder PJ, Kopperdahl DL, Stephens-Shields AJ, Ellenberg SS, Cauley JA, Ensrud KE, Lewis CE, Barrett-Connor E, Schwartz AV, Lee DC, Bhasin S, Cunningham GR, Gill TM, Matsumoto AM, Swerdloff RS, Basaria S, Diem SJ, Wang C, Hou X, Cifelli D, Dougar D, Zeldow B, Bauer DC, Keaveny TM. Effect of Testosterone Treatment on Volumetric Bone Density and Strength in Older Men With Low Testosterone: A Controlled Clinical Trial. JAMA Intern Med. 2017 Apr 1;177(4):471-479.)

Vitality

All men in The Testosterone Trials were evaluated for vitality and its converse, fatigue, by the Functional Assessment of Chronic Illness Therapy Fatigue Scale. In men who were judged to be fatigued at the outset, testosterone had no effect on fatigue.[6] In all men, testosterone was associated with a very small improvement, not likely of clinical import.

Cognitive Function

In the 493 men in The Testosterone Trials who had age-associated memory impairment, testosterone was not associated with a significant change in any aspect of cognition tested, including immediate or delayed paragraph recall, visual memory, spatial ability, or executive function.[14]

Lipids and Glucose

Testosterone treatment was associated with small decreases in total cholesterol, low-density lipoprotein cholesterol, and high-density lipoprotein cholesterol.[15] Testosterone treatment was also associated with small decreases in insulin and homeostatic model assessment insulin resistance, but not with fasting glucose or hemoglobin A1c concentrations. The clinical significance of these small changes is uncertain.

RISKS OF TESTOSTERONE TREATMENT OF OLDER HYPOGONADAL MEN

Several risks of testosterone treatment of older hypogonadal men have been proposed on the basis of theoretic grounds or observational studies. One, erythrocytosis, has been confirmed. The others have not been confirmed or refuted.

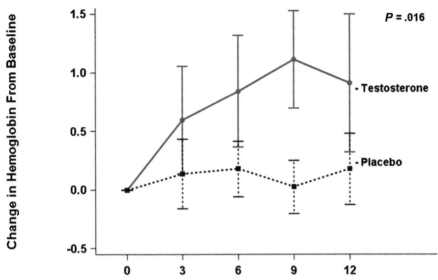

Fig. 3. The effect of testosterone treatment for 1 year on hemoglobin in older, hypogonadal men with unexplained anemia. (*From* Roy CN, Snyder PJ, Stephens-Shields AJ, Artz AS, Bhasin S, Cohen HJ, Farrar JT, Gill TM, Zeldow B, Cella D, Barrett-Connor E, Cauley JA, Crandall JP, Cunningham GR, Ensrud KE, Lewis CE, Matsumoto AM, Molitch ME, Pahor M, Swerdloff RS, Cifelli D, Hou X, Resnick SM, Walston JD, Anton S, Basaria S, Diem SJ, Wang C, Schrier SL, Ellenberg SS. Association of Testosterone Levels With Anemia in Older Men: A Controlled Clinical Trial. JAMA Intern Med. 2017 Apr 1;177(4):480-490. https://doi.org/10.1001/jamainternmed.2016.9540. Erratum in: JAMA Intern Med. 2019 Mar 1;179(3):457. Erratum in: JAMA Intern Med. 2021 May 1;181(5):727.)

Risk of Erythrocytosis

Testosterone stimulates erythropoiesis, and hypogonadism leads to anemia, which is then corrected by testosterone replacement, as described elsewhere in this article. Conversely, the administration of supraphysiologic doses of testosterone or other androgens, as occurs in androgen abuse, causes erythrocytosis. In The Testosterone Trials, in which the dose of testosterone was adjusted frequently to keep the serum testosterone concentration within the normal range, the development of erythrocytosis was uncommon, occurring in 7 of the 394 testosterone-treated men during the year of treatment.[6] In a meta-analysis of 51 randomized trials, testosterone was associated with an increase risk of erythrocytosis compared with placebo.[16]

Risk of Prostate Cancer

The possibility that testosterone treatment of older, hypogonadal men could increase their risk of developing prostate cancer or stimulate the growth of preexisting dormant prostate cancers is based on 2 observations. One is that the growth of prostate cancer is testosterone dependent, as dramatically demonstrated by the beneficial effects of severely decreasing testosterone in men who have metastatic prostate.[17] The second observation is that, as shown by an autopsy study, more than one-half of all men over the age of 50 years harbor an occult prostate cancer.[18] In The Testosterone Trials, only 1 man was diagnosed with prostate cancer during the 1 year of treatment.[6] In a meta-analysis of 51 randomized trials, testosterone treatment was not associated with an increased risk of prostate cancer.[16] The numbers of men in these trials, however, were too small, and the durations of observation were too short, to draw a conclusion about risk of testosterone treatment in stimulating prostate cancer.

Risk of Benign Prostatic Hypertrophy

The possibility that testosterone treatment of older, hypogonadal men could worsen benign prostatic hyperplasia is based on the observations that severe hypogonadism can retard the development of this condition and that blocking the conversion of testosterone to dihydrotestosterone reduces prostate volume in men who have this condition.[19] In The Testosterone Trials, symptoms of benign prostatic hyperplasia were evaluated by the International Prostate Symptoms Score; a score of more than 19 on this instrument indicates moderately severe lower urinary tract symptoms. During the 1 year of testosterone treatment, a similar number of men in the testosterone-treated group (n = 27) developed scores of more than 19, as did men in the placebo-treated group (n = 26).[6]

Risk of Sleep Apnea

A few small studies of testosterone administration in hypogonadal men seemed to show a worsening of sleep apnea, but a placebo-controlled trial of testosterone in older men showed no difference in apneic or hypopneic episodes in testosterone compared with placebo-treated men.[20]

Cardiovascular Risk

Two types of studies suggest that testosterone treatment of older men might increase their risk of cardiovascular disease. In 2 retrospective cohort studies, more men who were treated with testosterone experienced major adverse cardiovascular events than men who were not treated with testosterone.[21,22] One clinical trial of testosterone in men with mobility limitations was stopped by its data safety monitoring board because more men who received testosterone experienced cardiovascular events than those in the placebo group.[23] In the Cardiovascular Trial of The Testosterone Trials, in which 170 men were evaluated by computed tomographic angiography before and after 1 year of testosterone treatment, testosterone was associated with an increase in non-calcified coronary artery plaque volume of 40 mm^3, compared with 4 mm^3 with placebo treatment.[24]

Other studies, however, do not suggest an increased cardiovascular risk. A different retrospective cohort study did not show increased cardiovascular risk.[25] A different clinical trial in men with mobility limitations reported few adverse cardiovascular events.[10] In a different clinical trial, testosterone treatment for 3 years did not increase carotid intima media thickness more than placebo.[26] In The Testosterone Trials, the number of major adverse cardiovascular events was similar in testosterone- and placebo-treated men.[6] However, although The Testosterone Trial was the largest trial of testosterone to date, it was still not large enough or long enough to draw conclusions about cardiovascular risk.

SUMMARY OF BENEFITS AND RISKS OF TESTOSTERONE TREATMENT OF OLDER HYPOGONADAL MEN

Testosterone treatment of older hypogonadal men has clear benefits on sexual function, walking, mood, hemoglobin, and bone density. Because hypogonadism in older men is usually of a mild to moderate degree, the magnitude of the benefits is also of a mild to moderate degree. Testosterone had been postulated to benefit vitality, cognitive function and lipids and glucose metabolism, but these have not been confirmed.

Testosterone treatment may cause erythrocytosis, but this risk can be minimized by avoiding overtreatment. Testosterone has been postulated to increase the risk of prostate cancer, lower urinary tract symptoms owing to benign prostatic hypertrophy, and cardiovascular adverse events, but no trial yet completed has been large enough or long enough to confirm or refute these postulations. Although testosterone treatment has some clear benefits for older, hypogonadal men, decisions about administering this treatment should await the results of trials designed to determine long-term risk.

CLINICS CARE POINTS

- Testosterone treatment of older, hypogonadal men improves their sexual function, walking, mood, hemoglobin, and bone mineral density, all to a modest degree.
- Testosterone treatment of older, hypogonadal men does not improve vitality or cognition.
- The long-term risks of administering testosterone to older, hypogonadal men are not yet known.

REFERENCES

1. Deslypere JP, Vermeulen A. Leydig cell function in normal men: effect of age, lifestyle, residence, diet, and activity. J Clin Endocrinol Metab 1984;59:955–62.
2. Wu FC, Tajar A, Pye SR, et al. Hypothalamic-pituitary-testicular axis disruptions in older men are differentially linked to age and modifiable risk factors: the European Male Aging Study. J Clin Endocrinol Metab 2008;93:2737–45.
3. Harman SM, Metter EJ, Tobin JD, et al. Baltimore longitudinal study of A. longitudinal effects of aging on serum total and free testosterone levels in healthy men. Baltimore Longitudinal Study of Aging. J Clin Endocrinol Metab 2001;86:724–31.
4. Travison TG, Araujo AB, Kupelian V, et al. The relative contributions of aging, health, and lifestyle factors to serum testosterone decline in men. The J Clin Endocrinol Metab 2007;92:549–55.
5. Snyder PJ, Ellenberg SS, Cunningham GR, et al. The testosterone trials: seven coordinated trials of testosterone treatment in elderly men. Clin Trials 2014;11:362–75.
6. Snyder PJ, Bhasin S, Cunningham GR, et al. Effects of testosterone treatment in older men. New Engl J Med 2016;374:611–24.
7. Cunningham GR, Stephens-Shields AJ, Rosen RC, et al. Testosterone treatment and sexual function in older men with low testosterone levels. J Clin Endocrinol Metab 2016;101:3096–104.
8. Brock G, Heiselman D, Maggi M, et al. Effect of testosterone solution 2% on testosterone concentration, sex drive and energy in hypogonadal men: results of a placebo controlled study. J Urol 2016;195:699–705.
9. Bhasin S, Ellenberg SS, Storer TW, et al. Effect of testosterone replacement on measures of mobility in older men with mobility limitation and low testosterone concentrations: secondary analyses of the Testosterone Trials. Lancet Diabetes Endocrinol 2018;6:879–90.
10. Srinivas-Shankar U, Roberts SA, Connolly MJ, et al. Effects of testosterone on muscle strength, physical function, body composition, and quality of life in intermediate-frail and frail elderly men: a randomized, double-blind, placebo-controlled study. J Clin Endocrinol Metab 2010;95:639–50.

11. Travison TG, Basaria S, Storer TW, et al. Clinical meaningfulness of the changes in muscle performance and physical function associated with testosterone administration in older men with mobility limitation. J Gerontol Ser A, Biol Sci Med Sci 2011;66:1090–9.

12. Snyder PJ, Kopperdahl DL, Stephens-Shields AJ, et al. Effect of testosterone treatment on volumetric bone density and strength in older men with low testosterone: a controlled clinical trial. JAMA Intern Med 2017;177:471–9.

13. Roy CN, Snyder PJ, Stephens-Shields AJ, et al. Association of testosterone levels with anemia in older men: a controlled clinical trial. JAMA Intern Med 2017;177:480–90.

14. Resnick SM, Matsumoto AM, Stephens-Shields AJ, et al. Testosterone treatment and cognitive function in older men with low testosterone and age-associated memory impairment. JAMA 2017;317:717–27.

15. Mohler ER 3rd, Ellenberg SS, Lewis CE, et al. The effect of testosterone on cardiovascular biomarkers in the testosterone trials. J Clin Endocrinol Metab 2018;103:681–8.

16. Fernandez-Balsells MM, Murad MH, Lane M, et al. Clinical review 1: adverse effects of testosterone therapy in adult men: a systematic review and meta-analysis. J Clin Endocrinol Metab 2010;95:2560–75.

17. Iversen P, Christensen MG, Friis E, et al. A phase III trial of zoladex and flutamide versus orchiectomy in the treatment of patients with advanced carcinoma of the prostate. Cancer 1990;66:1058–66.

18. Sakr WA, Grignon DJ, Crissman JD, et al. High grade prostatic intraepithelial neoplasia (HGPIN) and prostatic adenocarcinoma between the ages of 20-69: an autopsy study of 249 cases. In Vivo 1994;8:439–43.

19. Gormley GJ, Stoner E, Bruskewitz RC, et al. The effect of finasteride in men with benign prostatic hyperplasia. The Finasteride Study Group. New Engl J Med 1992;327:1185–91.

20. Snyder PJ, Peachey H, Hannoush P, et al. Effect of testosterone treatment on bone mineral density in men over 65 years of age. J Clin Endocrinol Metab 1999;84:1966–72.

21. Finkle WD, Greenland S, Ridgeway GK, et al. Increased risk of non-fatal myocardial infarction following testosterone therapy prescription in men. PLoS One 2014;9:e85805.

22. Vigen R, O'Donnell CI, Baron AE, et al. Association of testosterone therapy with mortality, myocardial infarction, and stroke in men with low testosterone levels. JAMA 2013;310:1829–36.

23. Basaria S, Coviello AD, Travison TG, et al. Adverse events associated with testosterone administration. New Engl J Med 2010;363:109–22.

24. Budoff MJ, Ellenberg SS, Lewis CE, et al. Testosterone treatment and coronary artery plaque volume in older men with low testosterone. JAMA 2017;317:708–16.

25. Shores MM, Smith NL, Forsberg CW, et al. Testosterone treatment and mortality in men with low testosterone levels. J Clin Endocrinol Metab 2012;97:2050–8.

26. Basaria S, Harman SM, Travison TG, et al. Effects of testosterone administration for 3 years on subclinical atherosclerosis progression in older men with low or low-normal testosterone levels: a randomized clinical trial. JAMA 2015;314:570–81.

Testosterone, Diabetes Risk, and Diabetes Prevention in Men

Bu B. Yeap, MBBS, PhD[a,b,*], Gary A. Wittert, MBBCh, MD[c,d,e]

KEYWORDS

- Testosterone • Insulin resistance • Impaired glucose tolerance
- Metabolic syndrome • Diabetes • Prevention • Meta-analysis
- Randomized controlled trial

KEY POINTS

- There is a bidirectional association of lower testosterone concentrations with fat mass and insulin resistance in men
- Men with lower testosterone concentrations are at risk of developing metabolic syndrome and type 2 diabetes
- Testosterone treatment for 2 years reduces the risk of type 2 diabetes in men at high risk by 40%, beyond the effects of a lifestyle intervention
- The beneficial effect of testosterone on glucose metabolism reflects favorable changes in body composition

INTRODUCTION

Obesity is increasingly prevalent in developed and developing countries and contributes to increasing rates of type 2 diabetes (T2D) globally.[1,2] In addition, obesity is a central component of the metabolic syndrome, a cluster of risk factors for T2D and cardiovascular disease, which includes hypertension, elevated triglyceride, and reduced high-density lipoprotein cholesterol (HDL-C) concentrations, and abnormalities of glucose metabolism.[3] The presence of T2D in itself is associated with increased mortality risk, which is additive to the risk attributable to prevalent cardiovascular disease.[4] Intensive lifestyle interventions generally comprising weight loss,

[a] Medical School, University of Western Australia, Perth, Western Australia 6009, Australia; [b] Department of Endocrinology and Diabetes, Fiona Stanley Hospital, Perth, Western Australia 6150, Australia; [c] Freemasons Centre for Men's Health and Wellbeing, Medical School, University of Adelaide, Adelaide, South Australia 5000, Australia; [d] Department of Endocrinology, Royal Adelaide Hospital, Adelaide, South Australia 5000, Australia; [e] South Australian Health and Medical Research Institute, North Terrace, Adelaide, South Australia 5000, Australia
* Corresponding author. Medical School, M582, University of Western Australia, 35 Stirling Highway, Crawley, Perth, WA 6009, Australia.
E-mail address: bu.yeap@uwa.edu.au

Endocrinol Metab Clin N Am 51 (2022) 157–172
https://doi.org/10.1016/j.ecl.2021.11.004
0889-8529/22/© 2021 Elsevier Inc. All rights reserved.

nutrition management, and increased physical activity reduce T2D risk.[5–7] However, such interventions are difficult to implement and sustain in the general population, thus the global diabetes prevalence is estimated to increase to 10.2% (578 million people) by 2030.[2] Therefore, new therapeutic approaches are needed to prevent T2D and reduce its associated therapeutic and disease burdens.[8]

TESTOSTERONE AND ITS RELATIONSHIP WITH OBESITY AND INSULIN RESISTANCE
Testosterone and Obesity

In cross-sectional studies of middle-aged and older men, circulating testosterone is inversely associated with body mass index (BMI).[9–13] Total testosterone concentrations are greater than 20% lower in men with BMI 30 kg/m[2] or more, compared with those with BMI in the normal range.[9,10] In a cross-sectional analysis of 208,677 men from the UK Biobank aged 40 to 69 years, in whom median total testosterone measured using immunoassay was 11.6 nmol/L (334 ng/dL), the inverse association of serum testosterone with BMI was stronger than with age. Compared with 50-year-olds, in 70-year-old men serum testosterone level was ~0.5 nmol/L (~14 mg/dL) lower, whereas it was ~1.5 nmol/L (~43 ng/dL) lower in men with BMI 30 versus 25 kg/m[2] and ~3 nmol/L (~86 ng/dL) lower in men with BMI 40 versus 25 kg/m[2].[13] In longitudinal studies, obesity, weight gain, or increases in waist circumference, rather than age itself, were associated with decreases in testosterone concentrations.[14–16] In 2736 men aged 40 to 79 years from the European Male Aging Study, with mean total testosterone concentration measured using mass spectrometry of 16.9 nmol/L (487 mg/dL), a loss of 10% or more to less than 15% of body weight was associated with a 2.0 nmol/L (58 ng./dL) increase, and a loss of 15% or more with a 5.8 nmol/L (167 ng/dL) increase in testosterone concentrations.[15] In interventional studies of diet and/or exercise, loss of 6% to 17% of total weight resulted in total testosterone concentration increasing by 1.2 to 5.1 nmol/L (35–147 ng/dL), whereas bariatric surgery with loss of 29% to 36% of total weight resulted in total testosterone concentration increasing by 7.8 to 10.7 nmol/L (225–308 ng/dL).[17] Therefore, men who successfully reduce excess weight can expect to increase their endogenous testosterone concentrations, proportionate to the degree of weight loss.

Testosterone, Obesity, and Sex Hormone-Binding Globulin

Differences in total testosterone concentrations in relation to obesity are mediated in part via the association of obesity with lower circulating sex hormone-binding globulin (SHBG) concentrations.[9,10,13] SHBG is the major carrier protein for testosterone in the circulation, and concentrations of total testosterone and SHBG are correlated with coefficients of ~0.5 to 0.6.[9,18,19] Of note, the association may not be linear across the range of SHBG concentrations, with the increase in total testosterone concentrations leveling off with SHBG greater than 80 nmol/L in UK Biobank men.[13] Thus, men who are obese or insulin resistant can have low SHBG and testosterone concentrations, in the absence of pathologic hypogonadism.[20]

Circulating SHBG is primarily synthesized in the liver, and low SHBG concentrations are associated with the presence of insulin resistance and the metabolic syndrome.[21,22] Earlier experiments suggested a direct role of insulin to inhibit SHBG production in hepatoma cells.[23] More recent studies suggest that SHBG is a marker of de novo hepatic lipogenesis. Increasing de novo hepatic lipogenesis is associated with a lower SHBG, and vice versa.[19,24] Although lower SHBG contributes to lower total testosterone concentrations in overweight or obese men, men with more severe obesity also show reductions in luteinizing hormone (LH) concentrations and LH pulse amplitude, consistent with functional inhibition of the hypothalamic-pituitary-testicular (HPT) axis[25,26]; this is consistent with the observation that when men lose 15% or more of body weight, the increase in total testosterone is proportionately higher than the increase in SHBG concentrations compared with lesser degrees of weight loss.[15]

Testosterone and Insulin Resistance

Men with lower total testosterone or SHBG concentrations are more likely to have metabolic syndrome and to manifest insulin resistance.[27–29] These associations are likely to be mediated in large part by the underlying relationship of low circulating total testosterone and SHBG with central obesity and excess adiposity.[9–16] Whether or not there is a direct association of lower testosterone concentrations with insulin resistance, independently of body composition, is more difficult to discern. Observational studies have reported that apparent associations of lower testosterone concentrations with insulin resistance (assessed by calculations based on circulating glucose and insulin concentrations, either the quick insulin sensitivity check index or the homeostatic model assessment of insulin resistance [HOMA-IR]) may be abrogated by adjustment for SHBG.[30–33] However, in one study of older men, after adjusting for age, BMI, waist circumference, and HDL-C and triglyceride levels, lower total testosterone concentrations were independently associated with HOMA-IR, whereas SHBG concentrations were not.[34] In a study of 21 men with normal glucose tolerance, impaired glucose tolerance, and diabetes, insulin sensitivity assessed using hyperinsulinemic-euglycemic clamps correlated with testosterone concentrations and with testicular responses to human chorionic gonadotropin, suggesting an effect of insulin resistance to decrease Leydig cell testosterone secretion.[35] In another study of 74 men, undergoing a 75-g oral glucose tolerance test (OGTT) was associated with a decrease in total testosterone concentrations at 30, 60, 90, and 120 minutes, without any change in SHBG or LH concentrations.[36] Furthermore, in a study of 12 men diagnosed with idiopathic hypogonadotropic hypogonadism based on serum total testosterone levels less than 3.47 nmol/L (<100 ng/dL) in association with inappropriately low gonadotropin concentrations, suspension of testosterone treatment for 2 weeks resulted in increased fasting insulin concentrations and HOMA-IR without changes in BMI, indicating an acute effect of testosterone withdrawal on insulin sensitivity.[37] In a study of 94 men with T2D, 44 had calculated free testosterone levels less than 226 pmol/L and were randomly allocated to testosterone or placebo treatment.[38] Glucose infusion rates during hyperinsulinemic-euglycemic clamp did not change when assessed at 3 weeks, but after 6 months of testosterone treatment glucose infusion rates increased by 32%, associated with favorable changes in body composition.[38]

Summary: Testosterone, Obesity, and Insulin Resistance

Thus obesity, manifesting with central and visceral adiposity and insulin resistance, can inhibit function of the HPT axis at multiple levels (**Fig. 1**).[13–16,19,22,24–35] Higher degrees of obesity, visceral adiposity, and insulin resistance are associated with both reduced HPT axis activity and lower SHBG concentrations, hence lower circulating total testosterone (see **Fig. 1**).

TESTOSTERONE AND THE RISK OF METABOLIC SYNDROME AND DIABETES
Testosterone and Risk of Metabolic Syndrome

Several epidemiologic studies have associated lower total testosterone or SHBG concentrations with higher risk of metabolic syndrome in men in both cross-sectional and

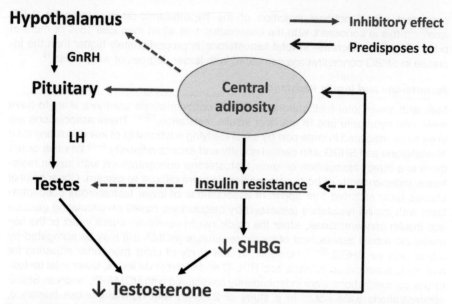

Fig. 1. Effects of central adiposity and insulin resistance on function of the hypothalamic-pituitary-testicular axis, and on testosterone and sex-hormone-binding globulin concentrations in men.

longitudinal analyses.[27–29,39–45] An individual participant data meta-analysis of 20 observational studies involving 14,025 men aged 18 years or older not using hormone therapy documented inverse associations of both total testosterone and SHBG with risk of prevalent and incident metabolic syndrome.[45] In the cross-sectional analysis, a quartile decrease in total testosterone concentration was associated with ~40% higher odds of metabolic syndrome, across categories of BMI, after adjusting for age, smoking, alcohol consumption, and physical activity. A quartile decrease in baseline total testosterone was associated with an ~25% higher risk of developing metabolic syndrome during follow-up, after adjusting for age and lifestyle factors, reducing to 14% higher risk after further adjustment for BMI.[45] Similarly, in that meta-analysis lower SHBG concentrations were associated with higher risk of both prevalent and incident metabolic syndrome. Thus, whereas obesity and central adiposity predispose to lower total testosterone and SHBG concentrations, the converse is also true, because men with lower total testosterone or SHBG concentrations are at increased risk of having or developing the metabolic syndrome.

Testosterone and Risk of Diabetes

Epidemiologic studies have consistently associated lower total testosterone or SHBG concentrations not only with insulin resistance[21,22,30–34] but also with higher risk of T2D in men.[31,43,46–50] In a systematic review and meta-analysis that included 43 observational studies with 6427 men, lower total testosterone concentrations were associated with higher risk of prevalent and incident T2D.[51] Men with T2D had a mean total testosterone concentration 2.7 nmol/L (78 ng/dL) lower than those of nondiabetic men. Furthermore, in prospective studies, men who developed diabetes had a baseline mean total testosterone concentration 2.5 nmol/L (72 ng/dL) lower than those of men who did not.[51] In that meta-analysis, men who had baseline total testosterone concentrations of 15.6 to 21.0 nmol/L (450–605 ng/dL) had a relative risk of developing T2D of 0.58, compared with men with baseline total testosterone concentration of 7.4 to 15.5 nmol/L (213–447 ng/dL).[51] Other studies have further reinforced the finding of lower total testosterone concentrations in men with T2D, compared with nondiabetic men.[17,52,53] This association likely reflects inhibition of HPT axis function in the presence of central adiposity, a reduction in SHBG concentrations, and possible effects of insulin resistance or hyperglycemia on testicular function.[9,10,13–16,19,21–24,35,36] Of note, in a study of 195 men aged 70 years or older the presence of metabolic syndrome, but not lower total testosterone concentration in the absence of metabolic syndrome, was predictive of incident T2D.[54] Thus, in older men, obesity and metabolic syndrome, in association with lower testosterone concentrations and worsening body composition, may be the key predisposing factors for T2D.

EFFECTS OF TESTOSTERONE TREATMENT ON BODY COMPOSITION AND GLUCOSE CONCENTRATIONS
Effect of Testosterone Treatment on Body Composition

Some, but not all, studies have reported an inverse association of muscle mass or strength with diabetes risk in men.[55–59] Therefore, a potential mechanism by which testosterone treatment might reduce the risk of T2D would be via its anabolic effects to increase lean mass.[60–64] Together with increasing lean mass, testosterone treatment also reduces fat mass, potentially an important mechanism to reduce the risk of T2D.[64–66] In men with BMI 30 kg/m^2 or more and total testosterone concentrations 12 nmol/L or less ($\leq$346 ng/dL), testosterone treatment given in conjunction with calorie restriction mitigated the loss of lean mass, while potentiating the loss of fat mass.[67] A meta-analysis by Isidori and colleagues[68] of 29 testosterone randomized controlled trials (RCTs) involving 625 testosterone-treated men and 458 controls with durations ranging from 1 to 36 months with baseline mean total testosterone concentrations ranging from 7.5 to 19.0 nmol/L (216–548 ng/dL) indicated an effect of testosterone treatment to increase lean mass by 1.6 kg (+2.7%) and decrease fat mass by 1.6 kg (−6.2%). A more recent meta-analysis by Corona and colleagues[69] including 59 RCTs with 3029 testosterone-treated men and 2049 controls with duration ranging from 1 to 48 months with baseline mean total testosterone concentrations ranging from 2.3 to 21.1 nmol/L (66–608 ng/dL) confirmed the effect of testosterone to increase lean mass and reduce fat mass (standardized mean difference, +0.51 and −0.32 respectively). In an analysis of observational studies, testosterone supplementation was associated with a reduction of waist circumference of 6.2 cm at 24 months.[70]

Effect of Testosterone Treatment on Glucose Concentrations

Several RCTs have investigated the effect of testosterone treatment on fasting or postchallenge glucose concentrations, or measures of insulin sensitivity, with mixed results.[66,71–73] The previous analysis of observational studies reported that testosterone-treated men had a 0.47 mmol/L lower fasting glucose concentration and a HOMA-IR 2.8 lower.[70] However, these estimates were smaller, particularly for HOMA-IR, in the meta-analysis of RCTs by Corona and colleagues[69] in which testosterone treatment reduced fasting glucose concentrations by 0.34 mmol/L and HOMA-IR by 0.80. A review of 3 RCTs conducted specifically in men with T2D with baseline mean total testosterone concentrations of 12 to 15 nmol/L (346–432 ng/dL), suggested a mean reduction of fasting glucose of 1.2 mmol/L with testosterone treatment over durations of 3 to 12 months in that population.[74] A more recent meta-analysis of testosterone RCTs in men with T2D and/or metabolic syndrome included 7 RCTs involving 833 men with baseline mean total testosterone concentrations ranging from 6.7 to 10.1 nmol/L (193–291 ng/dL).[75] In that meta-analysis, testosterone treatment improved measures of insulin resistance, but did not lower hemoglobin A_{1c} (HbA_{1c}) values.

Summary: Testosterone and Risk of Type 2 Diabetes

Obesity, metabolic syndrome, low testosterone concentrations, and risk of T2D are closely interrelated (**Fig. 2**). Obesity per se, and the presence of metabolic syndrome, predispose to both lower testosterone concentrations and diabetes risk, with diabetes risk amplified by the presence of lower testosterone concentrations resulting in unfavorable changes to body composition (loss of lean mass and gain of fat) and alterations in insulin sensitivity (see **Fig. 2A**). This is consistent with lower testosterone concentrations being predictive of incident T2D in men.[46–51,76] In older men, obesity and metabolic syndrome, in association with lower testosterone concentrations and worsening body composition, may be the major contributors to risk of T2D (see **Fig. 2B**).

Testosterone treatment by increasing lean mass, reducing fat mass, and by reducing glucose concentrations would thus be expected to reduce the risk of T2D.[60–70] An uncontrolled, registry-based observational study of 316 men with baseline total testosterone concentrations 12.1 nmol/L or less (~350 ng/dL) followed for 8 years reported an improvement in HbA_{1c} in 229 testosterone-treated men, none of whom progressed to T2D, compared with 40% of the 87 untreated men who developed HbA_{1c} greater than 6.5%.[77] Collectively, these existing data on testosterone, obesity, metabolic syndrome, and T2D justify a large-scale, high-quality RCT to determine whether testosterone treatment prevents development of T2D in men at high risk.

TESTOSTERONE FOR THE PREVENTION OF TYPE 2 DIABETES MELLITUS
Overview

Testosterone for the Prevention of Type 2 Diabetes Mellitus (T4DM) was a randomized, double-blind, placebo-controlled, 2-year, phase 3b trial to determine whether

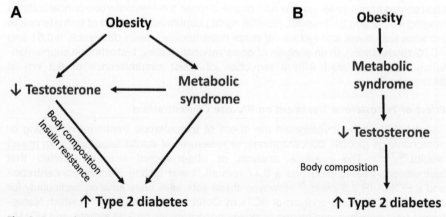

Fig. 2. Interrelationships between obesity, metabolic syndrome, low testosterone concentrations, and type 2 diabetes risk in men. (*A*) Obesity and metabolic syndrome contribute to lower testosterone, lower testosterone and metabolic syndrome contribute to risk of type 2 diabetes. (*B*) Lower testosterone in the presence of metabolic syndrome contributes to risk of type 2 diabetes.

testosterone treatment prevents or reverts T2D in men enrolled in a lifestyle program.[78] Important features of T4DM are summarized (**Box 1**). The trial randomized 1007 men across 6 centers in Australia, with a 2-year duration of intervention; all participating men also receiving a lifestyle intervention.[79] T4DM represents the largest testosterone RCT completed to date, with the key outcome of T2D and 2 years of safety data.

The T4DM Study Population

As T4DM was conceived as a prevention trial; only men without a previous history of diabetes were recruited. Eligible participants were men aged 50 to 74 years, with waist circumference 95 cm or more, who had either impaired glucose tolerance (OGTT 2-hour glucose $\geq$7.8 to <11.1 mmol/L) or newly diagnosed T2D (OGTT 2-hour glucose $\geq$11.1 to $\leq$15.0 mmol/L), for whom the primary intervention could reasonably be a lifestyle program, and who were willing to participate in such a program.[78,79] In addition, eligible participants were required to have a screening serum total testosterone concentration of 14.0 nmol/L (403 ng/dL) or less.[76] Exclusion criteria are reported.[78,79] Of note, men with major medical comorbidities, or with recent cardiovascular events or symptomatic cardiovascular disease, were excluded from T4DM.

Intervention

All participating men were enrolled into a free Weight Watchers program, with face-to-face participation via group sessions and online options available.[79] A lifestyle intervention was regarded as the expected standard of care for men with impaired glucose tolerance or newly diagnosed T2D without marked hyperglycemia.[5,6] Men were randomly allocated 1:1 to receive testosterone undecanoate 1000 mg or matching placebo, via intramuscular injection, at baseline, 6 weeks, and every 3 months thereafter for 2 years (9 injections in total). Of the participants, 20% of each arm had newly

---

Box 1
Testosterone for the Prevention of Type 2 Diabetes Mellitus (T4DM): a randomized controlled trial

Selection
    T4DM was an Australia-wide randomized clinical trial that recruited 1007 men aged 50 to 74 years, with waist 95 cm or more, baseline total testosterone concentration 14 nmol/L or less, and either impaired glucose tolerance or newly diagnosed type 2 diabetes.

Intervention
    All participating men were enrolled in a Weight Watchers program and randomly allocated to receive injections of testosterone undecanoate 1000 mg or matching placebo, at baseline, 6 weeks, and every 3 months thereafter for 2 years (9 injections in total).

Outcome of type 2 diabetes
    At the end of the 2-year intervention, the proportion of men with a 2-hour glucose on oral glucose tolerance testing 11.1 mmol/L or more was 12% in the testosterone group (55 of 443) and 21% in the placebo group (87 of 413), a relative risk reduction of 41%.

Change in body composition
    On average, men in the testosterone group gained 0.4 kg of muscle and lost 4.6 kg of fat, whereas men in the placebo group lost 1.3 kg of muscle and 1.9 kg of fat, after 2 years.

Safety considerations
    A safety trigger for hematocrit greater than 54% occurred in 1% of the placebo group and 22% of the testosterone group. There was no evidence of excess prostate cancer or cardiovascular adverse events.

diagnosed T2D based on the entry OGTT result. In 503 men randomized to placebo, 370 completed 2 years of treatment and 413 had outcome data available for primary analysis at 2 years. In the testosterone arm, 386 completed 2 years of treatment and 443 had outcome data for primary analysis at 2 years.[79]

Outcomes

At the end of the 2-year intervention, 55 of 443 (12%) of testosterone-treated men and 87 of 413 (21%) of men in the placebo arm had a 2-hour glucose on OGTT of 11.1 mmol/L or more (relative risk, 0.59; 95% confidence interval [CI], 0.43–0.80; P = .0007). For the second primary outcome, mean change from baseline in 2-hour glucose on OGTT was −1.70 mmol/L (SD 2.47) in the testosterone arm and −0.95 mmol/L (SD 2.78) in the placebo arm (mean difference −0.75 mmol/L; 95% CI, -1.10 to −0.40; P < .0001).[79]

Testosterone treatment resulted in a mean increase of 0.39 kg of total muscle mass, and a mean decrease of 4.60 kg of fat mass, whereas men in the placebo group had a mean reduction of 1.32 kg of muscle mass and 1.89 kg of fat mass, after 2 years. Hand grip strength improved with testosterone treatment. Testosterone treatment also resulted in a greater likelihood of having a normal 2-hour glucose on OGTT (<7.8 mmol/L; odds ratio, 1.20; 95% CI, 1.04–1.38; P = .012) and a lower fasting glucose concentration (−0.17 mmol/L; 95% CI, -0.29 to −0.06; P = .0036) at 2 years.[79] However, HbA$_{1c}$ was not different between the 2 groups at 2 years (treatment effect −0.02%; 95% CI, -0.07–0.03; P = .42). Rates of participation in the Weight Watchers program were similar in both arms of the trial. Testosterone treatment increased on-study testosterone concentrations, and suppressed LH, with a small reduction in SHBG concentrations.[79] In a sensitivity analysis, the benefit of testosterone treatment was similar for men with baseline testosterone concentrations less than 11 nmol/L and 11 nmol/L or more (317 ng/dL), confirming that this was a pharmacologic effect of testosterone treatment.

Adverse Events

At least one safety trigger occurred for 19% participants in the placebo arm and 38% of participants in the testosterone arm, including triggers for hematocrit of 54% or higher (1% in placebo versus 22% in the testosterone arm), and increase in level of prostate-specific antigen of 0.75 ng/mL or more (19% of the placebo and 23% of the testosterone arm). In most cases in which a trigger for raised hematocrit occurred, men were retested nonfasting, and some had study injections deferred, with one man in the placebo arm and 25 in the testosterone arm permanently discontinuing treatment. Serious adverse events (SAEs) were recorded in 7.4% of the placebo and 10.9% of the testosterone groups, in a total of 41 of 503 placebo recipients and 55 of 504 testosterone-treated men; these included 21 (4.2%) and 26 (5.2%) cardiovascular SAEs in placebo and testosterone arms, respectively. As noted earlier, men at high risk of cardiovascular adverse events were excluded from the study, leaving a lower risk population. In the placebo arm, 3 men had hospital admissions related to benign prostate hyperplasia and 5 men were diagnosed with prostate cancer, compared with 8 and 4 in the testosterone arm, respectively.

Significance of T4DM

The main result of T4DM, demonstrating an unequivocal effect of testosterone treatment to reduce the likelihood of having T2D in men at high risk is important conceptually and practically. First, in the context of the prior discussion of testosterone, obesity, metabolic syndrome, and diabetes risk (see **Figs. 1** and **2**), T4DM provides evidence of the bidirectional association. In this large, multicenter, double-blind, placebo-controlled RCT, with a background lifestyle intervention, the 2-year testosterone intervention reduced the risk of T2D, by preventing progression of impaired glucose tolerance or reverting newly diagnosed diabetes. The effect size was large, with a relative risk reduction of 40% for the outcome of T2D. Therefore, although obesity, metabolic syndrome, and T2D are associated with lower testosterone concentrations, the association is bidirectional, because low testosterone concentrations predispose to metabolic syndrome and T2D, and testosterone intervention improves body composition, reduces glucose concentrations, and reduces risk of T2D in the context of a concomitant lifestyle program.

Second, in the context of the worldwide increase in the prevalence of obesity and T2D, T4DM offers a new therapeutic option, that of testosterone pharmacotherapy in combination with a readily available lifestyle intervention. The lifestyle program was an intrinsic component of the study. Men who have pathologic hypogonadism merit testosterone treatment.[20,80–82] For these men, the metabolic benefits of testosterone now clearly include improvements in glucose tolerance and prevention of T2D. With regard to men with obesity and metabolic syndrome-related reductions in serum testosterone concentrations in the absence of pathologic hypogonadism, our findings suggest that testosterone treatment for 2 years, as an adjunct to a lifestyle program, can prevent or revert T2D. However, increases in hematocrit might be treatment limiting, and the minimum dose exposure, duration of treatment, durability of effect, and long-term safety and cardiovascular outcomes of testosterone treatment remain to be determined.[83] Thus, the benefit of testosterone treatment on the outcome of T2D as demonstrated in T4DM, needs to be carefully weighed against the limitations of the study, and the potential side effects that may be encountered. If such treatment is considered, a concomitant lifestyle program should be implemented, and there must be careful monitoring of hematocrit, cardiovascular risk factors, and prostate health.

Cardiovascular Effects of Testosterone Treatment

Whether testosterone treatment has beneficial, neutral, or adverse effects on the cardiovascular system remains a complex and debated issue (for review, see[84]). In brief, one RCT of testosterone in older men aged 65 years or more with baseline total testosterone 3.5 to 12.1 nmol/L (100–350 ng/dL) or calculated free testosterone less than 173 pmol/L with mobility limitations showed an excess of broadly defined cardiovascular adverse events; another similar RCT in frail or intermediate-frail older men aged 65 years or more with baseline total testosterone of 12 nmol/L or less (≤345 ng/dL) or calculated free testosterone of 250 pmol/L or less showed no such signal.[85,86] There was no excess of cardiovascular adverse events in T Trials, which recruited men with symptoms suggesting hypogonadism aged 65 years or more with baseline total testosterone levels less than 9.54 nmol/L (<275 ng/dL), and T4DM, the 2 largest testosterone RCTs.[79,87] Furthermore, recent large meta-analyses of testosterone RCTs have not shown evidence of excess cardiovascular adverse events.[88–90] Of note, the cardiovascular substudy of T Trials involving 138 men reported an increase in coronary atheroma measured as noncalcified plaque volume using cardiac computed tomography angiography in testosterone-treated men.[91] However, the groups were unbalanced: men in the placebo group (N = 65) had substantially more calcified and noncalcified plaque volume at baseline and at the end of the study compared with men in the testosterone group (N = 73), making the findings challenging to interpret.[84,92] Therefore, additional studies are needed to clarify the effect of testosterone on the cardiovascular system. Pending the outcomes of such studies, careful monitoring of cardiovascular risk factors and disease would be appropriate.

Holistic Evaluation and Optimizing Lifestyle, Behavioral, and Medical Factors

All men expressing concerns over their risk of obesity or T2D, whether or not there is concomitant concern over low testosterone concentrations related to these, should be offered a careful assessment and optimal management of medical risk factors and comorbidities.[93] Pathologic disorders affecting the HPT axis need to be excluded, or if identified, treated appropriately.[20,81,82] Men without HPT axis pathology who are overweight can be advised on losing excess weight, eating healthily, and exercising regularly. Depression and sleep disturbances, if present, should be managed appropriately.[94] As discussed earlier, losing excess weight should improve HPT axis function and raise endogenous testosterone levels, and thus represents an attractive nonpharmacologic approach with the potential to capture multiple health benefits. Only after a holistic evaluation and optimization of lifestyle and medical factors has been achieved should further discussion on testosterone pharmacotherapy be considered.[79]

SUMMARY

There is an intimate and bidirectional association of lower testosterone concentrations with obesity and the risk of T2D risk in middle-aged and older men. Men who are obese, or have metabolic syndrome or T2D, are more likely to have lower testosterone concentrations; conversely, lower testosterone concentrations predispose men to developing metabolic syndrome or T2D. Testosterone pharmacotherapy is effective in preventing or reverting newly diagnosed T2D in men at high risk, reducing the risk of T2D by 40% beyond the effect of a lifestyle intervention. However, the first step for improving men's health must remain a holistic evaluation of lifestyle, behavioral and medical factors, engagement in healthy dietary choices and physical activity, and optimal treatment of existing medical risk factors and comorbidities. Subsequently, men at high risk of diabetes can be counseled on the benefits versus risks of testosterone pharmacotherapy on top of a lifestyle program to prevent diabetes, based on the findings and also realizing the limitations of T4DM. In this context, it could be noted that neither metformin nor the glucagonlike peptide-1 receptor agonist class of drugs increase muscle mass nor do they improve bone and sexual health, as testosterone does.[79,87,95,96] If testosterone treatment is considered for prevention of T2D, a concomitant lifestyle program is necessary as is careful monitoring of hematocrit, cardiovascular risk factors, and prostate health. Further research is needed to clarify the effects of testosterone on the cardiovascular system.

CLINICS CARE POINTS

- Men who are overweight, or have metabolic syndrome or T2D, are likely to have lower testosterone concentrations compared with other men, even if no pituitary or testicular disorders are present.
- Men with lower testosterone concentrations are at greater risk of developing metabolic syndrome or T2D
- Reducing excess weight restores endogenous testosterone concentrations in obese men
- T4DM randomized 1007 men and demonstrated efficacy of testosterone treatment to prevent or revert newly diagnosed T2D

- In T4DM, 2 years of testosterone treatment on a background of lifestyle intervention reduced the risk of T2D by 40% in men with waist circumference of 95 cm or more and impaired glucose tolerance or newly diagnosed T2D.
- In relation to T4DM, durability of effect, long-term safety, and cardiovascular outcomes remain to be determined.
- Overweight men at risk of T2D should be offered a holistic evaluation, encouragement, and support to engage in healthy lifestyle behaviors, and optimized management of medical risk factors and conditions, before discussion of pharmacotherapy.

DISCLOSURE

B.B. Yeap has received speaker honoraria and conference support from Bayer, Lilly, and Besins and research support from Bayer, Lilly, and Lawley Pharmaceuticals and held advisory roles for Lilly, Besins, Ferring, and Lawley. G.A. Wittert has received speaker honoraria from Bayer and Besins and research support from Bayer, Lilly, and Lawley Pharmaceuticals and held an advisory role for Bayer.

REFERENCES

1. NCD Risk factor Collaboration. Trends in adult body-mass index in 200 countries from 1975 to 2014: a pooled analysis of 1698 population-based measurement studies with 19·2 million participants. Lancet 2016;387:1377–96.
2. Saeedi P, Petersohn I, Salpea P, et al. Global and regional diabetes prevalence estimates for 2019 and projections for 2030 and 2045: Results from the International Diabetes Federation Diabetes Atlas, 9th edition. Diabetes Res Clin Pract 2019;157:107843.
3. Alberti KGMM, Zimmet P, Shaw J, et al. The metabolic syndrome – a new worldwide definition. Lancet 2005;366:1059–62.
4. Emerging Risk Factors Collaboration, Di Angelantonio E, Kaptoge S, Wormser D, et al. Association of cardiometabolic multimorbidity with mortality. JAMA 2015;314:52–60.
5. Tuomilehto J, Lindstrom J, Eriksson JG, et al. Prevention of type 2 diabetes mellitus by changes in lifestyle among subjects with impaired glucose tolerance. N Engl J Med 2001;344:1343–50.
6. Knowler WC, Barrett-Connor E, Fowler SE, et al. Reduction in the incidence of type 2 diabetes with lifestyle intervention of metformin. N Engl J Med 2002;346:393–403.
7. Schellenberg ES, Dryden DM, Vandermeer B, et al. Lifestyle interventions for patients with and at risk for type 2 diabetes. Ann Intern Med 2013;159:543–51.
8. Chatterjee S, Khunti K, Davies MJ. Type 2 diabetes. Lancet 2017;389:2239–51.
9. Allen NE, Appleby PN, Davey GK, et al. Lifestyle and nutritional determinants of bioavailable androgens and related hormones in British men. Cancer Causes Control 2002;13:353–63.
10. Muller M, den Tonkelaar I, Thijssen JHH. Endogenous sex hormones in men aged 40-80 years. Eur J Endocrinol 2003;149:583–9.
11. Mohr BA, Guay AT, O'Donnell AB, et al. Normal, bound and nonbound testosterone levels in normally ageing men: results from the Massachusetts Male Ageing Study. Clin Endocrinol 2005;62:64–73.
12. Yeap BB, Alfonso H, Chubb SAP, et al. Reference ranges and determinants of testosterone, dihydrotestosterone, and estradiol levels measured using liquid

chromatography-tandem mass spectrometry in a population-based cohort of older men. J Clin Endocrinol Metab 2012;97:4030–9.

13. Yeap BB, Marriott RJ, Antonio L, et al. Sociodemographic, lifestyle and medical influences on serum testosterone and sex hormone-binding globulin in men from UK Biobank. Clin Endocrinol 2021;94:290–302.

14. Shi Z, Araujo AB, Martin S, et al. Longitudinal changes in testosterone over five years in community-dwelling men. J Clin Endocrinol Metab 2013;98:3289–97.

15. Camacho EM, Huhtaniemi IT, O'Neill TW, et al. Age-associated changes in hypothalamic-pituitary-testicular function in middle-aged and older men are modified by weight change and lifestyle factors: longitudinal results from the European Male Ageing Study. Eur J Endocrinol 2013;168:445–55.

16. Rastrelli G, Carter EL, Ahern T, et al. Development and recovery from secondary hypogonadism in aging men: prospective results from the EMAS. J Clin Endocrinol Metab 2015;100:3172–82.

17. Grossmann M. Low testosterone in men with type 2 diabetes: significance and treatment. J Clin Endocrinol Metab 2011;96:2341–53.

18. Orwoll E, Lambert LC, Marshall LM, et al. Testosterone and estradiol among older men. J Clin Endocrinol Metab 2006;91:1336–44.

19. Gyawali P, Martin SA, Heilbronn LK, et al. Cross-sectional and longitudinal determinants of serum sex hormone-binding globulin (SHBG) in a cohort of community-dwelling men. PLoS One 2018;13:e0200078.

20. Yeap BB, Grossmann M, McLachlan RI, et al. Endocrine Society of Australia position statement on male hypogonadism (part 1): assessment and indications for testosterone therapy. Med J Aust 2016;205:173–8.

21. Wallace IR, McKinley MC, Bell PM, et al. Sex hormone binding globulin and insulin resistance. Clin Endocrinol 2013;78:321–9.

22. Kalme T, Seppala M, Qiao Q, et al. Sex hormone-binding globulin and insulin-like growth factor-binding protein-1 as indicators of metabolic syndrome, cardiovascular risk, and mortality in elderly men. J Clin Endocrinol Metab 2005;90:1550–6.

23. Plymate SR, Matej LA, Jones RE, et al. Inhibition of sex hormone-binding globulin production in the human hepatoma (Hep G2) cell line by insulin and prolactin. J Clin Endocrinol Metab 1988;67:460–4.

24. Simo R, Saez-Lopez C, Barbosa-Desongles A, et al. Novel insights in SHBG regulation and clinical implications. Trends Endocrinol Metab 2015;26:376–83.

25. Vermeulen A, Kaufman JM, Deslypere JP, et al. Attenuated luteinizing hormone(LH) pulse amplitude but normal LH pulse frequency, and its relation to plasma androgens in hypogonadism of obese men. J Clin Endocrinol Metab 1993;76:1140–6.

26. Giagulli VA, Kaufman JM, Vermeulen A. Pathogenesis of the decreased androgen levels in obese men. J Clin Endocrinol Metab 1994;79:997–1000.

27. Muller M, Grobbee DE, den Tonkelaar I, et al. Endogenous sex hormones and metabolic syndrome in aging men. J Clin Endocrinol Metab 2005;90:2618–23.

28. Kupelian V, Hayes FJ, Link CL, et al. Inverse association of testosterone and the metabolic syndrome in men is consistent across race and ethnic groups. J Clin Endocrinol Metab 2008;93:3403–10.

29. Chubb SAP, Hyde Z, Almeida OP, et al. Lower sex hormone-binding globulin is more strongly associated with metabolic syndrome than lower total testosterone in older men: the Health In Men Study. Eur J Endocrinol 2008;158:785–92.

30. Simon D, Preziosi P, Barrett-Connor E, et al. Interrelationship between plasma testosterone and plasma insulin in healthy adult men: the Telecom Study. Diabetologia 1992;35:173–7.

31. Oh J-Y, Barrett-Connor E, Wedick NM, et al. Endogenous sex hormones and the development of type 2 diabetes in older men and women: the Rancho Bernardo Study. Diabetes Care 2002;25:55–60.
32. Tsai EC, Matsumoto AM, Fujimoto WY, et al. Association of bioavailable, free, and total testosterone with insulin resistance. Diabetes Care 2004;27:861–8.
33. Rajala UM, Keinanen-Kiukaanniemi SM, Hirsso PK, et al. Associations of total testosterone and sex hormone-binding globulin levels with insulin sensitivity in middle-aged Finnish men. Diabetes Care 2007;30:e13.
34. Yeap BB, Chubb SAP, Hyde Z, et al. Lower serum testosterone is independently associated with insulin resistance in non-diabetic older men: the Health In Men Study. Eur J Endocrinol 2009;161:591–8.
35. Pitteloud N, Hardin M, Dwyer AA, et al. Increasing insulin resistance is associated with a decrease in Leydig cell testosterone secretion in men. J Clin Endocrinol Metab 2005;90:2636–41.
36. Caronia LM, Dwyer AA, Hayden D, et al. Abrupt decrease in serum testosterone levels after an oral glucose load in men: implications for screening for hypogonadism. Clin Endocrinol 2013;78:291–6.
37. Yialamas MA, Dwyer AA, Hanley E, et al. Acute sex steroid withdrawal reduces insulin sensitivity in healthy men with idiopathic hypogonadotrophic hypogoadism. J Clin Endocrinol Metab 2007;92:4254–9.
38. Dhindsa S, Ghanim H, Batra M, et al. Insulin resistance and inflammation in hypogonadotrphic hypogonadism and their reduction after testosterone replacement in men with type 2 diabetes. Diabetes Care 2016;39:82–91.
39. Haring R, Volzke H, Felix SB, et al. Prediction of metabolic syndrome by low serum testosterone levels in men. Diabetes 2009;58:2027–31.
40. Li C, Ford ES, Li B, et al. Association of testosterone and sex hormone-binding globulin with metabolic syndrome and insulin resistance in men. Diabetes Care 2010;33:1618–24.
41. Yeap BB, Knuiman MW, Divitini ML, et al. Differential associations of testosterone, dihydrotestosterone and oestradiol with physical, metabolic and health-related factors in community-dwelling men aged 17-97 years from the Busselton Health Survey. Clin Endocrinol 2014;83:268–76.
42. Kupelian V, Page ST, Araujo AB, et al. Low sex hormone-binding globulin, total testosterone, and symptomatic androgen deficiencyare associated with development of the metabolic syndrome in nonobese men. J Clin Endocrinol Metab 2006;91:843–50.
43. Rodriguez A, Muller DC, Metter EJ, et al. Aging, androgens, and the metabolic syndrome in a longitudinal study of aging. J Clin Endocrinol Metab 2007;92:3568–72.
44. Laaksonen DE, Niskanen L, Punnonen K, et al. Testosterone and sex hormone-binding globulin predict the metabolic syndrome and diabetes in middle-aged men. Diabetes Care 2004;27:1036–41.
45. Brand JS, Rovers MM, Yeap BB, et al. Testosterone, sex hormone-binding globulin and the metabolic syndrome in men: an individual participant data meta-analysis of observational studies. PLoS One 2014;9:e100409.
46. Goodman-Gruen D, Barrett-Connor E. Sex differences in the association of endogenous sex hormone levels and glucose tolerance status in older men and women. Diabetes Care 2000;23:912–8.
47. Svartberg J, Jenssen T, Sundsfjord J, et al. The associations of endogenous testosterone and sex hormone-binding globulin with glycosylated haemoglobin

levels, in community-dwelling men. The Tromso Study. Diabetes Metab 2004;30: 29–34.

48. Haffner SM, Shaten J, Stern MP, et al. Low levels of sex hormone-binding globulin and testosterone predict the development of non-insulin-dependent diabetes mellitus in men. MRFIT Research Group. Am J Epidemiol 1996;143:889–97.

49. Stellato RK, Feldman HA, Hamdy O, et al. Testosterone, sex hormone-binding globulin, and the development of type 2 diabetes in middle-aged men: prospective results from the Massachusetts Male Aging Study. Diabetes Care 2000;23: 490–4.

50. Gyawali P, Martin SA, Heilbronn LK, et al. The role of sex hormone-binding globulin (SHBG), testosterone, and other sex steroids, on the development of type 2 diabetes in a cohort of community-dwelling middle-aged to elderly men. Acta Diabetol 2018;55:861–72.

51. Ding EL, Song Y, Malik VS, et al. Sex difference of endogenous sex hormones and risk of type 2 diabetes. JAMA 2006;295:1288–99.

52. Selvin E, Feinleib M, Zhang L, et al. Androgens and diabetes in men: results from the Third National Health and Nutrition Examination Survey (NHANES III). Diabetes Care 2007;30:234–8.

53. Grossmann M, Thomas MC, Panagiotopoulos S, et al. Low testosterone levels are common and associated with insulin resistance in men with diabetes. J Clin Endocrinol Metab 2008;93:1834–40.

54. Chen RYT, Wittert GA, Andrews GR. Relative androgen deficiency in relation to obesity and metabolic status in older men. Diabetes Obes Metab 2006;8:429–35.

55. Srikanthan P, Karlamangla AS. Relative muscle mass is inversely associated with insulin resistance and prediabetes. Findings from the third National Health and Nutrition Examination Survey. J Clin Endocrinol Metab 2011;96:2898–903.

56. Li JJ, Wittert GA, Vincent A, et al. Muscle grip strength predicts incident type 2 diabetes: population-based cohort study. Metabolism 2016;65:883–92.

57. Son JW, Lee SS, Kim SR, et al. Low muscle mass and risk of type 2 diabetes in middle-aged and older adults: findings from the KoGES. Diabetologia 2017;60: 865–72.

58. Yeung CHC, Au Yeung SL, Fong SSM, et al. Lean mass, grip strength, and risk of type 2 diabetes: a bi-directional Mendelian randomisation study. Diabetologia 2019;62:789–99.

59. Larsen BA, Wassel CL, Kritchevsky SB, et al. Association of muscle mass, area, and strength with incident diabetes in older adults: the Health ABC Study. J Clin Endocrinol Metab 2016;101:1847–55.

60. Bhasin S, Storer TW, Berman N, et al. The effects of supraphysiologic doses of testosterone on muscle size and strength in normal men. N Engl J Med 1996; 335:1–7.

61. Bhasin S, Woodhouse L, Casaburi R, et al. Older men are as responsive as younger men to the anabolic effects of graded doses of testosterone on the skeletal muscle. J Clin Endocrinol Metab 2005;90:678–88.

62. Page ST, Amory JK, Bowman FD, et al. Exogenous testosterone (T) alone or with finasteride increases physical performance, grip strength, and lean body mass in older men with low serum T. J Clin Endocrinol Metab 2005;90:1502–10.

63. Allan CA, Strauss BJG, Burger HG, et al. Testosterone therapy prevents gain in visceral adipose tissue and los of skeletal muscle in nonobese aging men. J Clin Endocrinol Metab 2008;93:139–46.

64. Snyder PJ, Peachey H, Hannoush P, et al. Effect of testosterone treatment on body composition and muscle strength in men over 65 years of age. J Clin Endocrinol Metab 1999;84:2647–53.

65. Wittert GA, Chapman IM, Haren MT, et al. Oral testosterone supplementation increases muscle and decreases fat mass in healthy elderly males with low-normal gonadal status. J Gerontol A Biol Sci Med Sci 2003;58:618–25.

66. Emmelot-Vonk MH, Verhaar HJJ, Nakhai Pour HR, et al. Effect of testosterone supplementation on functional mobility, cognition, and other parameters in older men. JAMA 2008;299:39–52.

67. Ng MTF, Prendergast LA, Dupuis P, et al. Effects of testosterone treatment on body fat and lean mass in obese men on a hypocaloric diet: a randomised controlled trial. BMC Med 2016;14:153.

68. Isidori AM, Giannetta E, Greco EA, et al. Effects of testosterone on body composition, bone metabolism and serum lipid profile in middle-aged men: a meta-analysis. Clin Endocrinol 2005;63:280–93.

69. Corona G, Giagulli VA, Maseroni E, et al. Testosterone supplementation and body composition: results from a meta-analysis study. Eur J Endocrinol 2016;174:R99–116.

70. Corona G, Giagulli VA, Maseroli E, et al. Testosterone supplementation and body composition: results from a meta-analysis of observational studies. J Endocrinol Invet 2016;39:967–81.

71. Simon D, Charles M-A, Lahlou N, et al. Androgen therapy improves insulin sensitivity and decreases leptin level in healthy adult men with low plasma total testosterone. Diabetes Care 2001;24:2149–51.

72. Basu R, Dalla Man CD, Campioni M, et al. Effect of 2 years of testosterone replacement on insulin secretion, insulin action, glucose effectiveness, hepatic insulin clearance, and postprandial glucose turnover in elderly men. Diabetes Care 2007;30:1972–8.

73. Mohler ER, Ellenberg SS, Lewis CE, et al. The effect of testosterone on cardiovascular biomarkers in the testosterone trials. J Clin Endocrinol Metab 2018;103:681–8.

74. Corona G, Monami M, Rastrelli G, et al. Type 2 diabetes mellitus and testosterone: a meta-analysis study. Int J Androl 2010;34:528–40.

75. Grossmann M, Hoermann R, Wittert G, et al. Effects of testosterone treatment on glucose metabolism and symptoms in men with type 2 diabetes and the metabolic syndrome: a systematic review and meta-analysis of randomized controlled clinical trials. Clin Endocrinol 2015;83:344–51.

76. Atlantis E, Fahey P, Martin S, et al. Predictive value of serum testosterone for type 2 diabetes risk assessment in men. BMC Endocr Disord 2016;16:26.

77. Yassin A, Haider A, Haider KS, et al. Testosterone therapy in men with hypogonadism prevents progression from prediabetes to type 2 diabetes: eight-year data from a registry study. Diabetes Care 2019;42:1104–11.

78. Wittert G, Atlantis E, Allan C, et al. Testosterone therapy to prevent type 2 diabetes mellitus in at-risk men (T4DM): Design and implementation of a double-blind randomized controlled trial. Diabetes Obes Metab 2019;21:772–80.

79. Wittert G, Bracken K, Robledo KP, et al. Testosterone treatment to prevent or revert type 2 diabetes in men enrolled in a lifestyle programme (T4DM): a randomised, double-blind, placebo-controlled, 2-year phase 3b trial. Lancet Diabetes Endocrinol 2021;9:32–45.

80. Yeap BB, Grossmann M, McLachlan RI, et al. Endocrine Society of Australia position statement on male hypogonadism (part 2): treatment and therapeutic considerations. Med J Aust 2016;205:228–31.

81. Bhasin S, Brito JP, Cunningham GR, et al. Testosterone therapy in men with hypogonadism: an Endocrine Society Clinical Practice Guideline. J Clin Endocrinol Metab 2018;103:1715–44.

82. Yeap BB, Wu FCW. Clinical practice update on testosterone therapy for male hypogonadism: contrasting perspectives to optimize care. Clin Endocrinol 2019;90: 56–65.

83. Sattar N, Boyle JG, Al-Ozairi E. Testosterone replacement to prevent type 2 diabetes? Not just yet. Lancet Diabetes Endocrinol 2021;9:5–6.

84. Yeap BB, Dwivedi G, Chih HJ, et al. Androgens and cardiovascular disease in men. In: Feingold KR, Anawalt B, Boyce A, et al, editors. Endotext (Internet). South Dartmouth (MA): MDText.com, Inc.; 2019. Available at: https://www.ncbi.nlm.nih.gov/books/NBK279151/.

85. Basaria S, Coviello AD, Travison TG, et al. Adverse events associated with testosterone administration. N Engl J Med 2010;363:109–22.

86. Srinivas-Shankar U, Roberts SA, Connolly MJ, et al. Effects of testosterone on muscle strength, physical function, body composition, and quality of life in intermediate-frail and frail elderly men: a randomized, double-blind, placebo-controlled study. J Clin Endocrinol Metab 2010;95:639–50.

87. Snyder PJ, Bhasin S, Cunningham GR, et al. Effects of testosterone treatment in older men. N Engl J Med 2016;374:611–24.

88. Alexander GC, Iyer G, Lucas E, et al. Cardiovascular risks of exogenous testosterone use among men: a systematic review and meta-analysis. Am J Med 2017; 130:293–305.

89. Elliott J, Kelly SE, Millar AC, et al. Testosterone therapy in hypogonadal men: a systematic review and network meta-analysis. BMJ Open 2017;7:e015284.

90. Corona G, Rastrelli G, Di Pasquale GD, et al. Testosterone and cardiovascular risk: meta-analysis of interventional studies. J Sex Med 2018;15:820–38.

91. Budoff MJ, Ellenberg SS, Lewis CE, et al. Testosterone treatment and coronary artery plaque volume in older men with low testosterone. JAMA 2017;317:708–16.

92. Yeap BB, Page ST, Grossmann M. Testosterone treatment in older men: clinical implications and unsolved questions from the Testosterone Trials. Lancet Diabetes Endocrinol 2018;6:659–72.

93. Grossmann M, Matsumoto AM. A perspective on middle-aged and older men with functional hypogonadism: focus on holistic management. J Clin Endocrinol Metab 2017;102:1067–75.

94. Wittert G. The relationship between sleep disorders and testosterone. Curr Opin Endocrinol Diabetes Obes 2014;21:239–43.

95. Snyder PJ, Kopperdahl DL, Stephens-Shields AJ, et al. Effect of testosterone treatment on volumetric bone density and strength in older men with low testosterone. JAMA Intern Med 2017;177:471–9.

96. Ng MTF, Hoermann R, Bracken K, et al. Effect of testosterone treatment on bone microarchitecture and bone mineral density in men: a two-year RCT. J Clin Endocrinol Metab 2021;106:e3143–58.

Testicular Dysfunction Among Cancer Survivors

Angel Elenkov, MD, PhD[a,b], Aleksander Giwercman, MD[a,b],*

KEYWORDS

- Cancer • Testicular cancer • Fertility • Hypogonadism • Cancer therapy
- Irradiation • Chemotherapy

KEY POINTS

- Testicular function is an important aspect of quality of life of young male cancer survivors
- Impairment of both sperm production and Leydig cell function may be due to cancer *per se* as well as cancer therapy
- Male cancer survivors are at increased risk of long-term morbidity including cardio-metabolic disease and low bone mineral density
- Pretreatment evaluation and posttreatment follow-up of testicular function are important parts of the management of male patients with cancer

INTRODUCTION

Securing the survival of patients with cancer disease is traditionally considered the main task of clinical oncologists. However, for many types of malignant disease, the survival rates have steadily increased. Thus, due to improved diagnostic as well as therapeutic procedures physicians are more likely to be confronted with young cancer survivors. One of the examples is testicular cancer, the most common malignancy of young males, with survival rates, in many centers, exceeding the level of 95%. Very high cure rates are also seen for those suffering from childhood cancer or lymphomas.

For those young cancer survivors, the issue of quality of life (QoL) plays a crucial role. Many studies have demonstrated that, among young men treated for malignant disease, well-preserved testicular function represents one of the most important aspects of the QoL.

Furthermore, as the age at first parenthood is gradually increasing, the demand for the preservation of reproductive function has been extended to men at a more advanced age, and may be relevant for a proportion of patients treated for common malignancies as colon or prostate cancer.

[a] Department of Translational Medicine, Lund University, CRC; Jan Waldenströms gata 35, SE 214 28 Malmö, Sweden; [b] Reproductive Medicine Centre, Skane University Hospital, Östra Varvsgatan 11F, SE 205 02 Malmö, Sweden
* Corresponding author. CRC 91-10-058; Jan Waldenströms gata 35, SE 214 28 Malmö, Sweden.
E-mail address: aleksander.giwercman@med.lu.se

Endocrinol Metab Clin N Am 51 (2022) 173–186
https://doi.org/10.1016/j.ecl.2021.11.014
0889-8529/22/© 2021 The Author(s). Published by Elsevier Inc. This is an open access article under the CC BY license (http://creativecommons.org/licenses/by/4.0/).
endo.theclinics.com

Both cancer *per se*, but also different modalities of oncological treatment, can be harmful to gonadal function. For many decennia, most attention has been given to impairment of fertility in young cancer survivors.[1] However, there is increasing evidence showing that those patients are at increased risk of developing both primary and secondary hypogonadism.[2–5]

Testicular damage can be due to testicular disease, surgery of the gonads, or radiation therapy directed to the testes and adjacent tissues, as well as systemic chemotherapy. Secondary hypogonadism can be induced by surgery or radiotherapy of tumors in the central nervous system, foremost in the pituitary region. In addition, testosterone levels naturally decrease with age, and men being eugonadal in early adulthood can develop androgen deficiency in more advanced age[6,7] (**Table 1**).

This article focuses on the direct and indirect impact of most common cancer treatments on testicular function leading to the impairment of:

a. Testosterone production
b. Fertility

POSSIBLE MECHANISMS BEHIND TESTICULAR DYSFUNCTION IN PATIENTS WITH CANCER

Testicular function can be negatively affected by cancer disease *per se* and/or by its treatment, the pathogenesis including impairment of function at either pretesticular (pituitary/hypothalamic) or testicular level (**Box 1**).

Impact of disease per se

This effect is most pronounced in men with testicular germ cell cancer (TGCC). Patients with TGCC have a poor testicular function.

- because of etiological and pathologic links between the development of TGCC and gonadal dysfunction.[8]
- due to the fact that the disease is localized in the testis

According to the *testicular dysgenesis syndrome* (TDS) hypothesis[8,9] TGCC, poor semen quality, Leydig cell dysfunction, testicular maldescent, and hypospadias are part of a syndrome caused by early fetal exposure to environmental and/or lifestyle-related factors combined with genetically determined susceptibility to the adverse effects of these exposures.[8] Ten per cent of the patients with TGCC have a history of testicular maldescent. Severe histologic abnormalities were reported in about 25% of the biopsies from the contralateral testis in men who were orchidectomized for unilateral TGCC.[10]

For that reason, it is obvious to expect the patients with TGCC having an impairment of spermatogenesis which may also be associated with deficient Leydig cell function.

Accordingly, significantly lower Leydig cell response to hCG stimulation was seen in men unilaterally orchidectomized due to TGCC, as compared with those in whom one testis was removed due to torsion or trauma.[11] Furthermore, in 33% of patients with TGCC—before orchidectomy—the LH/testosterone ratio was reported to be outside the 97.5 percentile suggesting subtle disturbances of the pituitary-Leydig cell axis already present at the time of diagnosis.[12]

Data on decreased semen quality in TGCC men are more solid. Half of the patients with TGCC has sperm concentration less than 10 to 15 mill/mL before any treatment has been given.[13] In the general population, median levels are about 50 to 100 mill/mL.[14,15] Thus, TGCC implies a more pronounced impairment of sperm production than it could be explained by the fact that one testis harbors a tumor. Patients with

Table 1
Clinical and laboratory characteristics, causes and level of damage in relation to cancer treatment-related impairment of fertility and androgen production

Level of Damage	Cause	Clinical/laboratory Characteristics
Hypothalamic/pituitary	• Cranial irradiation • Surgery in hypothalamic/ pituitary region	• Low levels of FSH/LH • Low testosterone and ejaculate volume • Often azoospermia
Testes	• Due to cancer (eg, testicular) • Surgery – total or partial orchidectomy • Radiation[a] (directly or as scattered irradiation) Chemotherapy[a]	• High levels of FSH/LH • Low testosterone and ejaculate volume • Often oligozoospermia or azoospermia
Ejaculatory process	• Surgery in the pelvic area Radiation	• Normal hormone levels • Often anejaculation or aspermia (eg, due to retrograde ejaculation)

[a] For a list of impact of different cancer treatments on fertility – see **Box 1**.

TGCC have higher follicle-stimulating hormone (FSH) and lower Inhibin B levels as compared with healthy men,[13] which points to testicular dysfunction as a cause of impaired semen quality.

It is still unclear to which degree other malignancies are associated with impaired semen quality. In patients with Hodgkin's disease or sarcomas some studies have reported sperm counts comparable to or only slightly lower than age-matched healthy donors.[16,17] However, a recent study including 4500 patients with cancer indicated that even men with leukemias, lymphomas, sarcomas, and brain tumors do have significantly decreased sperm counts as well as impairment of sperm motility and morphology.[18]

Secondary hypogonadism, due to the impairment of GnRH/gonadotropin secretion may be seen in case of relatively uncommon expansively growing tumors in the pituitary gland, hypothalamus, or their vicinity including prolactinomas.[19]

Impact of cancer therapy

Surgery

Orchidectomy, standard treatment in men with TGCC seems not to imply an immediate decline in testosterone levels but an increase in LH concentration indicates a reduction in Leydig cell capacity.[14] In patients with TGCC treated with surgery only,

Box 1
How can cancer treatment affect male fertility

• Oligozoospermia or Azoospermia – reduced sperm concentration/number or no sperms in the ejaculate

• Impairment of sperm motility/morphology

• Anejaculation/retrograde ejaculation

• Impairment of sperm DNA integrity

• Other functional defects

long-term follow-up has shown a doubling in the prevalence of hypogonadism in—as compared to controls.[20]

Semen quality expressed by sperm concentration and total sperm count per ejaculate is apparently poorer after orchidectomy as compared with the preorchidectomy level.[21] From a clinical point of view it is worth to note that 10% of patients with TGCC with sperms in the ejaculate azoospermic after orchidectomy.[21] In patients treated with orchidectomy alone for stage I testicular cancer some compensatory improvement of semen quality seems to occur during the first 2 years after surgery, with some deterioration during subsequent years.[22]

Also, other types of surgical treatment may have a negative impact on the fertility of cancer survivors:

- Pelvic surgery in men with TGCC (retroperitoneal lymph node dissection), rectal or prostate cancer may, due to the damage of nerve fibers lead to disturbed ejaculation and/or erectile dysfunction;
- Gonadotropin deficiency and, due to that, disturbed sperm production may be caused by the impairment of hypothalamic/pituitary function.

Radio- and chemotherapy

The risk of androgen deficiency seems to be dependent on treatment intensity. Almost 30% of 10 years survivors given chemotherapy in doses above the standard treatment present with increased LH and/or subnormal testosterone levels.[20]

It also seems that some of the men given standard-dose chemotherapy or retroperitoneal irradiation may develop hypogonadism 6 to 12-months posttreatment.[23]

The risk of hypogonadism was found to be 1.5 times higher in TGCC survivors more than 45 years as compared with those in the younger age group. This finding may be explained by the age-related deterioration of Leydig cell function.[20]

Increased risk of hypogonadism was also reported in childhood cancer survivors (CCS). Decreased testosterone and/or high LH were seen in 25% of them who reach early adulthood, which corresponded to 5 to 7 times increased odds ratio as compared with age-matched healthy controls.[4]

In CCS - hypophysectomy and testicular irradiation (eg, as part of leukemia treatment or total body irradiation before bone marrow transplantation) are obvious causes of secondary and primary hypogonadism, respectively. Other treatment modalities were also found to increase the risk of testosterone deficiency[4]:

- Hypogonadism was seen in 20% of CCS following brain surgery (not close to the pituitary), but not in those receiving cranial irradiation or with extracranial surgery alone.
- Chemotherapy, alone or in combination with nontesticular radiation therapy was also associated with higher risk of hypogonadism. Most pronounced risk increase seen in patients with CCS treated with alkylating drugs, but was even observed for other types of cytotoxic drugs.

Two per cent of men develop rectal cancer (RC) and 60% of them are cured. Preoperative radiotherapy implies scattered or even direct irradiation of the testes which results in three times increased risk of subnormal testosterone levels in patients with RC given irradiation as compared with those treated with surgery only.[24,25]

Primary Leydig cell dysfunction may also become a clinical problem in men treated for hematological malignancies. Nonmyeloablative bone marrow transplantation resulted in Leydig cells damage with a significant increase in LH levels (median LH pretransplant, 5.4 IU/L; median LH posttransplant, 9.6 IU/L) and reduced testosterone/LH ratio (2.6 pretransplant vs 1.6 posttransplant).[26] In patients with lymphoma also chemotherapy seems deleterious to Leydig cell function. Thus, 25% of men treated with COPP (cyclophosphamide, oncovin, procarbazine, and prednisone) had elevated levels of LH and the GnRH-stimulated LH response was increased in 90% of them.[27]

Similarly to what is the case for the impact of chemotherapy on spermatogenesis, the treatment regimens not including alkylating drugs and/or irradiation seem less deleterious to testosterone production.[4]

The effects of single-dose irradiation on spermatogenesis in normal men are well studied and show irreversible azoospermia if testicular dose exceeds 6 to 8 Gy.[28] Permanent azoospermia is seen following total body irradiation, given before bone marrow transplantation, or direct testicular irradiation given to boys with acute lymphoblastic leukemia.

Radiotherapy given in fractionated schedules is known to be more toxic to the germ cells than the bio-equivalent dose given as a single dose. TGCC men treated with infradiaphragmatic irradiation will receive scattered irradiation (approximately 0.5 Gy) on the residual testis despite a gonadal shield. This treatment was shown to cause an initial decline in sperm concentration, which returned to pretreatment levels 2 to 5 years after therapy (28). However, although at group level the mean sperm counts, following radiotherapy, return to the postorchidectomy level, it cannot be excluded that some subjects may develop permanent or long-term azoospermia. Adjuvant abdominal radiotherapy, with an estimated testicular dose of less than 0.5 Gy, was shown to induce a transient increase in the proportion of sperms with DNA strand breaks, normalizing within 3 to 5 years.[29] Also in CCS, the percentage of spermatozoa with DNA strand breaks was increased following extragonadal irradiation.[30]

Irradiation of the prostate bed in patients with prostate cancer results in a pronounced dose into the testicles. The calculated projected doses into the testicles made on a standard series of 40 fractions of external-beam radiotherapy were 196 cGy ($\pm$145 cGy). In this patient group, direct irradiation (15–35 cGy) causes oligozoospermia; doses between 35 cGy and 50 cGy cause reversible azoospermia. The nadir of sperm count occurs 4 to 6 months after the end of treatment, and 10 to 18 months are required for complete recovery. However, doses more than 120 cGy are associated with a reduced risk of recovery of spermatogenesis. Cumulative doses of fractionated radiotherapy more than 250 cGy generally result in prolonged and likely permanent azoospermia.

The effects of brachytherapy given as treatment of prostate cancer, with irradiation doses received by the testes usually being less than 20 cGY, seems to be less harmful to fertility than external radiotherapy[31].

Gonadotoxicity caused by chemotherapy is due to the fact that it targets rapidly proliferating cells. The effect of chemotherapy on gonadal function is dependent on the type of treatment as well as the dose given. **Table 2** gives an overview of the risk of azoospermia in relation to different types of cytotoxic treatments. Generally, the harmful effect on spermatogenesis is most pronounced in alkylating drugs and cisplatin.

Most data are available for the treatment of TGCC, as this is the most common type of cancer in young males and the treatment is relatively standardized.

Patients with TGCC treated with 1 to 2 cycles of chemotherapy exhibit no or only a slight decrease in sperm concentration, 6-months posttreatment with a following return to the same level before cytotoxic treatment. The risk of developing long-term or persisting azoospermia following this treatment is considered to be close to zero. On the other hand, 3 to 4 cycles of cisplatin-based chemotherapy induce gonadal dysfunction with azoospermia in significant proportion of patients with TGCC and a

Table 2
Risk of azoospermia in relation to different types and doses of cancer treatment

Agent	Cumulative Dose	Azoospermia	Additive effect with other Cytotoxic Drugs	Comments
Radiation				
Testes	2,5 Gy/0,6 Gy	Permanent/Temporary	Yes	Fractionated treatment worse than single dose
Total body	8 Gy single/12 Gy fractionated	Permanent	Yes	
Chemotherapy				
Cyclophosphamide	19 g/m²	Yes		
Chlorambucil	1,4 g/m²	Yes		
Cisplatin	500 mg/m²	Yes		
Procarbazine	4 g/m²	Yes		
Carboplatin	>2 g/m²	Likely		
Nitrosoureas				
Busulfan	>600 mg/kg	Likely		
Ifosfamide	>30 g/m²	Likely	+ cyclophosphamide	
Carmustine	1 g/m²	Likely		
Lomustine	500 mg/m²	Likely		
Nitrogen mustard		Unknown		Used with other highly gonadotoxic agents
Melphalan		Unknown		Same
Actinomycin D		Unknown		Same
Doxorubicin	770 mg/m²	Yes	Yes	Azoospermia in combination with other cytotoxics
Cytosine arabinoside	1 g/m²	Temporary oligozoospermia	Yes	Azoospermia in combination with other cytotoxics
Vinblastine	50 g/m²	Temporary oligozoospermia	Yes	Azoospermia in combination with other cytotoxics

Vinkristin	8 g/m²	Temporary oligozoospermia	Yes	Azoospermia in combination with other cytotoxics. Less toxic than vinblastine
Pacliatxel		Unknown		
Docetaxel		Unknown		
Gemicitabine		Unknown		
Trastuzumab		Unknown		
Irinotecan		Unknown		
Oxaliplatin		Unknown		

Adapted from Puscheck E, Philip PA, Jeyendran RS. Male fertility preservation and cancer treatment. *Cancer Treat Rev.* 2004;30(2):173-180.

simultaneous rise in FSH levels is seen in most of them. Recovery of spermatogenesis is seen in most patients during the 2 to 5 years after chemotherapy.[32] After this follow-up period, approximately 8% of TGCC men remain azoospermic, this proportion being as high as 65% in those who have received a cumulative dose of cisplatin at 600 mg/m^2 or more.[33,34] Possibly there is a genetic variability explaining the intraindividual sensitivity observed.

Among the CCS, approximately 20% present with azoospermia, this risk being approximately 15% in those treated with chemotherapy only and 33% in patients who had received a combination of chemotherapy and radiotherapy[35].

Of the CCS who had received potentially sterilizing doses of cisplatin / alkylating agents (**Table 2**), but no radiotherapy, the proportion of men with azoospermia is as high as 80% but 5% only if cisplatin / alkylating agents were given in doses less than the anticipated threshold doses.

In both patient groups mentioned above, chemotherapy was not shown to affect sperm DNA.

In Hodgkin's Lymphoma (HL) until the late 1970s MOPP (mustargen, oncovin, procarbazine, prednisone) was the cornerstone of HL treatment, this regimen implying long-term azoospermia in 70% to 80% of patients. However, the introduction of ABVD (adriamycin, bleomycin, vinblastine, dacarbazine) reduced this side effect to almost zero, without worsening the survival prognosis.[36] However, in more advanced cases of HL, the standard ABVD treatment is substituted by mixed regimens as BEACOPP (bleomycin, etoposide, adriamycin, cyclophosphamide, oncovin procarbazine, prednisone), COPP/ABVD, OPP/ABVD, or MOPP. Patients given 6 or more cycles of these treatments were found to have a permanent absence of sperm in the seminal fluid, while following a low number of cycles (<6), spermatogenesis recovered after 3 to 5 years but semen quality was highly impaired[16].

Modern treatment regimens

Modern cancer therapy includes the use of biological or targeted therapies that often involve small molecule inhibitors or monoclonal antibodies. There is only limited information regarding the effect of those treatment modalities on testicular function and the available data focus on their impact on semen quality.[37]

Men treated with imatinib, a tyrosine kinase inhibitor, produce normal pregnancies and offspring although there may be some negative effects on spermatogenesis.[38]

The use of rapamycin (sirolimus) – mTOR inhibitor –as cancer treatment in humans has been shown to imply elevated FSH, indicating spermatogenic dysfunction; sperm counts on one patient did show oligozoospermia, reversed within 6 months of cessation of treatment (30).

Chronic treatment of adult male patients with cancer with interferon-alpha did not affect sperm counts.[37]

In general, data in patients obtained so far with most of the biological targeted therapies are compatible with the men being either naturally fertile or having some sperm for use to achieve pregnancies by assisted reproductive techniques. However, most targeted therapies are new, and newer targets and therapies are constantly under development but have not been evaluated in humans for reproductive effects.

POSSIBLE LINK BETWEEN HYPOGONADISM AND LATE MORBIDITIES

CCS face higher risks to develop non–cancer-related chronic, disabling, or life-threatening conditions in the years and decades following the therapy.[39] Similar results have been presented for the adolescence and early young adult groups showing higher mortality risks independently of cancer progression and recurrence.[40] Biochemical signs of testosterone deficiency are well-known markers for decreased life expectancy and CVD. Young childhood and germ cancer survivors have been shown to be at particularly high risk for hypogonadism especially after testicular irradiation or after receiving more than 4 cycles of cisplatin-based radiotherapy.[41] Furthermore, germ cell cancer survivors have been shown to have higher risk to develop CVD 1 year after bleomycin–etoposide–cisplatin treatment and mildly higher 10 years afterward when compared with healthy individuals.[42]

Effects of low testosterone levels are particularly visible in patients with prostate cancer on long-term androgen deprivation therapy (ADT). In these patients, lifelong castrational levels of testosterone need to be maintained to prevent recurrence and/ or progression of the disease. ADT has been associated with high risk for diabetes mellitus, CVD, and myocardial infarction even only after 6 months after initiation.[43] Meta-analysis of reports presenting observational data link GNRH agonist treatment to fatal, nonfatal myocardial infarction, and stroke.[44] Metabolic syndrome is more represented among men during ADT when compared with non-ADT treated men.[45] Neurologic consequences of ADT include stroke, depression, cognitive decline, and Alzheimer disease.[46]

Bone mineral density is negatively affected by a large number of cytotoxic agents and radiation regimens, making the cancer survivors a vulnerable group for fragility fractures and osteoporosis with a negative effect on life expectancy and life quality. Bone metabolism is controlled by sex hormones. Hypogonadal state among child and germ cell cancer survivors have indeed been shown to further reduce the bone mineral density.[47] ADT in prostate cancer-treated men is well known to lead to higher fracture risk.[48]

Screening and treatment of hypogonadism among cancer-treated men are therefore important not only to provide better QoL but also possibly to prevent or reduce the risk of future adverse health events.

CLINICAL MANAGEMENT BEFORE AND AFTER CANCER DIAGNOSIS
Prepubertal and pubertal boys

In the management of prepubertal and pubertal boys diagnosed with cancer, most attention has been given to fertility preservation.

Semen cryopreservation has to be considered in boys who have not yet reached full pubertal development. In boys aged 12 to 18 years, almost 90% had spermatozoa in the ejaculate. Approximately 15% of the boys were unable to deliver a semen sample by masturbation why penile vibration or electroejaculation was applied. The youngest patient with an ejaculate containing motile spermatozoa was 12.2 years old, and the smallest testicular volumes in boys associated with motile spermatozoa in the ejaculate were 6 to 7 mL. It was, therefore, concluded that regardless of their age, adolescent boys with testicular volumes of more than 5 mL should be offered semen banking before gonadotoxic treatment or other procedures that could potentially damage future fertility.[49]

Cryopreservation of testicular tissue from prepubertal boys represents a medical as well as ethical challenge. Attempts to in vivo and in vitro maturation of prepubertal human testicular tissue are ongoing and despite such procedure cannot yet be offered as a clinical routine, it has been suggested that—as part of research project—storage of testicular tissue should be offered to boys before cancer treatment implying a high risk of sterility.[50]

Posttreatment follow-up in CCS should primarily focus on diagnosing them with delayed or absent pubertal development. These should be part of routine follow-up of those boys, mainly if they belong to one of the groups being at highest risk for developing androgen deficiency (please, see above).

Also, the issue of posttreatment sperm production should be discussed with the patient. In those who received the most gonadotoxic types of treatment, postpubertal semen analysis and cryopreservation of spermatozoa in those with severe oligozoospermia, should be considered. Although solid scientific evidence is still lacking, the rational is a potential risk age-related deterioration of sperm production implying azoospermia.

Postpubertal men

When cancer treatment is initiated after puberty, the patient should be referred for seminal cryopreservation as soon as possible and promptly informed of the associated risks for infertility and hypogonadism following the treatment. Also, levels of reproductive hormones—testosterone, LH, and FSH—as well as SHBG should be checked. Having information on the endocrine status before cancer therapy may help in posttreatment evaluation of possible testicular damage caused by the treatment given.

In some cases, however, the patient might not be able to deposit a sperm sample before the initiation of cancer treatment. This might be due to one or more of the following mechanisms: severe stress, bad overall physical state, functional illness-related hypogonadism, inability to ejaculate due to neurologic impairment from metastasis or gonadal tumor (testicular cancer, lymphoma, etc.). In these cases, if logistically possible and after patients' consent a testicular biopsy might be performed to cryopreserve testicular tissue for subsequent sperm extraction. In cases of azoospermia and testicular cancer, the so-called onco-TESE can be performed simultaneously with the orchiectomy. In these cases, testicular tissue is obtained from multiple areas surrounding the testicular tumor.

Posttreatment follow-up of males treated for cancer should also include assessment of testosterone production and—if there is a potential future wish of fatherhood—even spermatogenesis.

In patients with TGCC, reproductive hormone levels should be checked annually for at least 5 years after treatment. Due to increased risk of late development of hypogonadism, the patient should be encouraged to seek andrological expertise if he develops symptoms of this condition. For other cancer forms, the andrological follow-up of endocrine testicular function should be tailored according to the cancer treatment given. The indication for androgen replacement therapy is similar to that for other hypogonadal men. However, in young cancer survivors, the potential wish of fatherhood should be taken into consideration.

Several posttreatment options exist if pretreatment cryopreservation was not conducted. In cases of isolated hypothalamic/pituitary dysfunction and unaffected testicular function, long-term treatment with gonadotropins may restore fertility and testosterone levels. If paternity is not desired, testosterone replacement therapy might be initiated according to available guidelines.

However, in cases of gonadotoxic treatment, the patients often present with high LH and FSH and sperm counts may vary from normozoospermia to azoospermia. In the latter case, the treatment options are often limited to testicular biopsy, either conventional or micro-TESE. Focal preservation of spermatogenesis has been described even after aggressive cytotoxic treatments followed by bone marrow transplantation.[51]

In some cases, fertility might be impaired due to anejaculation or retrograde ejaculation. This complication is common in men who undergo retroperitoneal lymph node dissection due to nonseminoma testicular cancer. In these cases, if pharmacologic

Table 3
Summary of andrological procedures to be routinely offered to patients with cancer

Procedure	Before Treatment	6–12 mo Post-treatment	Long-Term Follow-up
Andrological counseling	X	X	X[a]
Semen analysis	X		X[a]
Cryopreservation of semen or testicular tissue (pubertal and post-pubertal)	X		
Hormonal evaluation	X	X	X

[a] if the patient needs fertility counseling or have symptoms/biochemical signs of hypogonadism.

treatment with adrenergic α-receptor stimulators fails, use of urinary spermatozoa—in case of retrograde ejaculation—or testicular biopsy might be an option for retrieving sperms to be used for assisted reproduction.

Andrological procedures to be offered to male patients with cancer, before and after the treatment, are summarized in **Table 3**.

RESEARCH NEEDS

As the number of young cancer survivors is steadily increasing and the importance of the reproductive aspect for the QoL of those subjects, there is an urgent need for understanding the biology and clinical aspects of the impact of cancer disease- and treatment on testicular function. This information is needed to develop evidence-based guidelines for the proper management of those patients.

New treatment modalities need to be tested for potential gonadotoxic effect. Even for the existing cancer therapies, their impact on Leydig cell function needs to be more thoroughly investigated. From both research and clinical point of view, it is important to elucidate the direction of causality in the established link between hypogonadism and cardio-metabolic disturbances in cancer survivors. In this context, the low-grade inflammation may be one of the pathogenetic key players.

A special and demanding problem is the possibility of fertility preservation in prepubertal subjects.

Taking into consideration, the multitude of diseases and different treatment options to be studied, establishing multi-centre international consortia for research on testicular dysfunction among cancer survivors is highly warranted.

CLINICS CARE POINTS

- Semen cryopreservation, before cancer treatment, should be offered to men and pubertal boys
- Hypogonadism is frequently seen in boys/men treated for malignant disease and checking levels of reproductive hormones should be a mandatory part of posttreatment follow-up of men treated for cancer.
- Male cancer survivors are at increased long-term risk of osteoporosis, as well as cardiovascular and metabolic disease which may be associated with hypogonadism.

DISCLOSURE

This work was supported by grants from the Swedish Cancer Society, Swedish Society of Childhood Cancer; Malmo University Hospital Cancer Fund; Swedish

Governmental Fund for Clinical Research; Region Skane Research Fund, and Repro-Union (Interreg V program). ReproUnion has received an unrestricted research grant from Ferring Pharmaceuticals. Aleksander Giwercman has served as a consultant for Besins Healthcare.

REFERENCES

1. Giwercman A, Petersen PM. Cancer and male infertility. Baillieres Best Pract Res Clin Endocrinol Metab 2000;14(3):453–71.
2. Greenfield DM, Walters SJ, Coleman RE, et al. Prevalence and consequences of androgen deficiency in young male cancer survivors in a controlled cross-sectional study. J Clin Endocrinol Metab 2007;92(9):3476–82.
3. Fung C, Fossa SD, Williams A, et al. Long-term Morbidity of Testicular Cancer Treatment. Urol Clin North Am 2015;42(3):393–408.
4. Romerius P, Stahl O, Moell C, et al. Hypogonadism risk in men treated for child-hood cancer. J Clin Endocrinol Metab 2009;94(11):4180–6.
5. Oldenburg J. Hypogonadism and fertility issues following primary treatment for testicular cancer. Urol Oncol 2015;33(9):407–12.
6. Harman SM, Metter EJ, Tobin JD, et al. Longitudinal effects of aging on serum to-tal and free testosterone levels in healthy men. Baltimore Longitudinal Study of Aging. J Clin Endocrinol Metab 2001;86(2):724–31.
7. Tajar A, Forti G, O'Neill TW, et al. Characteristics of secondary, primary, and compensated hypogonadism in aging men: evidence from the European Male Ageing Study. J Clin Endocrinol Metab 2010;95(4):1810–8.
8. Skakkebaek NE, Rajpert-De Meyts E, Main KM. Testicular dysgenesis syndrome: an increasingly common developmental disorder with environmental aspects. Hum Reprod 2001;16(5):972–8.
9. Sharpe RM, Skakkebaek NE. Testicular dysgenesis syndrome: mechanistic in-sights and potential new downstream effects. Fertil Steril 2008;89(2 Suppl): e33–8.
10. Berthelsen JG, Skakkebaek NE. Gonadal function in men with testis cancer. Fertil Steril 1983;39(1):68–75.
11. Willemse PH, Sleijfer DT, Sluiter WJ, et al. Altered Leydig cell function in patients with testicular cancer: evidence for bilateral testicular defect. Acta Endocrinol (Copenh) 1983;102(4):616–24.
12. Bandak M, Aksglaede L, Juul A, et al. The pituitary-Leydig cell axis before and after orchiectomy in patients with stage I testicular cancer. Eur J Cancer 2011; 47(17):2585–91.
13. Petersen PM, Giwercman A, Skakkebaek NE, et al. Gonadal function in men with testicular cancer. Semin Oncol 1998;25(2):224–33.
14. Petersen PM, Skakkebaek NE, Vistisen K, et al. Semen quality and reproductive hormones before orchiectomy in men with testicular cancer. J Clin Oncol 1999; 17(3):941–7.
15. Shoshany O, Shtabholtz Y, Schreter E, et al. Predictors of spermatogenesis in radical orchiectomy specimen and potential implications for patients with testic-ular cancer. Fertil Steril 2016;106(1):70–4.
16. Paoli D, Rizzo F, Fiore G, et al. Spermatogenesis in Hodgkin's lymphoma patients: a retrospective study of semen quality before and after different chemotherapy regimens. Hum Reprod 2016;31(2):263–72.

17. Caponecchia L, Cimino G, Sacchetto R, et al. Do malignant diseases affect semen quality? Sperm parameters of men with cancers. Andrologia 2016;48(3): 333–40.

18. Auger J, Sermondade N, Eustache F. Semen quality of 4480 young cancer and systemic disease patients: baseline data and clinical considerations. Basic Clin Androl 2016;26:3.

19. Littley MD, Shalet SM, Beardwell CG, et al. Hypopituitarism following external radiotherapy for pituitary tumours in adults. Q J Med 1989;70(262):145–60.

20. Nord C, Bjoro T, Ellingsen D, et al. Gonadal hormones in long-term survivors 10 years after treatment for unilateral testicular cancer. Eur Urol 2003;44(3):322–8.

21. Petersen PM, Skakkebaek NE, Rorth M, et al. Semen quality and reproductive hormones before and after orchiectomy in men with testicular cancer. J Urol 1999;161(3):822–6.

22. Hansen PV, Trykker H, Svennekjaer IL, et al. Long-term recovery of spermatogenesis after radiotherapy in patients with testicular cancer. Radiother Oncol 1990; 18(2):117–25.

23. Eberhard J, Stahl O, Cwikiel M, et al. Risk factors for post-treatment hypogonadism in testicular cancer patients. Eur J Endocrinol 2008;158(4):561–70.

24. Buchli C, Martling A, Arver S, et al. Testicular function after radiotherapy for rectal cancer–a review. J Sex Med 2011;8(11):3220–6.

25. Buchli C, Tapper J, Bottai M, et al. Testosterone and body composition in men after treatment for rectal cancer. J Sex Med 2015;12(3):774–82.

26. Kyriacou C, Kottaridis PD, Eliahoo J, et al. Germ cell damage and Leydig cell insufficiency in recipients of nonmyeloablative transplantation for haematological malignancies. Bone Marrow Transplant 2003;31(1):45–50.

27. Bramswig JH, Heimes U, Heiermann E, et al. The effects of different cumulative doses of chemotherapy on testicular function. Results in 75 patients treated for Hodgkin's disease during childhood or adolescence. Cancer 1990;65(6): 1298–302.

28. Rowley MJ, Leach DR, Warner GA, et al. Effect of graded doses of ionizing radiation on the human testis. Radiat Res 1974;59(3):665–78.

29. Stahl O, Eberhard J, Jepson K, et al. Sperm DNA integrity in testicular cancer patients. Hum Reprod 2006;21(12):3199–205.

30. Romerius P, Stahl O, Moell C, et al. Sperm DNA integrity in men treated for childhood cancer. Clin Cancer Res 2010;16(15):3843–50.

31. Tran S, Boissier R, Perrin J, et al. Review of the Different Treatments and Management for Prostate Cancer and Fertility. Urology 2015;86(5):936–41.

32. Eberhard J, Stahl O, Giwercman Y, et al. Impact of therapy and androgen receptor polymorphism on sperm concentration in men treated for testicular germ cell cancer: a longitudinal study. Hum Reprod 2004;19(6):1418–25.

33. Petersen PM, Hansen SW, Giwercman A, et al. Dose-dependent impairment of testicular function in patients treated with cisplatin-based chemotherapy for germ cell cancer. Ann Oncol 1994;5(4):355–8.

34. Isaksson S, Eberhard J, Stahl O, et al. Inhibin B concentration is predictive for long-term azoospermia in men treated for testicular cancer. Andrology 2014; 2(2):252–8.

35. Romerius P, Stahl O, Moell C, et al. High risk of azoospermia in men treated for childhood cancer. Int J Androl 2011;34(1):69–76.

36. Viviani S, Santoro A, Ragni G, et al. Gonadal toxicity after combination chemotherapy for Hodgkin's disease. Comparative results of MOPP vs ABVD. Eur J Cancer Clin Oncol 1985;21(5):601–5.

37. Meistrich ML. Effects of chemotherapy and radiotherapy on spermatogenesis in humans. Fertil Steril 2013;100(5):1180–6.
38. Szakacs Z, Hegyi PJ, Farkas N, et al. Pregnancy outcomes of women whom spouse fathered children after tyrosine kinase inhibitor therapy for chronic myeloid leukemia: A systematic review. PLoS One 2020;15(12):e0243045.
39. Oeffinger KC, Mertens AC, Sklar CA, et al. Chronic health conditions in adult survivors of childhood cancer. N Engl J Med 2006;355(15):1572–82.
40. Suh E, Stratton KL, Leisenring WM, et al. Late mortality and chronic health conditions in long-term survivors of early-adolescent and young adult cancers: a retrospective cohort analysis from the Childhood Cancer Survivor Study. Lancet Oncol 2020;21(3):421–35.
41. Isaksson S, Bogefors K, Stahl O, et al. High risk of hypogonadism in young male cancer survivors. Clin Endocrinol (Oxf) 2018;88(3):432–41.
42. Lauritsen J, Hansen MK, Bandak M, et al. Cardiovascular Risk Factors and Disease After Male Germ Cell Cancer. J Clin Oncol 2020;38(6):584–92.
43. Keating NL, O'Malley A, Freedland SJ, et al. Diabetes and cardiovascular disease during androgen deprivation therapy: observational study of veterans with prostate cancer. J Natl Cancer Inst 2012;104(19):1518–23.
44. Bosco C, Bosnyak Z, Malmberg A, et al. Quantifying observational evidence for risk of fatal and nonfatal cardiovascular disease following androgen deprivation therapy for prostate cancer: a meta-analysis. Eur Urol 2015;68(3):386–96.
45. Braga-Basaria M, Dobs AS, Muller DC, et al. Metabolic syndrome in men with prostate cancer undergoing long-term androgen-deprivation therapy. J Clin Oncol 2006;24(24):3979–83.
46. Nead KT, Gaskin G, Chester C, et al. Androgen Deprivation Therapy and Future Alzheimer's Disease Risk. J Clin Oncol 2016;34(6):566–71.
47. Isaksson S, Bogefors K, Akesson K, et al. Risk of low bone mineral density in testicular germ cell cancer survivors: association with hypogonadism and treatment modality. Andrology 2017;5(5):898–904.
48. Smith MR, Boyce SP, Moyneur E, et al. Risk of clinical fractures after gonadotropin-releasing hormone agonist therapy for prostate cancer. J Urol 2006;175(1):136–9.
49. Hagenas I, Jorgensen N, Rechnitzer C, et al. Clinical and biochemical correlates of successful semen collection for cryopreservation from 12-18-year-old patients: a single-center study of 86 adolescents. Hum Reprod 2010;25(8):2031–8.
50. Jahnukainen K, Stukenborg JB. Clinical review: Present and future prospects of male fertility preservation for children and adolescents. J Clin Endocrinol Metab 2012;97(12):4341–51.
51. Jacobsen FM, Fode M, Sønksen J, et al. Successful extraction of sperm cells after autologous bone marrow transplant: a case report. Scand J Urol 2019;53(2–3):174–5.

Testosterone Treatment As a Function-Promoting Therapy in Sarcopenia Associated with Aging and Chronic Disease

Marcelo Rodrigues Dos Santos, PhD[a], Thomas W. Storer, PhD[b],*

KEYWORDS

- Androgens • Body composition • Muscle strength • Physical function

KEY POINTS

- Sarcopenia is characterized by the loss of muscle mass, muscle, strength, and physical ability because of aging and/or chronic disease.
- The prevalence of sarcopenia among older people with chronic disease is generally greater than in healthy older people.
- Low serum testosterone level has been associated with age-related loss of muscle mass and strength.
- Treatment with testosterone or other anabolic steroids has been investigated as a countermeasure to muscle wasting and loss of muscle strength and physical function associated with aging and chronic diseases.

INTRODUCTION

Although testosterone and its derivatives are approved only for treating symptomatic hypogonadism, they have been used off-label at least since the mid-1950s in the United States to promote athletic performance, physical appearance, and myriad complaints of age- and or disease-related loss of skeletal muscle mass, muscle strength, and physical function in men. Indeed, low total testosterone and free

Financial Support: This work was supported in part by grants from the NIA (1RO1-AG-14369-01), an NIA cooperative agreement (1UO1AG14369), and Boston Claude D. Pepper Older Americans Independence Center grants (5P30AG031679 and P30AG3167). Additional support was provided by Boston University Clinical and Translational Science Institute grant (1UL1RR025771) and resources and facilities of the VA Boston Healthcare System.

[a] Instituto do Coração (InCor), Hospital das Clínicas HCFMUSP, |Faculdade de Medicina, Universidade de São Paulo, Av. Dr. Enéas de Carvalho Aguiar, 44, Sao Paulo 05403-900 Brazil; [b] Research Program in Men's Health: Aging and Metabolism, Brigham and Women's Hospital, 221 Longwood Avenue, 5th Floor, Boston, MA 02115, USA
* Corresponding author.
E-mail address: tstorer@bwh.harvard.edu

Endocrinol Metab Clin N Am 51 (2022) 187–204
https://doi.org/10.1016/j.ecl.2021.11.012
0889-8529/22/© 2021 Elsevier Inc. All rights reserved.

endo.theclinics.com

testosterone (FT) concentrations have been associated with reduced muscle mass and upper and lower extremity strength, and increased risk of mobility limitation, falls, and fractures.[1] Here we present evidence from randomized controlled trials (RCT) for the use of testosterone for reducing the effects of age- and chronic disease-related sarcopenia.

Hypotheses Underlying the Use of Testosterone As a Function-Promoting Therapy for Sarcopenia

The term sarcopenia was introduced by Rosenberg in 1988 to describe muscle loss in older people.[2] Over the ensuing 33 years, the term has received worldwide attention and has undergone several iterations to clarify its defining features. Expert opinion has generally agreed that measures of muscle strength and physical performance should be included in the definition. Recent evidence-based position statements from the Sarcopenia Definition and Outcomes Consortium have emphasized low handgrip strength and slow gait speed as the most important defining features of sarcopenia.[3]

Recommendations for management of sarcopenia have consistently included resistance exercise training, high-protein diets, and increased caloric intake.[4] Despite its known anabolic effects and demonstrated safety in many randomized trials,[5] the long-term efficacy and safety of testosterone treatment in improving physical function and reducing physical disability, falls, and fractures in older adults with sarcopenia is still uncertain.[6]

Because testosterone administration in older, healthy men is associated with dose- and concentration-dependent increases in fat-free mass (FFM) and maximal voluntary muscle strength (**Fig. 1**),[7] its use in patients with sarcopenia has biologic rationale. In an experimental model, testosterone supplementation was associated with stimulation of cellular metabolism and regenerative potential of aged-satellite cells and it blunted skeletal muscle apoptosis.[8] In a single-center RCT, testosterone therapy in intermediate-frail and frail elderly men seemed to prevent age-associated loss of muscle strength and improved body composition, quality of life, and physical function.[9] However, these findings are not universal. One 6-month study of testosterone undecanoate administration in older men with low testosterone levels did not increase these outcomes.[10] However, mean handgrip strength (43–47 kg) and timed up-and-go time (4.24 seconds) in these subjects were well higher than current cut points for sarcopenia.

Mechanistic Indicators of Testosterone As a Function-Promoting Therapy

Testosterone acts on anabolic and catabolic pathways to induce dose-related hypertrophy of type 1 and type 2 skeletal muscle fibers.[11] Testosterone treatment increases the numbers of muscle satellite cells and myonuclei but does not alter the myonuclear domain or the number of muscle fibers.[11] The mechanisms of testosterone action are not fully understood but involve increased expression of androgen receptor protein and insulin-like growth factor 1 in skeletal muscle.[12] Liganded androgen receptor associates with β-catenin and other coactivators, translocates into the nucleus where it binds T-cell factor 4, and induces the transcription of several Wnt-target genes including follistatin.[13,14] Follistatin blocks signaling through the transforming growth factor-β pathway and plays an important role in mediating testosterone's effects in promoting myogenic differentiation and inhibiting adipogenic differentiation of mesenchymal muscle progenitor cells.[13,15] Testosterone has also been reported to stimulate Akt, a regulatory kinase, which is involved in protein synthesis via the mammalian target of rapamycin (mTOR) and protein degradation repressing via the transcription factors of the FoxO family.[8,16]

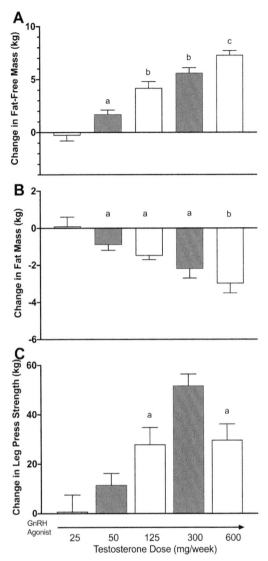

Fig. 1. Changes in fat-free mass (*A*) and fat mass (*B*) derived from dual-energy X-ray absorptiometry scans and changes in one-repetition maximum leg press strength (*C*). Men 60 to 75 years of age with normal serum testosterone at baseline received a long-acting GnRH agonist to suppress endogenous testosterone and 25 mg (n = 13), 50 mg (n = 12), 125 mg (n = 12), 300 mg (n = 14), or 600 mg (n = 10) testosterone enanthate weekly for 20 weeks. Data are mean ± standard error of the mean. [a] $P < .05$ versus 25-mg group; [b] $P < .05$ versus the 25- and 50-mg groups; [c] $P < .05$ versus all other groups. GnRH, gonadotropin-releasing hormone. (*Data from* Bhasin S, Woodhouse L, Casaburi R, et al. Older men are as responsive as young men to the anabolic effects of graded doses of testosterone on the skeletal muscle. *J Clin Endocrinol Metab.* 2005;90(2):678-688.)

Testosterone treatment increases the numbers of muscle satellite cells likely by regulating Notch signaling, Wnt/β-catenin, and myogenic regulatory factors leading to hypertrophy of type I and II muscle fibers.[8,11] Testosterone also stimulates myoblast proliferation by upregulating ornithine decarboxylase 1, the rate-limiting step in polyamine pathway, and increasing polyamines.[17]

TESTOSTERONE AS A FUNCTION-PROMOTING THERAPY IN SARCOPENIA ASSOCIATED WITH AGING
Older Men with Low Testosterone

The Endocrine Society Clinical Practice Guideline defines low testosterone as total testosterone lower than 9.2 nmol/L.[18] In the European Male Aging Study, only sexual symptoms had a syndromic association with total testosterone concentrations lower than 11 nmol/L and FT lower than 220 pmol/L.[19] In epidemiologic studies, low levels of FT at baseline are associated with lower muscle mass and muscle strength, and a greater risk of incident or worsening mobility limitation and falls in community-dwelling older men.[20] However, whether testosterone replacement can reverse this functional abnormality is not completely known.

In a randomized, double-blinded controlled trial, 108 men older than 65 years of age were allocated to receive either testosterone patch or placebo for 36 months.[21] The study found a significant reduction in fat mass, whereas lean body mass (LBM) increased by an average of 1.9 kg in the testosterone group. However, strength of knee extension and flexion, as measured by an isokinetic dynamometer, did not differ significantly between testosterone and placebo.

The TEAAM Trial was one of the largest long-term studies of testosterone intervention in older men.[22] This 3-year study was designed to investigate the effects of long-term testosterone treatment on atherosclerosis progression in older men with low and low-normal testosterone. The study also reported testosterone's effects on measures of body composition, muscle performance, and physical function. Testosterone-treated men showed significantly greater improvements in LBM, muscle strength and power, stair climbing power, and aerobic capacity ($\dot{V}O_2peak$) than placebo-treated men. The improvements in muscle strength, stair climbing power, and $\dot{V}O_2peak$ were modest and tended to wane over time.

Older Men with Low Testosterone and Mobility Limitation

The Testosterone in Older Men with Mobility Limitations (TOM) Trial[23] included older men with testosterone deficiency and mobility limitation at baseline. The primary outcome of this 6-month RCT was to determine whether testosterone therapy improves maximal voluntary muscle strength. Testosterone administration was associated with greater gains in leg press strength, chest press strength and power, skeletal muscle mass, and loaded stair-climbing power when compared with patients assigned to placebo. Walking speed did not change significantly in either group. A separate, secondary analysis examined changes in $\dot{V}O_2peak$, a measure of aerobic capacity.[24] Men receiving testosterone had significantly greater improvements in $\dot{V}O_2peak$ versus placebo. The clinical meaningfulness and the durability of the small 1.7 mL/kg/min between-group difference requires further investigation.

The Testosterone Trials, a set of seven coordinated trials, included 790 men aged 65 years or older and with an average of two total testosterone concentrations less than 275 ng/dL (9·5 nmol/L), of whom 390 had mobility limitation and a walking speed less than 1·2 m/s and were enrolled in the Physical Function Trial.[25] Testosterone treatment consistently improved self-reported walking ability, modestly improved 6-

minute-walking distance across all participants relative to placebo, but did not affect falls. The effect of testosterone on mobility measures was related to baseline gait speed and self-reported mobility limitation, and changes in testosterone and hemoglobin concentrations.

In aggregate, testosterone supplementation in older men with low testosterone improves LBM, maximum voluntary muscle strength and power, and stair climbing power but the improvement in peak $\dot{V}O_2$[24] and walking speed has been small and inconsistent across trials.

Older Women

Only a few clinical trials of testosterone therapy in older women are available. Studies investigating testosterone's effects in older women tend to be focused on female sexual dysfunction,[26] psychological outcomes, and bone health, with few studies evaluating body composition[27] or other indices of sarcopenia per se.

The Testosterone Dose Response in Surgically Menopausal Women (TDSM Trial) was a randomized trial in surgically menopausal women with low testosterone allocated to one of four weekly doses of testosterone enanthate for 24 weeks.[28] All participants received transdermal estradiol starting 12 weeks before testosterone treatment. The principal outcome was change in sexual behavior. Secondary measures included body composition, muscle strength and power, and physical function. There were significant dose-dependent gains in the 25 mg/wk group relative to placebo in some domains of sexual function, LBM, and upper body measures of muscle power and stair climbing power while carrying a load. Adverse events were not statistically different among treatment groups but generally more frequent in the 25 mg/wk group. This 6-month study in middle-aged women saw few androgenic adverse effects. Larger trials of longer duration are needed to determine the long-term efficacy and safety of testosterone administration in older women with functional limitations.

Frailty

Frailty often coexists with sarcopenia with shared features, such as lower lean mass and poorer physical function[29]; both are associated with negative health outcomes. There is no consensus definition of frailty, although characteristics include extreme vulnerability to stressors, risk of decreased functional reserves, and negative health-related outcomes.[30,31] Observational studies have shown that low FT and high levels of luteinizing hormone and sex hormone binding globulin are associated with increased risk of frailty.[32] Longitudinal studies suggest that a decline in FT over time is associated with frailty progression.[33] Large cohort studies in frail older men suggest that serum testosterone alone may not be a major contributor to physical frailty.[34]

One RCT evaluated testosterone gel (5 mg/d) or placebo for its effects on muscle performance and physical function in frail, older men with low bone mass and low bioavailable testosterone.[35] No changes in muscle strength, power, or physical function were observed after 12 or 24 months of treatment, although the low adherence rate may have impacted outcomes. Similarly, in another trial, testosterone and a high-calorie nutritional supplement did not improve frailty levels in undernourished older people.[36] Additionally, a comprehensive review of interventional studies with testosterone therapy including frail older men, reported modest improvements on lean mass, conflicting results on muscle strength, and weak evidence for effects on physical function.[34] The characteristics of physical frailty suggest that testosterone might be effective in overcoming associated physical deficits, but data are scant, presenting an opportunity for future research with improved research designs.

TESTOSTERONE AS A COUNTERMEASURE TO SARCOPENIA IN CHRONIC DISEASE

Testosterone-induced improvements in LBM, muscle strength, and to a lesser degree, physical function, in healthy older individuals provide rationale for their use in sarcopenia associated with aging and chronic disease. Several RCTs with small samples and short study durations provide some insight into therapeutic effects of testosterone and other anabolic steroids in treating the loss of muscle mass and strength in a variety of chronic diseases.

Chronic Obstructive Pulmonary Disease

Systemic effects that often accompany chronic obstructive pulmonary disease (COPD) include weight loss, sarcopenia, and skeletal muscle dysfunction that have multiple etiologies. Low testosterone levels are frequently observed in men with COPD with prevalence estimates ranging from 22% to 69%.[37] Countermeasures usually include exercise training, especially resistance exercise training. Testosterone and its analogues are also attractive because of their demonstrated effects on muscle anabolism.

An 8-week RCT investigated the effects nandrolone decanoate (ND), with or without daily nutritional supplementation in adults with COPD.[38] The participants received biweekly doses of ND (50 mg for men and 25 mg for women), or placebo. Patients were stratified according to severity of weight loss and/or FFM. All participants were actively exercising. Individuals in the more severe tissue loss group who received nutritional supplementation with or without ND gained significantly more body mass (2.6 kg vs 0.4 kg in placebo). The ND group gained 1.4 kg FFM, whereas weight gain in the supplement-only group was primarily from fat accretion. Participants in the comparison group experienced less weight gain but greater increases in FFM, especially the 1.4-kg increase in those receiving ND. Twelve-minute-walk distance increased significantly (by 173 m and 147 m for those in the more severe tissue loss and comparison group, respectively), without significant differences between treatment groups. Importantly, respiratory muscle strength increased in the depleted group. These data suggest that an anabolic steroid when added to pulmonary rehabilitation and supplemental nutrition in adults with COPD can increase FFM, respiratory muscle strength, and walking distance.

In another RCT, depot injections of 250 mg testosterone enanthate or placebo every 4 weeks for 26 weeks were used to evaluate testosterone effects on pulmonary function and body composition in 29 eugonadal men with COPD.[39] Pulmonary function measures were not different between groups after 26 weeks but increases in FFM and decreases in fat mass were significantly greater in men receiving testosterone than in those receiving placebo.

Casaburi and colleagues[40] determined the effects of progressive resistance exercise training (PRT) and testosterone supplementation alone or in combination in men with COPD. Fifty-three participants with moderate to severe COPD and low testosterone were randomized to placebo controls, each intervention alone (testosterone or PRT), or the combined intervention (testosterone + PRT). After 10 weeks, serum testosterone increased to the mid-normal range in testosterone-treated men; those receiving placebo injections did not change. This study reported significantly greater increases in LBM and significantly greater decreases in fat mass in groups receiving testosterone compared with the nontestosterone arms (**Fig. 2**). The changes in body composition in testosterone + PRT were additive, equaling the sum of the changes in groups receiving testosterone alone or PRT alone. Additionally, leg strength increased by 22% in the combined group, 16% in those receiving PRT alone,

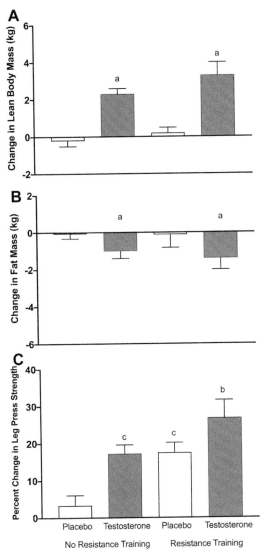

Fig. 2. Changes in lean body mass (A) and fat mass (B) derived from dual-energy X-ray absorptiometry scans and changes in one-repetition maximum leg press strength (C). Participants were men aged 55 to 80 years with moderate to severe chronic obstructive pulmonary disease and serum testosterone levels were less than 400 mg/dL. The men were randomized to receive one of four treatments for 10 weeks: placebo plus no resistance exercise training (n = 12), testosterone enanthate (100 mg/wk) plus no resistance exercise training (n = 12), placebo plus resistance exercise training (n = 12), and testosterone plus resistance exercise training (n = 11). Data are mean ± standard error. [a] P < .05 versus non-testosterone groups; [b] P < .05 versus nontraining groups; [c] P < .05 versus placebo + no training group. (Data from Casaburi R, Bhasin S, Cosentino L, et al. Effects of testosterone and resistance training in men with chronic obstructive pulmonary disease. Am J Respir Crit Care Med. 2004;170(8):870-878.)

and 12% in men assigned to testosterone alone. The 22% improvement in the combined group was significantly greater than the nonexercise groups and the three groups receiving at least one intervention had significantly greater strength increases than control subjects. This 10-week study provided short-term evidence of significant improvements in muscle mass and strength in men with COPD when replacement doses of testosterone are used alone or augmented with PRT.

The oral androgen stanozolol was studied for 6 months in 23 undernourished, eugonadal men with COPD for changes in body mass and LBM.[41] Participants received either 12 mg per day stanozolol after a loading dose of 250 mg Durateston, or placebo. Patients received inspiratory muscle training during weeks 9 to 18 and cycle exercise training during the last 9 weeks of the study. Control subjects lost 0.4 (0.2) kg body weight versus a significant 1.8 (0.5) kg weight gain in 9 out of 10 androgen-treated men. LBM did not change in the control group but increased significantly in treated men; the increases were sustained through Week 27. However, the difference in change between groups was not significant. Fat mass, exercise capacity, and inspiratory pressure did not change significantly in either group. This small study of malnourished, functionally impaired men added to the growing body of evidence supporting androgen use for weight gain and increased lean mass in people with COPD.

Thus, limited evidence suggests that testosterone treatment improves muscle mass and maximal voluntary strength in adults with COPD and its effects on muscle mass and strength are augmented by progressive resistance exercise; however, testosterone has not been shown to improve pulmonary function or long-term health outcomes. The current statement on limb muscle dysfunction in COPD from the American Thoracic Society/European Respiratory Society[42] indicates that testosterone supplementation should not be recommended as a routine treatment of muscle wasting in COPD because of the potential for adverse events and the lack of long-terms studies evaluating clinical outcomes, durability, quality of life, safety, and survival.

Chronic Kidney Disease

The prevalence of sarcopenia in people with chronic kidney disease (CKD) ranges from 4% to 42% depending on the definition used and CKD stage[43] and a 33% higher hazard of mortality in those with sarcopenia compared with those without.[44] The men with CKD have a higher prevalence of low testosterone levels than the general population.[45] The cause of alterations in the hypothalamic-pituitary-gonadal axis in men with CKD is multifactorial; the contributing factors include the uremic toxins, advanced age, chronic inflammation, malnutrition, accelerated atherosclerosis, and a chronic catabolic milieu.[46]

Individuals with end-stage renal disease (ESRD) exhibit significant skeletal muscle atrophy and weakness[47–49] and have abnormal muscle morphology.[50,51] Strength and physical function are approximately 60% to 70% of age-matched healthy individuals.[51,52] Low exercise tolerance[53,54] and poor physical functioning are common features. Excitation-contraction coupling, central activation, and specific tension are not different between patients with ESRD and control subjects.[48,51] This suggests that muscle atrophy is a major cause of muscle weakness and the ensuing decrements in physical function.

The high prevalence of sarcopenia and the associated hypogonadism in men with ESRD has provided the rationale for the evaluation of anabolic hormones as adjunctive therapies. In a 12-month longitudinal study of 440 men receiving hemodialysis, 17% of whom had sarcopenia (low handgrip strength and slow walking speed),[55] the men with lower calculated FT concentration had 1.55-fold greater odds of having sarcopenia and 1.72-fold greater odds of developing sarcopenia. However, only a few small studies have investigated whether anabolic hormones would mitigate androgen deficiency and provide anabolic and functional benefits in patients with CKD.

ND has been administered alone or in combination with exercise training to men and women with CKD in only a few RCTs.[52,56,57] Nandrolone doses in studies spanning 12 to 24 weeks have ranged between 50 and 200 mg/wk for men[52,56,57] and 25 and 100 mg/wk for women. [56,57] The most common changes were significantly increased LBM[52,56] and skeletal muscle mass[57] versus zero change and significant differences in the change in LBM versus placebo. Other significant ND versus placebo group changes have been seen in skeletal muscle mass and quadriceps cross-sectional area, but inconsistent outcomes for muscle strength and objectively measured physical function.

Seventy-nine people (49 men) on hemodialysis were randomly allocated to receive ND (100 mg/wk for women and 200 mg/wk for men) or placebo with or without PRT for 12 weeks.[56] Individuals receiving ND alone significantly increased body mass, LBM, and fat mass relative to baseline. Similar, but not significant, changes were seen in the ND plus resistance training group, but not in the other two groups. Other changes in the intervention groups included significant increases in quadriceps cross-sectional area (CSA) in the single intervention groups relative to control subjects; improvement was additive in the combined treatment group. Leg strength improved only in the groups receiving PRT; no changes were observed in objectively measured physical function. Insufficient statistical power and the short study duration may not have allowed sufficient time for neuromuscular adaptations needed for translation of muscle mass and strength gains into functional improvements. This is an issue in need of further study.

The effects of oxymetholone, an oral androgen, were studied for 24 weeks in 41 individuals with sarcopenia (25 men) undergoing hemodialysis.[58] Baseline testosterone was in the normal range. Individuals were randomly assigned to receive 50-mg tablets of oxymetholone or placebo twice daily. Body mass and FFM increased and fat mass decreased significantly more in the oxymetholone group relative to control subjects. Handgrip strength, type I but not type II, vastus lateralis CSA, and muscle mRNA levels for several growth factors all increased significantly more in those receiving oxymetholone compared with control subjects. Changes in quality-of-life scores (Short Form-36) were not different between groups. Liver enzymes rose significantly in the oxymetholone group, a specific concern with oral androgens.

Small sample sizes, few RCTs, varying definitions of sarcopenia, differing baseline serum testosterone levels, and inconsistent outcome measures have led to uncertainty about the efficacy of anabolic hormones in CKD. These issues need resolution.

HIV Infection

Lower testosterone concentration in men living with HIV is associated with loss of LBM[59] and poor outcomes.[60,61] The prevalence of testosterone deficiency in this population is high (34.5%) and increases when comorbidities, such as type 2 diabetes, are associated.[60]

Testosterone effects on body composition in more than 700 individuals from 14 RCTs including four with HIV-infected women were recently analyzed in a systematic review/meta-analysis.[62] Studies were conducted over 8 weeks to 18 months using testosterone injections, transdermal patches, or oral androgens in varying doses. The analysis revealed that relative to control subjects, participants receiving testosterone in any form had significantly greater increases in body mass and LBM. These increases were substantially greater with intramuscular injections (1.83 kg) versus oral administration (1.43 kg) or transdermal patch (1.33 kg). In addition, the meta-analysis reported no significant testosterone effect on fat mass regardless of gender or androgen type.

An older meta-analysis of eight RCT included analysis of anabolic hormone therapy on exercise functional capacity in HIV-infected individuals with weight loss.[63] Four studies used testosterone injections, three used testosterone patches, and one study used oxandrolone tablets. Studies also used different methods to assess functional capacity and muscle strength, which, according to authors, make "...meta-analysis of continuous variables impossible." However, three studies reported improved physical function or muscle strength in treatment groups compared with control subjects. Conversely, three studies reported no changes. The combined treatment with testosterone and PRT was more likely to produce better results on muscle function, especially strength.[64] Similar results were observed in eugonadal men with AIDS wasting syndrome.[65]

Combining testosterone supplementation with or without resistance exercise training has also been studied in men living with HIV. Bhasin and colleagues[64] reported changes in body composition muscle strength in 49 HIV-infected men using the same 2×2 factorial design described previously for men with COPD and illustrated in **Fig. 2**. The men were 18 to 50 years of age, with self-reported weight loss of greater than or equal to 5% in the previous 6 months. Baseline serum testosterone was less than or equal to 349 ng/dL. Outcomes after 16 weeks of treatment for the four groups are displayed in **Fig. 3**. Body mass increased significantly in men who exercised alone (2.6 kg), received testosterone alone (2.2 kg), but did not change in the other two groups. Men receiving testosterone alone or testosterone and exercise increased FFM by 2.3 kg ($P = .004$) and 2.6 kg ($P < .001$), respectively, but did not change in men receiving placebo alone (0.9 kg; $P = .21$). Fat mass did not change in any group (data not shown). Leg press strength increased significantly in mean receiving testosterone alone (16%), resistance training alone (28%), or testosterone plus resistance training (22%). There was no change in the placebo, no exercise group. These data suggest the potential use of testosterone therapy to increase body mass, FFM, and leg strength in men living with HIV. The addition of resistance exercise training may contribute to these improvements.

Testosterone therapy typically increases muscle mass in HIV-infected men, but the effect of this treatment on changes in physical function are less clear.[66] Knapp and collaborators[67] set out to determine whether a supraphysiologic dose of testosterone enanthate (300 mg/wk) administered for 16 weeks improved physical function in addition to leg strength (see **Fig. 3**). The functional measures, gait speed, stair-climbing power, and load carrying ability did not change. Leg strength significantly increased in the testosterone group but not in placebo; the differences in change between groups were not significant. Significant increases in FFM and decreases in fat mass were noted for the testosterone group but not for men allocated to placebo. Nevertheless, the difference between groups was not significant.

Chronic Heart Failure

Chronic heart failure, the late stage of many cardiovascular diseases, affects millions of people across the globe with exercise intolerance as its hallmark; cardiac dysfunction[68] and peripheral muscle wasting[69,70] are principal contributors to this intolerance. Evidence suggests that testosterone deficiency contributes to chronic heart failure and its progression.[71] Patients with heart failure and testosterone deficiency have higher mortality rate and increased hospital readmissions when compared with eugonadal patients.[72,73]

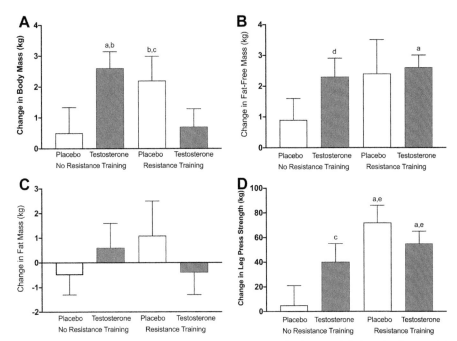

Fig. 3. Changes (mean ± standard error of the mean) in body mass (A), lean body mass (B), and fat mass (C) derived from dual-energy X-ray absorptiometry scans. (D) Changes in one-repetition maximum leg press strength. Participants were 61 men living with HIV, 18 to 50 years of age, with greater than or equal to 5% weight loss in the previous 6 months. Baseline serum testosterone levels were less than 205 ng/dL. The men were randomly allocated to one of four treatments for 24 weeks: placebo plus no resistance exercise training (n = 14), testosterone enanthate (100 mg/wk) plus no resistance exercise training (n = 17), placebo plus resistance exercise training (n = 15), and testosterone plus resistance exercise training (n = 15). [a] P < .001 versus zero change; [b] P < .01 versus placebo, no exercise; [c] P = .02; versus zero change; [d] P = .004 versus zero change; [e] P < .05 versus placebo, no exercise. (*Data from* Bhasin S, Storer TW, Javanbakht M, et al. Testosterone replacement and resistance exercise in HIV-infected men with weight loss and low testosterone levels. *JAMA.* 2000;283(6):763-770.)

Four RCTs revealed that compared with placebo, testosterone replacement substantially improved exercise capacity and symptoms in patients with heart failure.[74–77] A subsequent meta-analysis that included these studies showed a significant improvement in exercise capacity of approximately 54 m in the 6-minute-walk test and 2.7 mL/kg/min (23%) in peak oxygen uptake after 12 to 52 weeks of testosterone supplementation relative to control subjects.[78] Left ventricular ejection fraction did not change in any of the studies. Hence, improvement in exercise capacity after testosterone therapy seems to rely on peripheral adaptations. Testosterone is a vasodilator and improves oxygen delivery to the exercised muscles, stimulates skeletal muscle hypertrophy, and improves some measures of physical function, all of which could contribute to improved exercise tolerance and lower fatigability.[79]

Spinal Cord Injury

Low serum testosterone in patients with spinal cord injury (SCI) presents in 12.7% to 43.3% of this population.[80–82] The prevalence of testosterone deficiency is significantly greater in patients with motor complete injuries than those with motor incomplete injuries.[80] Their hypogonadism does not result primarily from classic primary gonadal failure. Testicular paracrine factors and/or alteration of hypothalamus-pituitary-testicular axis may be involved in the pathogenesis of their hypogonadism.[81]

Studies in experimental models of SCI suggest that testosterone therapy is effective in attenuating alterations in myofibrillar proteins in affected skeletal muscles.[83] In humans, testosterone replacement therapy significantly improved lean tissue mass and energy expenditure in hypogonadal men with SCI.[84,85]

The overall ability to perform activities of daily living was assessed in patients with SCI and the findings suggest that negative androgen status might be prominent, specifically in the first year after injury.[86] In a retrospective study, men with SCI and testosterone replacement therapy showed strength gains in the affected muscle when compared with control subjects.[87]

Testosterone therapy alone is unlikely to improve physical function optimally in individuals with SCI. However, as demonstrated in healthy young and older men[7] and men with COPD,[40] testosterone therapy associated with PRT has shown impressive results. The few studies that have used this approach with individuals with SCI have revealed significantly greater improvements relative to placebo in lean mass, knee extensor cross-sectional area,[88] muscle quality[89] and vastus lateralis cross-sectional area, protein synthesis, and mitochondrial function.[90] The prevalence of low testosterone, muscle atrophy, and loss of strength in SCI and the limited evidence for successfully ameliorating these outcomes suggests a value in screening men with SCI for low testosterone. Additional research is needed to understand appropriate use of testosterone as an adjunctive therapy to improve health and function in people with SCI.

SUMMARY

Sarcopenia is an important clinical problem in aging men and women, and in patients with chronic diseases, that may lead to mobility limitation and loss of independence. Therefore, assessment of sarcopenia should be incorporated into clinical practice guidelines in specialties that care for such patients.[34] Data from RCT, systematic reviews, and meta-analyses have revealed consistent improvements in LBM among men who are treated with testosterone compared with placebo. However, this has not consistently translated into improvements in physical function. Moreover, participants in these studies were not systematically screened for sarcopenia. Because of the lack of adequately powered, long-term clinical trials in older adults with sarcopenia with or without chronic disease, efficacy trials to determine the long-term benefits of testosterone in improving mobility, function, quality of life, and survival are a fertile area for future investigation.

CLINICS CARE POINTS

Sarcopenia is an important clinical problem in aging men and women, in patients with chronic diseases, and is often associated with low serum testosterone. Left untreated, sarcopenia can lead to mobility limitation and loss of independence.

- Specialties that care for such individuals should incorporate clinical practice guidelines to assess for the presence of sarcopenia.[3]

- Endocrine Society Guidelines for Testosterone Therapy in Men with Hypogonadism should be used to screen men over age 65 who have symptoms associated with testosterone deficiency.[19]

- Testosterone treatment, monitored for adverse effects, may be considered on a case-by-case basis as a function promoting therapy for the losses of skeletal muscle strength, muscle mass, and physical function associated with sarcopenia and frailty due to aging and some chronic diseases.
- Clinicians may consider well designed and monitored progressive resistance exercise training as an initial countermeasure to improve muscle strength, muscle mass, and physical function.
- Combining testosterone treatment with progressive resistance exercise training has been shown to produce additive effects for increasing muscle strength and muscle size.

DISCLOSURE

The authors have nothing to disclose.

REFERENCES

1. Bhasin S, Storer T. Anabolic applications of androgens for functional limitations associated with aging and chronic illness. Front Horm Res 2009;37:163–82.
2. Rosenberg IH. Sarcopenia: origins and clinical relevance. J Nutr 1997;127(5): 990S–1S.
3. Bhasin S, Travison TG, Manini TM, et al. Sarcopenia definition: the position statements of the Sarcopenia Definition and Outcomes Consortium. J Am Geriatr Soc 2020;68(7):1410–8. https://doi.org/10.1111/jgs.163722.
4. Bauer J, Morley JE, Schols AMWJ, et al. Sarcopenia: a time for action. An SCWD Position Paper. J Cachexia Sarcopenia Muscle 2019;10(5):956–61.
5. De Spiegeleer A, Beckwée D, Bautmans I, et al. Sarcopenia Guidelines Development group of the Belgian Society of Gerontology and Geriatrics (BSGG). Pharmacological interventions to improve muscle mass, muscle strength and physical performance in older people: an umbrella review of systematic reviews and meta-analyses. Drugs Aging 2018;35(8):719–34.
6. Dent E, Morley JE, Cruz-Jentoft AJ, et al. Physical frailty: ICFSR international clinical practice guidelines for identification and management. J Nutr Health Aging 2019;23(9):771–87.
7. Bhasin S, Woodhouse L, Casaburi R, et al. Older men are as responsive as young men to the anabolic effects of graded doses of testosterone on the skeletal muscle. J Clin Endocrinol Metab 2005;90(2):678–88.
8. Kovacheva EL, Hikim APS, Shen R, et al. Testosterone supplementation reverses sarcopenia in aging through regulation of myostatin, c-Jun NH2-terminal kinase, Notch, and Akt signaling pathways. Endocrinology 2010; 151(2):628–38.
9. Srinivas-Shankar U, Roberts SA, Connolly MJ, et al. Effects of testosterone on muscle strength, physical function, body composition, and quality of life in intermediate-frail and frail elderly men: a randomized, double-blind, placebo-controlled study. J Clin Endocrinol Metab 2010;95(2):639–50.
10. Emmelot-Vonk MH, Verhaar HJJ, Nakhai Pour HR, et al. Effect of testosterone supplementation on functional mobility, cognition, and other parameters in older men: a randomized controlled trial. JAMA 2008;299(1):39–52.
11. Sinha-Hikim I, Cornford M, Gaytan H, et al. Effects of testosterone supplementation on skeletal muscle fiber hypertrophy and satellite cells in community-dwelling older men. J Clin Endocrinol Metab 2006;91(8):3024–33.

12. Ferrando AA, Sheffield-Moore M, Yeckel CW, et al. Testosterone administration to older men improves muscle function: molecular and physiological mechanisms. Am J Physiol Endocrinol Metab 2002;282(3):E601–7.

13. Singh R, Bhasin S, Braga M, et al. Regulation of myogenic differentiation by androgens: cross talk between androgen receptor/beta-catenin and follistatin/transforming growth factor-beta signaling pathways. Endocrinology 2009;150(3): 1259–68.

14. Braga M, Bhasin S, Jasuja R, et al. Testosterone inhibits transforming growth factor-β signaling during myogenic differentiation and proliferation of mouse satellite cells: potential role of follistatin in mediating testosterone action. Mol Cell Endocrinol 2012;350(1):39–52.

15. Singh R, Artaza JN, Taylor WE, et al. Androgens stimulate myogenic differentiation and inhibit adipogenesis in C3H 10T1/2 pluripotent cells through an androgen receptor-mediated pathway. Endocrinology 2003;144(11):5081–8.

16. Schiaffino S, Mammucari C. Regulation of skeletal muscle growth by the IGF1-Akt/PKB pathway: insights from genetic models. Skelet Muscle 2011;1(1):4.

17. Jasuja R, Costello JC, Singh R, et al. Combined administration of testosterone plus an ornithine decarboxylase inhibitor as a selective prostate-sparing anabolic therapy. Aging Cell 2014;13(2):303–10.

18. Bhasin S, Storer TW, Asbel-Sethi N, et al. Effects of testosterone replacement with a nongenital, transdermal system, Androderm, in human immunodeficiency virus-infected men with low testosterone levels. J Clin Endocrinol Metab 1998;83(9): 3155–62.

19. Bhasin S, Brito JP, Cunningham GR, et al. Testosterone therapy in men with hypogonadism: an Endocrine Society clinical practice guideline. J Clin Endocrinol Metab 2018;103(5):1715–44.

20. Krasnoff JB, Basaria S, Pencina MJ, et al. Free testosterone levels are associated with mobility limitation and physical performance in community-dwelling men: the Framingham Offspring Study. J Clin Endocrinol Metab 2010;95(6):2790–9.

21. Snyder PJ, Peachey H, Hannoush P, et al. Effect of testosterone treatment on body composition and muscle strength in men over 65 years of age. J Clin Endocrinol Metab 1999;84(8):2647–53.

22. Basaria S, Harman SM, Travison TG, et al. Effects of testosterone administration for 3 years on subclinical atherosclerosis progression in older men with low or low-normal testosterone levels: a randomized clinical trial. JAMA 2015;314(6): 570–81.

23. Travison TG, Basaria S, Storer TW, et al. Clinical meaningfulness of the changes in muscle performance and physical function associated with testosterone administration in older men with mobility limitation. J Gerontol A Biol Sci Med Sci 2011;66(10):1090–9.

24. Storer TW, Bhasin S, Travison TG, et al. Testosterone attenuates age-related fall in aerobic function in mobility limited older men with low testosterone. J Clin Endocrinol Metab 2016;101(6):2562–9.

25. Bhasin S, Ellenberg SS, Storer TW, et al. Effect of testosterone replacement on measures of mobility in older men with mobility limitation and low testosterone concentrations: secondary analyses of the Testosterone Trials. Lancet Diabetes Endocrinol 2018;6(11):879–90.

26. Davis SR, Worsley R, Miller KK, et al. Androgens and female sexual function and dysfunction: findings from the Fourth International Consultation of Sexual Medicine. J Sex Med 2016;13(2):168–78.

27. Elraiyah T, Sonbol MB, Wang Z, et al. Clinical review: the benefits and harms of systemic testosterone therapy in postmenopausal women with normal adrenal function: a systematic review and meta-analysis. J Clin Endocrinol Metab 2014; 99(10):3543–50.

28. Huang G, Basaria S, Travison TG, et al. Testosterone dose-response relationships in hysterectomized women with or without oophorectomy: effects on sexual function, body composition, muscle performance and physical function in a randomized trial. Menopause 2014;21(6):612–23.

29. Cesari M, Landi F, Vellas B, et al. Sarcopenia and physical frailty: two sides of the same coin. Front Aging Neurosci 2014;6:192.

30. Cesari M, Prince M, Thiyagarajan JA, et al. Frailty: an emerging public health priority. J Am Med Dir Assoc 2016;17(3):188–92.

31. Thompson MQ, Yu S, Tucker GR, et al. Frailty and sarcopenia in combination are more predictive of mortality than either condition alone. Maturitas 2021;144: 102–7.

32. Mohr BA, Bhasin S, Kupelian V, et al. Testosterone, sex hormone-binding globulin, and frailty in older men. J Am Geriatr Soc 2007;55(4):548–55.

33. Afilalo J. Androgen deficiency as a biological determinant of frailty: hope or hype? J Am Geriatr Soc 2014;62(6):1174–8.

34. Hsu B, Cumming RG, Handelsman DJ. Testosterone, frailty and physical function in older men. Expert Rev Endocrinol Metab 2018;13(3):159–65.

35. Kenny AM, Kleppinger A, Annis K, et al. Effects of transdermal testosterone on bone and muscle in older men with low bioavailable testosterone levels, low bone mass, and physical frailty. J Am Geriatr Soc 2010;58(6):1134–43.

36. Theou O, Chapman I, Wijeyaratne L, et al. Can an intervention with testosterone and nutritional supplement improve the frailty level of under-nourished older people? J Frailty Aging 2016;5(4):247–52.

37. Balasubramanian V, Naing S. Hypogonadism in chronic obstructive pulmonary disease: incidence and effects. Curr Opin Pulm Med 2012;18(2):112–7.

38. Schols AM, Soeters PB, Mostert R, et al. Physiologic effects of nutritional support and anabolic steroids in patients with chronic obstructive pulmonary disease. A placebo-controlled randomized trial. Am J Respir Crit Care Med 1995;152(4 Pt 1):1268–74.

39. Svartberg J, Aasebø U, Hjalmarsen A, et al. Testosterone treatment improves body composition and sexual function in men with COPD, in a 6-month randomized controlled trial. Respir Med 2004;98(9):906–13.

40. Casaburi R, Bhasin S, Cosentino L, et al. Effects of testosterone and resistance training in men with chronic obstructive pulmonary disease. Am J Respir Crit Care Med 2004;170(8):870–8.

41. Ferreira IM, Verreschi IT, Nery LE, et al. The influence of 6 months of oral anabolic steroids on body mass and respiratory muscles in undernourished COPD patients. Chest 1998;114(1):19–28.

42. Maltais F, Decramer M, Casaburi R, et al. An official American Thoracic Society/ European Respiratory Society statement: update on limb muscle dysfunction in chronic obstructive pulmonary disease. Am J Respir Crit Care Med 2014; 189(9):e15–62.

43. Chatzipetrou V, Bégin M-J, Hars M, et al. Sarcopenia in chronic kidney disease: a scoping review of prevalence, risk factors, association with outcomes, and treatment. Calcif Tissue Int 2021. https://doi.org/10.1007/s00223-021-00898-1.

44. Wilkinson TJ, Mikzsa J, Yates T, et al. Association of sarcopenia with mortality and end-stage renal disease in those with chronic kidney disease: a UK Biobank study. J Cachexia Sarcopenia Muscle 2021;12(3):586–98.

45. Skiba R, Matyjek A, Syryło T, et al. Advanced chronic kidney disease is a strong predictor of hypogonadism and is associated with decreased lean tissue mass. Int J Nephrol Renovasc Dis 2020;13:319–27.

46. Dousdampanis P, Trigka K, Fourtounas C, et al. Role of testosterone in the pathogenesis, progression, prognosis and comorbidity of men with chronic kidney disease. Ther Apher Dial 2014;18(3):220–30.

47. Adams GR, Vaziri ND. Skeletal muscle dysfunction in chronic renal failure: effects of exercise. Am J Physiol Ren Physiol 2006;290(4):F753–61.

48. Johansen KL, Shubert T, Doyle J, et al. Muscle atrophy in patients receiving hemodialysis: effects on muscle strength, muscle quality, and physical function. Kidney Int 2003;63(1):291–7.

49. Kouidi E, Albani M, Natsis K, et al. The effects of exercise training on muscle atrophy in haemodialysis patients. Nephrol Dial Transpl 1998;13(3):685–99.

50. Diesel W, Knight BK, Noakes TD, et al. Morphologic features of the myopathy associated with chronic renal failure. Am J Kidney Dis 1993;22(5):677–84.

51. Fahal IH, Bell GM, Bone JM, et al. Physiological abnormalities of skeletal muscle in dialysis patients. Nephrol Dial Transpl 1997;12(1):119–27.

52. Johansen KL. Physical functioning and exercise capacity in patients on dialysis. Adv Ren Replace Ther 1999;6(2):141–8.

53. Painter P, Zimmerman SW. Exercise in end-stage renal disease. Am J Kidney Dis 1986;7(5):386–94.

54. Storer TW, Casaburi R, Sawelson S, et al. Endurance exercise training during haemodialysis improves strength, power, fatigability and physical performance in maintenance haemodialysis patients. Nephrol Dial Transpl 2005;20(7): 1429–37.

55. Chiang JM, Kaysen GA, Segal M, et al. Low testosterone is associated with frailty, muscle wasting and physical dysfunction among men receiving hemodialysis: a longitudinal analysis. Nephrol Dial Transpl 2019;34(5):802–10.

56. Johansen KL, Painter PL, Sakkas GK, et al. Effects of resistance exercise training and nandrolone decanoate on body composition and muscle function among patients who receive hemodialysis: a randomized, controlled trial. J Am Soc Nephrol 2006;17(8):2307–14.

57. Macdonald JH, Marcora SM, Jibani MM, et al. Nandrolone decanoate as anabolic therapy in chronic kidney disease: a randomized phase II dose-finding study. Nephron Clin Pract 2007;106(3):c125–35.

58. Supasyndh O, Satirapoj B, Aramwit P, et al. Effect of oral anabolic steroid on muscle strength and muscle growth in hemodialysis patients. CJASN 2013;8(2): 271–9.

59. Grinspoon S, Corcoran C, Lee K, et al. Loss of lean body and muscle mass correlates with androgen levels in hypogonadal men with acquired immunodeficiency syndrome and wasting. J Clin Endocrinol Metab 1996;81(11):4051–8.

60. Postel N, Wolf E, Balogh A, et al. Functional hypogonadism and testosterone deficiency in aging males with and without hiv-infection. Exp Clin Endocrinol Diabetes 2021. https://doi.org/10.1055/a-1210-2482.

61. De Vincentis S, Decaroli MC, Fanelli F, et al. Health status is related to testosterone, estrone and body fat: moving to functional hypogonadism in adult men with HIV. Eur J Endocrinol 2021;184(1):107–22.

62. Zhou T, Hu Z-Y, Zhang H-P, et al. Effects of testosterone supplementation on body composition in hiv patients: a meta-analysis of double-blinded randomized controlled trials. Curr Med Sci 2018;38(1):191–8.

63. Kong A, Edmonds P. Testosterone therapy in HIV wasting syndrome: systematic review and meta-analysis. Lancet Infect Dis 2002;2(11):692–9.

64. Bhasin S, Storer TW, Javanbakht M, et al. Testosterone replacement and resistance exercise in HIV-infected men with weight loss and low testosterone levels. JAMA 2000;283(6):763–70.

65. Grinspoon S, Corcoran C, Parlman K, et al. Effects of testosterone and progressive resistance training in eugonadal men with AIDS wasting. A randomized, controlled trial. Ann Intern Med 2000;133(5):348–55.

66. Bross R, Casaburi R, Storer TW, et al. Androgen effects on body composition and muscle function: implications for the use of androgens as anabolic agents in sarcopenic states. Baillieres Clin Endocrinol Metab 1998;12(3):365–78.

67. Knapp PE, Storer TW, Herbst KL, et al. Effects of a supraphysiological dose of testosterone on physical function, muscle performance, mood, and fatigue in men with HIV-associated weight loss. Am J Physiol Endocrinol Metab 2008; 294(6):E1135–43.

68. Hirai DM, Musch TI, Poole DC. Exercise training in chronic heart failure: improving skeletal muscle O2 transport and utilization. Am J Physiol Heart Circ Physiol 2015;309(9):H1419–39.

69. Suzuki T, Palus S, Springer J. Skeletal muscle wasting in chronic heart failure. ESC Heart Fail 2018;5(6):1099–107.

70. von Haehling S, Garfias Macedo T, Valentova M, et al. Muscle wasting as an independent predictor of survival in patients with chronic heart failure. J Cachexia Sarcopenia Muscle 2020;11(5):1242–9.

71. Volterrani M, Rosano G, Iellamo F. Testosterone and heart failure. Endocrine 2012; 42(2):272–7.

72. Jankowska EA, Biel B, Majda J, et al. Anabolic deficiency in men with chronic heart failure: prevalence and detrimental impact on survival. Circulation 2006; 114(17):1829–37.

73. Santos MR dos, Sayegh ALC, Groehs RVR, et al. Testosterone deficiency increases hospital readmission and mortality rates in male patients with heart failure. Arq Bras Cardiol 2015;105(3):256–64.

74. Pugh PJ, Jones RD, West JN, et al. Testosterone treatment for men with chronic heart failure. Heart 2004;90(4):446–7.

75. Malkin CJ, Pugh PJ, West JN, et al. Testosterone therapy in men with moderate severity heart failure: a double-blind randomized placebo controlled trial. Eur Heart J 2006;27(1):57–64.

76. Caminiti G, Volterrani M, Iellamo F, et al. Effect of long-acting testosterone treatment on functional exercise capacity, skeletal muscle performance, insulin resistance, and baroreflex sensitivity in elderly patients with chronic heart failure a double-blind, placebo-controlled, randomized study. J Am Coll Cardiol 2009; 54(10):919–27.

77. Iellamo F, Volterrani M, Caminiti G, et al. Testosterone therapy in women with chronic heart failure: a pilot double-blind, randomized, placebo-controlled study. J Am Coll Cardiol 2010;56(16):1310–6.

78. Toma M, McAlister FA, Coglianese EE, et al. Testosterone supplementation in heart failure: a meta-analysis. Circ Heart Fail 2012;5(3):315–21.

79. Dos Santos MR, Sayegh ALC, Bacurau AVN, et al. Effect of exercise training and testosterone replacement on skeletal muscle wasting in patients with heart failure with testosterone deficiency. Mayo Clin Proc 2016;91(5):575–86.

80. Durga A, Sepahpanah F, Regozzi M, et al. Prevalence of testosterone deficiency after spinal cord injury. PM R 2011;3(10):929–32.

81. Wang YH, Huang TS, Lien IN. Hormone changes in men with spinal cord injuries. Am J Phys Med Rehabil 1992;71(6):328–32.

82. Schopp LH, Clark M, Mazurek MO, et al. Testosterone levels among men with spinal cord injury admitted to inpatient rehabilitation. Am J Phys Med Rehabil 2006; 85(8):678–84.

83. Gregory CM, Vandenborne K, Huang HFS, et al. Effects of testosterone replacement therapy on skeletal muscle after spinal cord injury. Spinal Cord 2003;41(1):23–8.

84. Bauman WA, Cirnigliaro CM, La Fountaine MF, et al. A small-scale clinical trial to determine the safety and efficacy of testosterone replacement therapy in hypogonadal men with spinal cord injury. Horm Metab Res 2011;43(8):574–9.

85. Nightingale TE, Moore P, Harman J, et al. Body composition changes with testosterone replacement therapy following spinal cord injury and aging: a mini review. J Spinal Cord Med 2018;41(6):624–36.

86. Celik B, Sahin A, Caglar N, et al. Sex hormone levels and functional outcomes: a controlled study of patients with spinal cord injury compared with healthy subjects. Am J Phys Med Rehabil 2007;86(10):784–90.

87. Clark MJ, Petroski GF, Mazurek MO, et al. Testosterone replacement therapy and motor function in men with spinal cord injury: a retrospective analysis. Am J Phys Med Rehabil 2008;87(4):281–4.

88. Gorgey AS, Khalil RE, Gill R, et al. Low-dose testosterone and evoked resistance exercise after spinal cord injury on cardio-metabolic risk factors: an open-label randomized clinical trial. J Neurotrauma 2019;36(18):2631–45.

89. Holman ME, Gorgey AS. Testosterone and resistance training improve muscle quality in spinal cord injury. Med Sci Sports Exerc 2019;51(8):1591–8.

90. Gorgey AS, Graham ZA, Chen Q, et al. Sixteen weeks of testosterone with or without evoked resistance training on protein expression, fiber hypertrophy and mitochondrial health after spinal cord injury. J Appl Physiol (1985) 2020;128(6): 1487–96.

Body Image Disorders and Anabolic Steroid Withdrawal Hypogonadism in Men

Harrison G. Pope Jr, MD[a,b,*], Gen Kanayama, MD, PhD[a,b]

KEYWORDS

- Anabolic steroids • Hypogonadism • Testosterone • Human chorionic gonadotropin
- Clomiphene • Men

KEY POINTS

- Anabolic-androgenic steroid (AAS)-withdrawal hypogonadism is common and underrecognized.
- AAS-withdrawal hypogonadism is often prolonged and sometimes perhaps irreversible.
- Human chorionic gonadotropin and clomiphene are useful for helping to restore hypothalamic-pituitary-testicular function in men with AAS-withdrawal hypogonadism.

INTRODUCTION AND HISTORICAL BACKGROUND

The anabolic-androgenic steroids (AAS) are a family of hormones that includes the natural hormone testosterone together with its many analogs (**Box 1**). Testosterone was originally isolated in the 1930s and synthetic derivatives quickly followed.[1] By the early 1950s, elite athletes had discovered the potential of these drugs, and AAS use spread rapidly through the Olympics and other high-level sporting events. However, it was not until the 1980s and 1990s that AAS use began to spread from the elite athletic world and into the general population. Most of these new general-population AAS users were young men who simply wanted to get bigger, often purely for personal appearance, and who had no plans to use AAS for competitive athletics. Today, probably about 80% of the world's AAS users fall into this latter category, with only about 20% representing competitive athletes.[2–4] However, many clinicians, and many members of the general public, still think of AAS as largely a problem of doping by athletes, and remain unaware of the much larger, less visible population of nonathlete AAS users.[5] Most of these latter men are relatively young; even the older members

[a] Biological Psychiatry Laboratory, McLean Hospital, 115 Mill Street, Belmont, MA 02478, USA;
[b] Harvard Medical School, Boston, MA, USA
* Corresponding author. Biological Psychiatry Laboratory, McLean Hospital, 115 Mill Street, Belmont, MA 02478.
E-mail address: hpope@mclean.harvard.edu

Endocrinol Metab Clin N Am 51 (2022) 205–216
https://doi.org/10.1016/j.ecl.2021.11.007
0889-8529/22/© 2021 Elsevier Inc. All rights reserved.

endo.theclinics.com

> **Box 1**
> **Commonly used anabolic-androgenic steroids**
>
> *Oral preparations*
> Methandienone (Dianabol)
> Oxandrolone (Anavar)
> Oxymetholone (Anadrol)
> Stanozolol (Winstrol)
>
> *Depot preparations for intramuscular injection*
> Testosterone esters (eg, testosterone cypionate, enanthate, propionate)
> Nandrolone decanoate (Deca-Durabolin)
> Boldenone undecylenate (Equipoise)
> Trenbolone hexahydrobenzylcarbonate (Parabolan)
> Drostanolone propionate (Masteron)

of this group—those who first started using AAS as youths in the late 1980s or early 1990s—are only now reaching middle-age, and thus entering the age of risk for long-term consequences of AAS use, including persistent hypogonadism.

Other historical trends in the last few decades have helped to further potentiate AAS use. One of these developments has been the rise of the Internet.[6] Unlike other drugs of abuse, such as cocaine and heroin, AAS can be legally purchased without a doctor's prescription in many countries, such as in Latin America, former Eastern Bloc countries, and various countries in Asia. Thus, AAS dealers located in one of these countries can purchase any amount of AAS and then sell them via the Internet to buyers in countries where possession of nonprescribed AAS is illegal. In the authors' anecdotal experience with numerous studies of AAS users in the United States, such illicit purchases are really interdicted.

Even in countries where they are illegal, AAS are nevertheless present in a substantial percentage of "dietary supplements," sold over the counter in nutrition stores or on the Internet.[7-10] In some cases, these supplements contain AAS that represent small chemical variations on illegal AAS molecules, but which can still be sold openly because they are not technically outlawed. These variant compounds may be identified on the label of the supplement bottle, or a supplement may contain legal or illegal AAS that are not disclosed on the label at all. Men using these supplements are often not aware that they are ingesting AAS and unwittingly exposing themselves to AAS-induced toxicity.

Also starting roughly in the 1980s, another important historical trend began to develop, namely an increasing focus on male body image, and particularly male muscularity, throughout many Western societies.[11] Over the last 4 decades, people have seen more and more images of ideal muscular male bodies in movies, television, advertising, and even in children's "action toys" (**Fig. 1**). For example, the American "G.I. Joe" toy, when he first appeared on the market in the 1960s, had an ordinary looking male body, but by the 1970s he had become distinctly more muscular, and by the 1990s more muscular still.[12] A similar trend occurred with the smaller versions of G.I. Joe, culminating in the "G.I. Joe extreme," who, if he were extrapolated to the height of an actual man, sported biceps bigger than those of any natural human being. Similarly, the toys representing Luke Skywalker and Han Solo from "Star Wars," when they first appeared in the late 1970s, portrayed normal looking male bodies—but the equivalent figures 20 years later were dramatically more muscular. Similar trends have

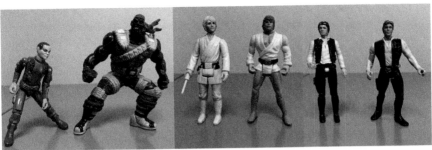

Fig. 1. The increasing muscularity of boys' action toys. Left panel: the 1982 G.I. Joe "Grunt" versus the 1997 G.I. Joe "Extreme"; center panel: Luke Skywalker 1977 versus 1997; right panel: Han Solo 1977 versus 1997. See reference 12 for details.

appeared in many other settings.[11,13] The possible causes of this mounting cultural focus on muscularity have been discussed elsewhere.[11,14–17]

These 2 parallel developments—the increasing availability of AAS and the growing cultural focus on male muscularity—have created a fertile soil for the development of AAS use, especially in younger men concerned about their body image. Particularly vulnerable are men who have developed so-called muscle dysmorphia, a form of body dysmorphic disorder in which the individual develops a pathologic concern that he is not sufficiently muscular. Men with muscle dysmorphia may devote long hours to weightlifting and other exercises, often with meticulous attention to diet.[18–20] Even when they become markedly muscular, these men may still feel that they are too small and will avoid being seen in situations where their bodies are visible, such as at the beach or in a locker room. Not surprisingly, such men are strongly attracted by AAS, and may indeed develop an AAS dependence syndrome, wherein they continue to use these drugs for years, often persisting despite adverse effects.[21,22] A recent study of adult male weightlifters found that men who retrospectively reported prominent body image concerns in early adolescence (between the ages of 13 and 16 years) were significantly more likely to have gone on to initiate AAS use than were men reporting lower levels of adolescent body image concern (**Fig. 2**).[23]

One study estimated that as of 2013, between 2.9 and 4.0 million men in the United States alone had used AAS at some time in their lives, and that about 1 million of these

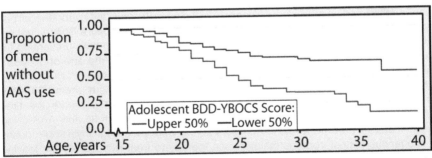

Fig. 2. Kaplan-Meier curves showing time to onset of first AAS use in men scoring in the lower 50% (upper curve) versus men in the upper 50% (lower curve) on the Body Dysmorphic Disorder Modification of the Yale-Brown Obsessive-Compulsive Scale (BDD-YOCS), based on their retrospective self-ratings for the period when they were 13 to 16 years old. See reference 23 for details.

men had developed an AAS dependence syndrome.[24] Notably, these estimates did not include the substantial number of additional men who may have used "dietary supplements" containing AAS, as described earlier. About 98% of all AAS users are men, as women rarely aspire to become extremely muscular, and are also vulnerable to the virilizing effects of AAS, such as beard growth, deepening of the voice, and masculinization of secondary sexual characteristics.[24] Thus, the present article refers only to male AAS users unless specified otherwise.

AAS-WITHDRAWAL HYPOGONADISM

All AAS suppress the hypothalamic-pituitary-testicular (HPT) axis via feedback inhibition. Thus, men who have used AAS for a few months or more will typically exhibit hypogonadism upon AAS withdrawal. AAS-withdrawal hypogonadism, like hypogonadism due to other causes, is associated with loss of libido, sometimes loss of erectile function, and occasionally, symptoms of depression. Interestingly, hypogonadism-associated depressive episodes appear to be idiosyncratic, with most men experiencing few depressive symptoms while a minority may develop prominent depression, sometimes even associated with suicidal ideation.[25,26] This idiosyncratic pattern of depressive symptoms has been found in laboratory studies where hypogonadism was deliberately induced in male volunteers by administration of depot leuprolide acetate,[27] in men administered reversible chemical castration for treatment of prostate cancer,[28] and in men undergoing AAS withdrawal.[29–31]

AAS withdrawal hypogonadism has been noted in the literature at least since the 1980s, and by 1989 was cited as a possible mechanism contributing to AAS dependence, whereby AAS users would be tempted to resume AAS in order to self-treat the dysphoric symptoms attendant on AAS withdrawal.[32] Nevertheless, before the last decade, most of the literature on AAS-withdrawal hypogonadism consisted of individual case reports or small case series (eg, see Refs. 33–39), with little to suggest that this phenomenon might be widespread, persistent, and sometimes perhaps irreversible.

Recent years, however, have seen reports from urologists, endocrinologists, and substance-abuse researchers demonstrating that AAS-induced hypogonadism is potentially a more serious problem than was once supposed. For example, Coward and colleagues[40] reviewed a database of 6033 cases of men seeking treatment for hypogonadism of any etiology. Of these men, 97 (1.6%) displayed profound hypogonadism, defined as a total testosterone level of 50 ng/dL or less. Remarkably, 42 (43%) of these severe cases were attributed to prior AAS use. The investigators subsequently conducted an anonymous survey of 382 men in their current hypogonadal patient population and found that 80 (21%) reported prior AAS exposure. These findings suggest the importance of seeking a history of AAS exposure in men presenting for treatment of hypogonadism, especially in cases of men under the age of 50 years and in men exhibiting profound hypogonadism as defined earlier.

Kanayama and colleagues[30] assessed indices of hypogonadism among 24 long-term AAS users who had discontinued AAS at least 3 months before the time of evaluation (mean, 58.9 months) and compared this group with 36 non–AAS-using weightlifters. Five of the former AAS users (21%) were receiving physiologic doses of exogenous testosterone as maintenance therapy to treat hypogonadism, leaving 19 untreated former AAS users for comparison with the 36 nonusers. Among these former users, 5 (26%) displayed testosterone levels of less than 200 ng/dL despite abstinence from AAS for 3, 7, 8, 16, and 26 months, respectively. On the "sexual desire" subscale of the International Index of Erectile Function, 7 former users (37%) scored 4 or less, indicating moderate to severe impairment. Five displayed major depressive disorder during AAS withdrawal; 3 of these 5 had never displayed major depressive disorder at any other time in their lives.

Rasmussen and colleagues[41] compared 37 current AAS users, 30 former users (mean duration of abstinence 2.5 years), and 30 nonusers. The men in all groups were aged 18 to 50 years and engaged in recreational strength training. Among the former AAS users, 28% displayed plasma testosterone levels below the reference limit of 12.1 nmol/L (350 ng/dL) as compared to none of the nonusers ($P<.01$). The former AAS users also displayed higher levels of depressive symptoms, erectile dysfunction, and decreased libido when compared with either of the other 2 groups.

These reports, together with other recent studies[42] and reviews,[43,44] suggest that AAS-induced hypogonadism is common but underrecognized, and may often be persistent and severe. Thus, it seems likely that as more of today's long-term AAS users begin to enter middle age, such cases of hypogonadism will become increasingly common, presenting in the clinics of primary care physicians, urologists, endocrinologists, and mental health clinicians involved in substance abuse treatment.

DIAGNOSIS AND DETECTION

The diagnosis and detection of AAS-induced hypogonadism is complicated by the fact that AAS users may be reluctant to disclose their AAS use to the clinician. In our experience, AAS use is arguably the most secret of the major forms of substance use disorders, perhaps for several reasons. First, AAS are illicit drugs in many countries. Second, if a man admits that he is using, say, illicit cocaine or opiates, he is simply revealing an illegal activity. But if he admits to using AAS, he is not only revealing illegal behavior but also admitting that his muscular prowess is merely a result of taking chemicals—a confession that he may be loath to make. Third, AAS users often have disdain for medical professionals. They recall that the medical community claimed for years, well into the 1970s and even 1980s, that AAS were ineffective for muscle gains or athletic improvement, even though athletes everywhere knew that these claims were false.[1] If doctors had been so misinformed, why should a patient confide to them about his AAS use?

This mistrust of physicians is illustrated by one study of 43 AAS users who were asked questions about how they trusted various sources of information about AAS.[45] Remarkably, 41% of these men users reported that they would trust information from their local drug dealer at least as much as information from their physicians, and 56% reported that they had never disclosed their AAS use to any physician that they had ever seen. Other writers have commented similarly on the physician's difficult task of securing trust with an AAS-using patient.[46,47] In light of the above, clinicians should use a careful, nonjudgmental approach with men reporting AAS use, as well as men who appear likely to have used AAS, but who are reluctant to disclose this fact.

Signs and Symptoms

If a patient does not initially disclose AAS use, several signs and symptoms may heighten the clinician's index of suspicion. First, does the patient exhibit marked muscularity? There is a clear upper limit to the amount of muscularity that a lean man can achieve without AAS use. We have developed and published a formula for calculating the so-called fat-free mass index in men, together with data suggesting that a man with low body fat (say <10%) cannot exceed a fat-free mass index of about 26 kg/m^2 without the use of drugs.[48]

It should be remembered that a man might exceed 26 kg/m^2 with low body fat, even though he has not knowingly taken AAS, because he may have used "nutritional supplements" containing surreptitious AAS or other anabolic substances, as discussed earlier in this article. Thus, clinicians should question carefully about supplement use when encountering an unusually muscular man who denies AAS consumption.

In addition to muscularity, various clinical signs and symptoms, such as truncal acne, gynecomastia, striae above the pectoralis muscles, and testicular atrophy may suggest AAS use.[49] Certain laboratory findings may also heighten the clinician's index of suspicion (**Table 1**).[3,50,51] Clinicians should be particularly alert upon finding abnormally low testosterone in conjunction with low follicle-stimulating hormone (FSH) and luteinizing hormone (LH) (ie, hypogonadotropic hypogonadism), in a young man who appears muscular. Any of these clues should prompt a gentle and sympathetic attempt to elicit a possible history of AAS use and to assess whether the patient is willing to discontinue future AAS use and consider treatment.

Laboratory Detection of AAS Use

A substantial literature has addressed the detection of AAS use by laboratory methods, but this approach is often of limited value to practicing clinicians. The only AAS detectable in blood samples with commercial testing is testosterone, and thus individuals taking multiple AAS in the absence of testosterone will be missed. Urine testing, on the other hand, can detect a wide range of AAS, but this testing is much more expensive (in the range of hundreds of dollars per sample), and available

Table 1
Laboratory abnormalities in anabolic-androgenic steroid users

Blood chemistries	
Muscle enzymes	Increased CK, ALT, AST, and LDH
Liver function tests	Increased ALT, AST, LDH, GGT & total bilirubin (caution: increased ALT, AST, & LDH are often muscular in origin and do not indicate liver disease)
Cholesterol levels	Decreased HDL-C, increased LDL-C Increase or no change in total cholesterol & triglycerides
Hormonal levels	Increased testosterone (in individuals currently using testosterone) Decreased testosterone (in individuals using other AAS but not testosterone) Decreased FSH & LH (in individuals currently using any AAS)
Hematology	Increased RBC count, hemoglobin & hematocrit
Urine testing	Positive for AAS in individuals currently or recently using AAS May be positive for other drugs of abuse as well
Electrocardiogram	Left ventricular hypertrophy (seen in intensive weight trainers also)
Echocardiogram	
Systolic function:	Decreased left ventricular ejection fraction
Diastolic function:	Decreased left ventricular relaxation velocity
Semen analysis	Decreased sperm count & motility, abnormal morphology

Abbreviations: AAS, anabolic-androgenic steroids; ALT, alanine aminotransferase; AST, aspartate aminotransferase; CK, creatine kinase; FSH, follicle-stimulating hormone; GGT, gamma-glutamyl transferase; HDL-C, high-density lipoprotein cholesterol; LDH, lactate dehydrogenase; LDL-C, low-density lipoprotein cholesterol; LH, luteinizing hormone; RBC, red blood cell.

in only a few reference laboratories. Also, urine testing can detect only current or relatively recent use of many AAS, such as orally administered compounds—although long-acting depot preparations (eg, nandrolone decanoate) may sometimes be detected many months after last use. Furthermore, commercial urine testing may fail to detect novel "designer" AAS, such as those sometimes present in "nutritional supplements," as described earlier.

TREATMENT

The literature on the treatment of AAS-induced hypogonadism remains limited. Most cases appear to be associated with low levels of gonadotropic hormones, LH, and FSH. This may be addressed by administering clomiphene, which stimulates the pituitary to secrete these 2 hormones, thus, in turn, stimulating testicular production of testosterone and spermatozoa. One early article[52] reported successful use of clomiphene, 100 mg per day for 2 months, to restore HPT function in a 30-year-old man with AAS-induced hypogonadism. Other articles have also described success with this medication in various cases of hypogonadism (eg, see Refs. 53,54). Importantly, Tan and Scally[55] have noted that clomiphene has 2 enantiomers with different actions. The *trans* enantiomer, enclomiphene, is an estradiol antagonist, whereas the *cis* enantiomer, zuclomiphene, is an estradiol agonist. Therefore, these authors have suggested that the addition of an estrogen receptor blocker, such as tamoxifen, might increase the overall antagonism of the estradiol receptor and hence improve the net effect of clomiphene on pituitary function, and secondarily on testicular function.

Another treatment for AAS-induced hypogonadism is human chorionic gonadotropin (hCG), which simulates the effect of pituitary gonadotropins by stimulating testicular Leydig cells to produce testosterone. Unfortunately, hCG must be administered parenterally and has a relatively short half-life, thus requiring injections every second day. However, for men prepared to self-administer hCG on a regular basis, this substance can fairly quickly increase serum testosterone levels. Moreover, hCG can be combined with clomiphene to achieve a dual stimulus on the HPT axis, hopefully resulting in more rapid return of testicular function in AAS users undergoing withdrawal. Various authorities (eg, see Refs. [44,56]) have proposed combination treatment protocols of this nature for attempting to restore both testosterone levels and fertility in men with AAS-induced hypogonadism.

Clinicians should be aware that many AAS users are already familiar with these treatments via their own personal research on the Internet. Karavolos and colleagues[57] have noted the vast number of Web sites providing information for users on how to self-treat AAS-withdrawal hypogonadism. These Web sites typically recommended the same compounds described in the scientific literature—hCG, selective estrogen receptor modulators such as clomiphene, and aromatase inhibitors. In our experience, users often obtain these compounds on the black market and self-treat their own cases of hypogonadism without coming to the attention of clinicians. Similarly, a well-known "underground" guide to AAS use[58] provides a detailed discussion of AAS-induced hypogonadism and offers a specific "postcycle therapy" program to treat AAS withdrawal, wherein the user takes 2000 international units of hCG every second today for 20 days, plus clomiphene citrate 50 mg twice a day for 30 days, and tamoxifen 20 mg twice a day for 45 days.

Practical Considerations

Patient motivation: In our experience, many AAS users, especially those under age 40 years, have little interest in stopping these drugs. This is particularly the case for men with body-image concerns or frank muscle dysmorphia, and who have become obsessed with looking lean and muscular. Such men may attempt to discontinue AAS but become panicky and resume the drugs when they perceive that they have lost even a few pounds of muscle.

However, symptoms of hypogonadism may eventually trump body-image concerns and bring the patient to the clinician. At this point, the clinician may be confronted with an ambivalent patient who recognizes that his loss of libido, erectile dysfunction, and possible depression are caused by AAS-induced hypogonadism, but who dreads stopping AAS entirely. Many such patients will ask for simple testosterone replacement therapy and will be content to self-administer physiologic or mildly supraphysiologic doses of testosterone (eg, 100–200 mg of testosterone cypionate intramuscularly once per week). However, maintenance testosterone represents an endless proposition, in that the patient's own HPT axis remains chronically suppressed and is never given the opportunity to recover on its own. AAS users, in our studies, are generally aware of this problem, and often report that they are resigned to taking testosterone for the remainder of their lives.

A happier alternative for willing AAS users is to attempt to regain their own HPT function and be freed from dependence on maintenance testosterone. Such men must be prepared to undergo a potentially prolonged regimen of drugs such as hCG, clomiphene, and antiestrogens, using protocols such as those cited earlier,[44,56] hoping that the HPT axis will recover and that the medication treatments can be gradually withdrawn. However, as discussed earlier, clinicians cannot assure users that they will be successful in this process. This is especially the case given our still incomplete knowledge of the pathophysiology of AAS-induced hypogonadism, which may have different subtypes and may reflect lesions at one or more different levels of the HPT axis (eg, in the hypothalamus, the pituitary, the testis, or the androgen receptor).

Psychiatric issues: As noted earlier, prominent depressive symptoms occur only in a minority of men with AAS-induced hypogonadism, but some depressive episodes are severe and require treatment with antidepressant medications.[29,59] One report has described a patient with suicidal depression attendant upon AAS withdrawal who failed to respond to successive trials of antidepressant medications but ultimately responded well to electroconvulsive therapy.[60] In cases of this nature, an endocrinologist should attempt to collaborate with a psychiatrist who can address these problems. Ideally, such a psychiatrist should be experienced in psychopharmacological interventions for major mood disorders, should have experience with substance use disorders in general, and should also be conversant with the particular psychiatric issues commonly encountered in AAS users, such as body-image disorders.

Patient commitment and compliance: Given the dysphoric symptoms associated with hypogonadism, together with the slow and difficult process of restoring normal HPT function, many AAS users will surreptitiously resume taking black-market AAS to supplement the drugs that they have been prescribed. In our anecdotal experience, as many as half of AAS users undergoing treatment for hypogonadism have engaged in at least some surreptitious AAS use in addition to prescribed medications. Clinicians who discover such behavior may be tempted to summarily refuse to treat the patient further. However, loss of medical treatment may plunge the patient back into repeated cycles of AAS use with worsening and more refractory symptoms of hypogonadism whenever he attempts to stop. In our experience, there is no simple answer in situations of this nature, and the physician will need to have a frank discussion with the patient about how to proceed. Again, it may be useful to seek the input of a psychiatrist familiar with substance use and body-image disorders.

SUMMARY

AAS are used by millions of men worldwide to achieve muscle growth for athletic performance or (more commonly) for personal appearance. The increasing availability of AAS, coupled with an increasing societal focus on male body image, has caused AAS use to spread widely since the 1980s and 1990s, especially in Western societies.

AAS suppress the HPT axis via feedback inhibition, thus resulting in AAS-induced hypogonadism after prolonged AAS exposure. Though little studied before the 21st century, AAS-induced hypogonadism has now been shown to be common, underrecognized, and often severe, persistent, and perhaps sometimes irreversible. As larger numbers of AAS users accumulate years of AAS exposure and begin to enter middle age, clinicians are likely to encounter increasing numbers of cases of this disorder.

The literature on treatment of AAS-induced hypogonadism remains limited, but strategies using hCG, selective estrogen receptor modulators, and estrogen receptor blockers may help to restore HPT axis function in men attempting to discontinue the use of AAS. However, treatment of such men involves several issues unique to this population, outlined earlier, that must be considered by endocrinologists and other clinicians who encounter such patients.

CLINICS CARE POINTS

- As AAS users are often reluctant to disclose their full drug history to a clinician, use a careful and nonjudgmental approach when evaluating the patient, while also looking for physical and laboratory evidence of AAS use and withdrawal.
- Assess the patient's motivation to discontinue AAS use, to engage in a potentially lengthy treatment regimen to restore his HPT function, and to avoid surreptitiously resuming AAS.
- Consider collaborating with a psychiatrist in patients exhibiting marked depression, anxiety, or body-image concerns during AAS withdrawal.

DISCLOSURE

Drs H.G. Pope and G. Kanayama are currently funded by a grant from the National Institute on Drug Abuse for research on the use of anabolic-androgenic steroids. Dr H.G. Pope testifies as an expert witness in cases involving anabolic-androgenic steroids approximately 1 to 2 times per year. Dr G. Kanayama declares no additional conflicts of interest.

REFERENCES

1. Kanayama G, Pope HG Jr. History and epidemiology of anabolic androgens in athletes and non-athletes. Mol Cell Endocrinol 2018;464:4–13.
2. Ip EJ, Barnett MJ, Tenerowicz MJ, et al. The Anabolic 500 survey: characteristics of male users versus nonusers of anabolic-androgenic steroids for strength training. Pharmacotherapy 2011;31(8):757–66.
3. Kanayama G, Hudson JI, Pope HG Jr. Anabolic-androgenic steroid use and body image in men: a growing concern for clinicians. Psychother Psychosom 2020; 89(2):65–73.
4. Parkinson AB, Evans NA. Anabolic androgenic steroids: a survey of 500 users. Med Sci Sports Exerc 2006;38(4):644–51.
5. Kanayama G, Pope HG. Misconceptions about anabolic-androgenic steroid abuse. Psychiatr Ann 2012;42(10):371–5.

6. Brennan BP, Kanayama G, Pope HG. Performance-enhancing drugs on the web: A growing public-health issue. Am J Addict 2013;22:158–61.

7. Baume N, Mahler N, Kamber M, et al. Research of stimulants and anabolic steroids in dietary supplements. Scand J Med Sci Sports 2006;16(1):41–8.

8. Geyer H, Parr MK, Koehler K, et al. Nutritional supplements cross-contaminated and faked with doping substances. J Mass Spectrom 2008;43(7):892–902.

9. Nasr J, Ahmad J. Severe cholestasis and renal failure associated with the use of the designer steroid Superdrol (methasteron): a case report and literature review. Dig Dis Sci 2009;54(5):1144–6.

10. Rahnema CD, Crosnoe LE, Kim ED. Designer steroids - over-the-counter supplements and their androgenic component: review of an increasing problem. Andrology 2015;3(2):150–5.

11. Pope H, Phillips K, Olivardia R. The Adonis complex: the secret crisis of male body obsession. New York: Simon & Schuster; 2000.

12. Pope HG, Olivardia R, Gruber A, et al. Evolving ideals of male body image as seen through action toys. Int J Eat Disord 1999;26(1):65–72.

13. Pope HG, Olivardia R, Borowiecki JJ 3rd, et al. The growing commercial value of the male body: a longitudinal survey of advertising in women's magazines. Psychother Psychosom 2001;70(4):189–92.

14. Field AE, Austin SB, Camargo CA Jr, et al. Exposure to the mass media, body shape concerns, and use of supplements to improve weight and shape among male and female adolescents. Pediatrics 2005;116(2):e214–20.

15. Hildebrandt T, Lai JK, Langenbucher JW, et al. The diagnostic dilemma of pathological appearance and performance enhancing drug use. Drug and alcohol dependence 2011;114(1):1–11.

16. Leit RA, Gray JJ, Pope HG Jr. The media's representation of the ideal male body: a cause for muscle dysmorphia? Int J Eat Disord 2002;31(3):334–8.

17. McCreary DR, Hildebrandt TB, Heinberg LJ, et al. A review of body image influences on men's fitness goals and supplement use. Am J Mens Health 2007;1(4): 307–16.

18. Pope HG, Gruber AJ, Choi P, et al. Muscle dysmorphia. An underrecognized form of body dysmorphic disorder. Psychosomatics 1997;38(6):548–57.

19. Hildebrandt T, Schlundt D, Langenbucher J, et al. Presence of muscle dysmorphia symptomology among male weightlifters. Compr Psychiatry 2006;47(2): 127–35.

20. Rohman L. The relationship between anabolic androgenic steroids and muscle dysmorphia: a review. Eat Disord 2009;17(3):187–99.

21. Brower KJ, Blow FC, Beresford TP, et al. Anabolic-androgenic steroid dependence. J Clin Psychiatry 1989;50(1):31–3.

22. Kanayama G, Brower KJ, Wood RI, et al. Anabolic-androgenic steroid dependence: an emerging disorder. Addiction 2009;104:1966–78.

23. Pope H, Kanayama G, Hudson J. Risk factors for illicit anabolic-androgenic steroid use in male weightlifters: A cross-sectional cohort study. Biol Psychiatry 2012;71:254–61.

24. Pope HG, Kanayama G, Athey A, et al. The lifetime prevalence of anabolic-androgenic steroid use and dependence in Americans: current best estimates. Am J Addict 2014;23:371–7.

25. Brower KJ, Blow FC, Eliopulos GA, et al. Anabolic androgenic steroids and suicide. Am J Psychiatry 1989;146(8):1075.

26. Thiblin I, Runeson B, Rajs J. Anabolic androgenic steroids and suicide. Ann Clin Psychiatry 1999;11(4):223–31.

27. Schmidt PJ, Berlin KL, Danaceau MA, et al. The effects of pharmacologically induced hypogonadism on mood in healthy men. Arch Gen Psychiatry 2004; 61(10):997–1004.

28. Almeida OP, Waterreus A, Spry N, et al. One year follow-up study of the association between chemical castration, sex hormones, beta-amyloid, memory and depression in men. Psychoneuroendocrinology 2004;29(8):1071–81.

29. Malone DA Jr, Dimeff RJ. The use of fluoxetine in depression associated with anabolic steroid withdrawal: a case series. J Clin Psychiatry 1992;53(4):130–2.

30. Kanayama G, Hudson J, DeLuca J, et al. Prolonged hypogonadism in males following withdrawal from anabolic-androgenic steroids: an underrecognized problem. Addiction 2015;110(5):823–31.

31. Pope HG, Katz DL. Psychiatric and medical effects of anabolic-androgenic steroid use. A controlled study of 160 athletes. Arch Gen Psychiatry 1994;51(5): 375–82.

32. Kashkin KB, Kleber HD. Hooked on hormones? An anabolic steroid addiction hypothesis. JAMA 1989;262(22):3166–70.

33. Boregowda K, Joels L, Stephens JW, et al. Persistent primary hypogonadism associated with anabolic steroid abuse. Fertil Steril 2011;96(1):e7–8.

34. Gazvani MR, Buckett W, Luckas MJ, et al. Conservative management of azoospermia following steroid abuse. Hum Reprod 1997;12(8):1706–8.

35. Jarow JP, Lipshultz LI. Anabolic steroid-induced hypogonadotropic hypogonadism. Am J Sports Med 1990;18(4):429–31.

36. Lloyd FH, Powell P, Murdoch AP. Anabolic steroid abuse by body builders and male subfertility. BMJ 1996;313(7049):100–1.

37. Menon DK. Successful treatment of anabolic steroid-induced azoospermia with human chorionic gonadotropin and human menopausal gonadotropin. Fertil Steril 2003;79(Suppl 3):1659–61.

38. Turek PJ, Williams RH, Gilbaugh JH 3rd, et al. The reversibility of anabolic steroid-induced azoospermia. J Urol 1995;153(5):1628–30.

39. Pirola I, Cappelli C, Delbarba A, et al. Anabolic steroids purchased on the Internet as a cause of prolonged hypogonadotropic hypogonadism. Fertil Steril 2010;94(6):2331.e1-3.

40. Coward RM, Rajanahally S, Kovac JR, et al. Anabolic steroid induced hypogonadism in young men. J Urol 2013;190(6):2200–5.

41. Rasmussen JJ, Selmer C, Ostergren PB, et al. Former abusers of anabolic androgenic steroids exhibit decreased testosterone levels and hypogonadal symptoms years after cessation: a case-control study. PLoS One 2016;11(8):e0161208.

42. Lykhonosov MP, Babenko AY, Makarin VA, et al. [Peculiarity of recovery of the hypothalamic-pituitary-gonadal (hpg) axis, in men after using androgenic anabolic steroids]. Probl Endokrinol (Mosk) 2020;66(1):104–12.

43. de Souza GL, Hallak J. Anabolic steroids and male infertility: a comprehensive review. BJU Int 2011;108(11):1860–5.

44. Rahnema CD, Lipshultz LI, Crosnoe LE, et al. Anabolic steroid-induced hypogonadism: diagnosis and treatment. Fertil Steril 2014;101(5):1271–9.

45. Pope HG, Kanayama G, Ionescu-Pioggia M, et al. Anabolic steroid users' attitudes towards physicians. Addiction 2004;99(9):1189–94.

46. Dawson R. Drugs in sport – the role of the physician. J Endocrinol 2001;170: 55–61.

47. Kutscher EC, Lund BC, Perry PJ. Anabolic steroids: a review for the clinician. Sports Med 2002;32(5):285–96.

48. Kouri EM, Pope HG Jr, Katz DL, et al. Fat-free mass index in users and nonusers of anabolic-androgenic steroids. Clin J Sport Med 1995;5(4):223–8.

49. Pope HG Jr, Wood RI, Rogol A, et al. Adverse health consequences of performance-enhancing drugs: an Endocrine Society scientific statement. Endocr Rev 2014;35(3):341–75.

50. Pope HG, Kanayama G. Can you tell if your patient is using anabolic steroids? Curr Psychiatry Prim Care 2005;1:28–34.

51. Pope HG, Kanayama G. Treatment of anabolic-androgenic steroid related disorders. In: Galanter M, Kleber H, Brady K, editors. The American Psychiatric Publishing Textbook of Substance Abuse Treatment. Fifth Edition. Washington, DC: American Psychiatric Association; 2015. p. 263–76.

52. Tan RS, Vasudevan D. Use of clomiphene citrate to reverse premature andropause secondary to steroid abuse. Fertil Steril 2003;79(1):203–5.

53. Alder NJ, Keihani S, Stoddard GJ, et al. Combination therapy with clomiphene citrate and anastrozole is a safe and effective alternative for hypoandrogenic subfertile men. BJU Int 2018;122(4):688–94.

54. Guay AT, Jacobson J, Perez JB, et al. Clomiphene increases free testosterone levels in men with both secondary hypogonadism and erectile dysfunction: who does and does not benefit? Int J Impot Res 2003;15(3):156–65.

55. Tan RS, Scally MC. Anabolic steroid-induced hypogonadism–towards a unified hypothesis of anabolic steroid action. Med Hypotheses 2009;72(6):723–8.

56. Tatem AJ, Beilan J, Kovac JR, et al. Management of Anabolic Steroid-Induced Infertility: Novel Strategies for Fertility Maintenance and Recovery. World J Mens Health 2020;38(2):141–50.

57. Karavolos S, Reynolds M, Panagiotopoulou N, et al. Male central hypogonadism secondary to exogenous androgens: a review of the drugs and protocols highlighted by the online community of users for prevention and/or mitigation of adverse effects. Clin Endocrinol 2015;82(5):624–32.

58. Llewellyn W. Anabolics. 11th edition. Jupiter (FL): Molecular Nutrition; 2017.

59. Malone DA Jr, Dimeff RJ, Lombardo JA, et al. Psychiatric effects and psychoactive substance use in anabolic-androgenic steroid users. Clin J Sport Med 1995; 5(1):25–31.

60. Allnutt S, Chaimowitz G. Anabolic steroid withdrawal depression: a case report. Can J Psychiatry 1994;39(5):317–8.

Optimized Use of the Electronic Health Record and Other Clinical Resources to Enhance the Management of Hypogonadal Men

Anna Goldman, MD[a],*, Martin Kathrins, MD[b]

KEYWORDS

• Electronic health record • EHR • Hypogonadism • Testosterone deficiency

KEY POINTS

• There are multiple benefits of an EHR, including increased accessibility of records, streamlining virtual care in an EHR system, clinical decision support, integration of artificial intelligence–driven algorithms, improved efficiency, and maintenance of privacy and confidentiality.

• Trade-offs and risks include cluttered notes, increased clinician burden and burnout, pop-up alert fatigue, and depersonalization of the physician-patient relationship.

• Strategies to eliminate these risks include integrated dictation technology, use of scribes, custom templates, clinician input into EHR design, access to technical help, and thoughtful changes in coding requirements.

INTRODUCTION

The implementation of the electronic health record (EHR) has allowed for the complete and accurate integration of a huge amount of data. EHR systems can improve communication between patients and providers to improve compliance, facilitate quality improvement, and reduce medical errors.[1] EHRs have also had some unintended consequences, including clinician burnout and depersonalization. Here, we discuss strategies to optimize the use of the EHR for the treatment of hypogonadal men while mitigating clinician burnout.

[a] Division of Endocrinology, Diabetes and Hypertension, Harvard Medical School, Brigham and Women's Hospital, 221 Longwood Avenue, RFB-2, Boston, MA 02115, USA; [b] Division of Urology, Harvard Medical School, Brigham and Women's Hospital, 45 Francis Street, ASB-II, Boston, MA 02115, USA
* Corresponding author.
E-mail address: Algoldman1@bwh.harvard.edu

Endocrinol Metab Clin N Am 51 (2022) 217–228
https://doi.org/10.1016/j.ecl.2021.11.008
0889-8529/22/© 2021 Elsevier Inc. All rights reserved.

endo.theclinics.com

HISTORY

EHRs have been commercially available since the 1970s, but their more recent, widespread implementation was driven in part by encouragement from the Office of the National Coordinator for Health Information and Technology (ONC) and other legislation. In 2009, President Obama signed into law the Health Information Technology for Economic and Clinical Health Act, (HITECH), which was part of the federal stimulus legislation known as the American Reinvestment and Recovery Act of 2009 (ARRA). This law was aimed at improving the quality, safety, and cost of health care by incentivizing adoption of health care information technology. In 2011, the Centers for Medicare & Medicaid Services (CMS) established the EHR Incentives Program to encourage the implementation and adoption of meaningful use of certified electronic health record technology (CEHRT). This program established requirements for the electronic capture of clinical data, continuous quality improvement, and improvement of health outcomes. To continue to promote interoperability, exchange of health care data, and patient access to their medical records, the program was renamed the Promoting Interoperability Program in 2018.

Outside of the United States, several countries have adopted universal EHRs. The Future Health Index commissioned a report in 2018, which focused on how health data are collected, shared, and used in 16 countries to improve value in health care.[2] It showed that universal EHR structures, in which every citizen's EHR is connected to a single national system, are linked to more trust in the health care system and higher value for patients.[2] The most significant success factor of a nationwide EHR system implementation process is to have the support and collaboration of all relevant stakeholders, including both health care professionals and the general population.[2,3] The 8 countries with universal EHRs had an average overall value measure of 47.29, whereas the countries without universal EHR coverage (including the United States), saw an average value measure of 39.67.[2] Resources to implement EHR, particularly universal EHR structures, may not be available in low-income and middle-income countries.

BENEFITS OF THE EHR
Billing Optimization

One of the benefits of EHR adoption has been the promise of more efficient and accurate billing. Although billing for professional services rendered remains the responsibility of the provider, the use of the EHR may increase the clarity and accuracy of this process. Reliance on the hand-written "Universal Billing Form" is for a bygone era, now with the availability of point-and-click interfaces and smart-sets to optimize selection of Current Procedural Terminology (CPT) coding and diagnoses. From the perspective of accurate diagnostic testing, implementation of a clinician codesigned EHR tool for disease coding showed significant promise in improving the quantity and consistency of disease codes recorded.[4] Overall, adoption of outpatient EHR is associated with increased administrative burden, but overall cost-effectiveness.[5] In previous years, insurance carriers were known to decline payment for services when copies of medical documentation were unavailable, a problem effectively solved by digitization of all records.[6] The future promises increased application of natural language processing (NLP) and map-assisted coding to increase speed, reliability, and accuracy of diagnostic coding.[7] However, EHR allows physicians relatively more transparent access to aggregate billing data than paper-based systems. However, these efficiencies do come at the cost of exposure to pop-up reminders to encourage proper billing contributing to physician burnout.[8]

Clinical Decision Support Systems

Clinicians increasingly have access to advanced clinical decision support systems (CDSSs) through EHR. CDSSs allow for evidence-based test selection, reinforcement of best practices and clinical guidelines, and cross-reference for drug allergy and medication interactions, which lead to better quality of care and improved clinical.[9,10] In 2015, a large cross-sectional study of men receiving testosterone within the Veterans Affairs (VA) found that only a small proportion had undergone appropriate testing, and some received testosterone therapy despite contraindications, including prostate cancer, obstructive sleep apnea, and a baseline elevated hematocrit.[11] The EHR can be used to promote a more uniform application of clinical guidelines in the diagnosis and management of hypogonadism to ensure the appropriate use of testosterone.

By facilitating access to best clinical practices, CDSSs can encourage, but not dictate, more efficacious prescribing patterns. For instance, one meta-analysis examining CDSS utilization and prescribing patterns for acute respiratory infections found that information technology significantly improved the level of prescribing.[12] Conversely, CDSSs' use can contribute to inefficient documentation, deteriorating patient-physician interactions, and increase in unnecessary referrals.[13]

Telehealth

Telehealth allows providers to evaluate, diagnose, and treat patients remotely using electronic and telecommunication technologies. In 2016, the Department of Health and Human Services estimated that 60% of all health care institutions and 40% to 50% of all hospitals in the United States used some form of telehealth.[14] To reduce the transmission risk of SARS-CoV-2 between health care personnel and patients and to preserve PPE during the COVID-19 pandemic, major changes had to be implemented quickly for health care to continue to be delivered to patients. In March 2020, in response to the pandemic, CMS greatly expanded coverage for telehealth services as many health systems transitioned to providing virtual care via video and telephone visits. In one large academic medical center, for instance, telehealth visits in the Department of Medicine increased from less than 1% to 55% in less than 50 days.[15] Telehealth will likely remain in some capacity even when the pandemic is ultimately declared to be over as high-quality care can still be delivered effectively in an EHR system for certain conditions. In addition, patients routinely report high satisfaction rates with virtual care services.[16]

Even before the pandemic, many patients saw telehealth as a convenient and discreet way of accessing testosterone therapy for hypogonadism. There is social stigma related to discussing and seeking help for issues related to men's health. Although approximately 50% of men will experience some form of ED,[17] only approximately 25% seek consultation.[18] Several for-profit centers provide a direct-to-consumer telehealth platform for the treatment of "Low T," offering home testing of testosterone and other hormone levels followed by virtual sessions with a physician who creates a personalized treatment plan. Such centers offer various forms of testosterone replacement therapy, though often without a clear, evidence-based indication.[19] There are minimal data to suggest that this strategy causes clear harm, but it remains to be seen if these for-profit centers, whose main goal is to monetize testosterone therapy, are accurately diagnosing and monitoring treatment for hypogonadism.

Artificial Intelligence–Driven Algorithms for Monitoring and Health Research

With the successful implementation of EHRs, there has been an increase in their use for biomedical research.[20] Clinical data from EHRs can be extracted with the potential for revealing previously unknown disease correlations and discovering new patterns for classification and prediction of patient outcomes.[20] Research using EHR has already led to several contributions to our understanding of male hypogonadism (**Box 1**). EHRs were not designed for population-based research and therefore researchers must consider selection bias, missing data, and phenotyping errors in their analysis.[21] Integration of advanced artificial intelligence (AI) and NLP algorithms into CDSS represents the future of EHR utilization. By applying AI processing to CDSS, many complicated surveillance protocols may be automated.

Statistical approach NLP uses probabilistic or machine-learning algorithms for text analysis. For instance, research indicates such tools may be used to monitor prostate cancer survivors for biochemical recurrence by incorporating prostate-specific antigen monitoring over time.[22] NLP can also extract numerous informational domains from narrative prostate pathology reports to create a prospective database containing accurate information on data points such as the number of biopsy cores positive for cancer and the grading Gleason score.[23] Advances in NLP technology are necessary for modeling temporal extraction. For example, capturing a diagnosis of erythrocytosis *before* or *after* initiation of testosterone supplementation therapy is of utmost importance in assisting clinicians monitoring such patients. Presently, NLP is not yet adept at incorporating comorbidities from unstructured clinical text for predictive algorithms nor does it well model the long-term course of patients with chronic disease.[24]

Although there is much work to be done, there is great potential for the application of NLP for the monitoring of patients with testosterone deficiency whether or not they are treated with testosterone supplementation therapy. Integrating EHR databases with genetic databases may also enable a more in-depth understanding of genotype-phenotype relationships. In the future, it could be possible for EHR data to be linked to genetic data to provide genotype-based decision support.

DISADVANTAGES ASSOCIATED WITH EHR AND STRATEGIES TO MITIGATE THESE
Information Clutter and the 2021 E&M Coding Changes

One of the benefits of EHR documentation is to maximize the billing potential for harried clinicians who are increasingly burdened with additional administrative tasks. Previous iterations of billing based on evaluation and management (E/M) services have relied on a complicated series of documentation requirements, which can be automatically populated into progress notes. However, this automated text creation may come at the expense of documentation clarity. EHR-created progress notes may contain

---

Box 1
Summary of contributions to our understanding of male hypogonadism from research conducted using EHR

Determination of testosterone replacement therapy (TRT) prescribing practices in large databases[11,47–49]

New and existing prevalence of patients with hypogonadism[48]

Follow-up evaluation of patients after TRT initiation[48]

Variables associated with hypogonadism[48,50,51]

Adverse outcomes associated with TRT[52,53]

Effects of TRT on hypogonadal men with other comorbidities[51,54,55]

Association of hypogonadism with other conditions[56–58]

significant repetition of information within the same note.[25] Furthermore, while the common copy-and-paste practice to expedite note population may also contribute to the propagation of inaccurate information. Such copy-and-paste practices can even contribute to documentation in the wrong patient's medical record.[26]

On January 1, 2021, the Centers for Medicare & Medicaid Services (CMS) updated the policy for Medicare payments under the Physician Fee Schedule (PFS), and other Medicare Part B issues. The 2021 Medicare Physician Fee Schedule (MPFS), and the subsequent Consolidated Appropriations Act of 2021, decreased the Medicare conversion factor and increased the work relative value units (RVUs) for common E&M office visits. For many years, the RVU associated with the outpatient E/M code was considered too low compared with other physician services—these changes addressed this and also reviewed coding and documentation guidelines for the first time in more than 25 years.

Since 1995, providers have been frustrated by the complexity of documentation requirements and "documenting for the sake of documenting." The new guidelines decrease the administrative burden of documentation and coding and should decrease unnecessary documentation/clutter in the medical record (**Box 2**). Starting in January 2021, E&M documentation now focuses on medical decision-making (MDM) or time; elements of the history and examination should only be documented when clinically appropriate and not to meet certain billing criteria. Providers can use either MDM or time to bill depending on which is most beneficial for the visit. With the new rules, total time is considered face-to-face and non–face-to-face on the date of the encounter by the "reporting" provider. Although the goal of these changes was not to redistribute payment between specialties, Medicare projected significant increases in reimbursement for specialties involving substantial office-based E&M services and decreasing reimbursement for specialists performing few to no office visits (see **Box 2**). Documentation is ultimately meant to communicate between clinicians, and future iterations of EMR and billing requirements may emphasize processes that support that goal. Indeed, these changes to documentation and coding may serve to limit the documentation burden for clinicians.

Depersonalization of the Physician-Patient Interaction During Office Visit

The requisites of time-intensive documentation in the EHR have added to clinician burden. When providers write notes while interviewing the patient to improve efficiency, this may be associated with reduced eye contact and make the office visit feel less personal to the patient. Reasonable concerns have been raised about the lack of eye contact during the patient consultation, and its potential to diminish the

---

Box 2
Guiding principles of the redesign of E&M codes

Decrease administrative burden for clinicians

Decrease the need for audits

Decrease unnecessary documentation

Ensure that payment for E&M is resource-based and has no direct goal of payment redistribution between specialties

Data from Levy, B.a.J., C. *2021 E/M Updates: EHR Workflow and Operational Considerations.* 2021; Available from: https://www.ama-assn.org/system/files/2021-03/ama-em-updates-ehr-workflow-white-paper.pdf.

traditional empathetic quality of the doctor-patient interaction. A Brown University study evaluated the attitude transformation of more than 2000 physicians since the introduction of the EHR. Physicians reported a substantial decrease in the time and the quality of interactions with their patients since the introduction of the EHR.[27] The patients also reported lower satisfaction when physicians spent more time looking at a computer during the patient-physician encounter.[28]

Given the rapid rise of telehealth during the COVID-19 pandemic, it is notable that the first encounter that many patients may have with their provider is now virtual. With a video visit, the elements of the traditional provider/patient visit can remain but certainly something quintessential is lost with just a telephone call. Patients infected with SARS-CoV-2 had to be quarantined during the pandemic, which may mean less contact with health practitioners. Lack of a physical examination or inadequacies of the examination have been shown to be a clear, preventable source of error, increasing diagnostic errors, reducing efficiency, and compromising the quality of clinical decision-making.[29] Physical disengagement from patients may also have other more profound effects on patient care and the experience of care as the disembodiment, "datafication."[30] The substitution of patient "charts" as surrogates for patients themselves also serves to remove the patient narrative and the personalization of care, diminishing and even "destroy(ing) … every kind of subjectivity"[31] and chances to develop interpersonal trust and empathy. Using in-person or video visits when possible, instead of telephone visits should be advised whenever possible; however, patients who lack access to technology should not be penalized as this may exacerbate disparities in access to health care.

Depersonalization is certainly a frustrating trade-off of the EHR.[32] Several steps can further reduce the risk of depersonalization: regular eye contact, frequent breaks from the screens, voicing of patient concerns, and active listening may improve the patient experience.[33] Other approaches include the use of professional scribes or increasingly accurate real-time software dictation programs.

Pop-Up Alert Fatigue

Although intended to optimize safe prescribing and cost-effective ordering practices, EHR clinician notifications, or "pop-ups," can be a source of consternation for the user. However, there is concern that an increasing volume of these alerts may go unheeded. Alerts have been unfortunately associated with clinician fatigue and cognitive weariness.[34] Desensitization to such pop-ups is referred to as alert fatigue. Although alert fatigue is well-described by-product of clinical practice in the intensive care unit with multiple auditory and visual alerts bombarding the senses, the major concern over alert fatigue in EHR is that a truly important alert may be missed or ignored. Research indicates that over time the frequency of such alerts is increasing steadily.[35]

Application of AI to CDSS may serve to reduce the frequency, and thus the burden, of pop-up alerts. One study applied machine learning models to predict clinician acceptance of the automatic advice provided by EHR. Their results indicate a path forward to both reduce the burden of alerts while still limiting wasteful clinical practices.[36] Future design modifications to CDSS, such as noninterrupting dynamically annotated visualization, may reduce the toll of such well-meaning notifications.[37]

Clinician Burden and Burnout

One major unwanted product of widespread EHR adoption is its contribution to increased clinician burnout. Rates of burnout approach 55% among US physicians.[38] Burnout due to EHR has been associated with insufficient time for documentation and generally negative perceptions of the EHR by providers.[39] Beyond the burden of documentation through EHR, physicians now must contend with "in-box" messages from patients. Although this new communication avenue would seem to increase patient access to clinician input, the impact on physicians, in particular, can be significant. In-box responses contribute to out-of-work time spent and increased physiologic stress.[40] Indeed, patient messages may be the component of EHR use, which is most associated with clinician burnout.[41] It is also clear that EHR contributes to burn-out for nonphysicians, extending to nurses working on inpatient units.[42] Some of these problems may be mitigated by spreading the workload to other members of the outpatient health care delivery team and encouraging the use of custom templates (**Fig. 1**).

Limitations on the Validity of EHR data

There may be a bias toward coding for more common diagnoses like hypogonadism when clinicians have difficulty finding codes for uncommon, related conditions or they may code for hypogonadism when evaluating a patient with suspected but not confirmed hypogonadism.

The research focused on patients presenting with malignancies indicates that practice setting and clinician type are associated with the accuracy of diagnostic coding.[43] This ascertainment bias may lead to real challenges when using EHR data for large-scale, pragmatic clinical trials studying men with hypogonadism, particularly with regards to recruitment.[44] Fragmentation of EHRs between health care systems is also a significant drawback. There is a concern of report bias; that is, available data of prescribing behaviors for the diagnosis of hypogonadism within a given institution may not be representative of "real-world" practice. Thus, EHR-based health services research should be viewed in a different lens than those based on government databases and national insurance claims databases which may not suffer from these biases. Although EHR-based retrospective studies may offer expediency, this may come at the risk of lower accuracy than detailed chart reviews.

Use of Scribes

The use of professional scribes is one way to lessen burnout and improve clinician productivity. Medical scribes enter information directly into patients' EHR so that doctors can focus all their attention on taking a thorough history and conducting a targeted but detailed physical examination. The use of scribes has been shown to improve provider efficiency, productivity, revenue, and satisfaction.[45] It can be a burden for a practice to invest in hiring and training scribes who will be relied upon to accurately document important patient data in the EHR.

Dependence on scribes for data entry is susceptible to variable quality, imprecision, and/or inaccuracy of documentation.[46] Patients may object to the presence of an additional person in the room, especially based on gender preference or, in the setting of the COVID-19 pandemic, the need for social distancing.

DISCUSSION

Widespread adoption of EHR carries new promises and perils. However, EHR may facilitate patient access through messaging portals, optimize billing, and encourage evidence-based and cost-effective care. The tradeoff is that the use of the EHR has created a new and severe source of clinician burnout through increased documentation burden and alert fatigue. Gone are the days of waiting for a faxed clinical report from another hospital; EHR has effectively allowed the communication of timely information across disparate health care systems. The future may rely on increased

Name:
MRN:
DOB:
Date of Consultation:

History of Present Illness: NAME is a AGE SEX here today for consultation regarding hypogonadism.

Reproductive history:
Birth/Growth Dev/Puberty:
Reproductive history/fertility:
Hair growth: started shaving at age ***, no decreased shaving frequency needs
Muscle mass/exercise tolerance:
Lack of energy/sleep problems:
Weight stable:
Libido:
Erectile Function: ***. He has/has not done a trial of a phosphodiesterase inhibitor.
Gynecomastia:
Vision Disturbance/Headaches/Anosmia:
History of mumps orchitis:
History of cryptorchidism:
Lower urinary tract symptoms:
Increased Stress:
Steroids, opiates, ETOH:
Radiation/Chemotherapy:
Fractures:
Liver disease:
Diabetes:
Finasteride use:

Past medical history:

Past surgical history:

Medications:

Allergies:

Family history:

Social history:

Review of systems:

Physical Examination:

Review of Tests:
Total and free testosterone and SHBG
Prolactin
FSH/LH
TSH
PSA
CBC
A1C
CMP
Lipids

Relevant imaging:

Assessment and Plan: AGE year-old man with past medical history significant for *
presenting today with possible hypogonadism.**

-Check fasting AM total testosterone by LC-MS/MS and free testosterone by Equilibrium
Dialysis:
-check LH, FSH
-CBC, Chem 10, fasting Lipids, PSA
-Additional Testing if needed (Prolactin, Thyroid function tests, GH, IGF-1, ACTH, cortisol, Fe
Studies), MRI pituitary protocol.

Fig. 1. Patient education and practice enhancement materials: Sample New Patient Template for Hypogonadism.

clinician user design input for EHR redesigns to maintain clinical accuracy and efficiency while mitigating the resultant emotional toll and burnout rate.

SUMMARY

EHR has multiple benefits for both clinicians and patients; however, there are multiple trade-offs. To optimize the use of the EHR, clinicians ought to familiarize themselves with technological innovations, including CDSS and AI-driven algorithms that improve safety and quality of care. The burden of documentation and fatigue from pop-up alerts should not be discounted as contributors to clinician burnout and institutions that use EHR should frequently solicit clinician input so that the efficiency and useability of the EHR can continue to improve over time. Investment in dictation technology, scribes, custom templates (see **Fig. 1**), and technical support do cost money upfront but may reduce burnout and clinician turnover overtime.

CLINICS CARE POINTS

- Adoption of EHR in a medical practice is associated with multiple benefits, including clinical decision support, integration of AI-driven algorithms, improved efficiency, and quality of care.

- Investment in dictation technology, medical scribes, custom templates, and technical support may reduce clinician burden and burnout.

- To reduce depersonalization and encourage empathic physician-patient relationships, eye contact, either in person or via a video virtual visit, is encouraged.

- It is important to understand and integrate the 2021 E&M coding changes into one's practice as this should lead to reduced burden of documentation and potentially increased reimbursement.

DISCLOSURE

The authors have nothing to disclose.

REFERENCES

1. Lo B. Professionalism in the age of computerised medical records. Singapore Med J 2006;47(12):1018–22.
2. Index FH. Delivering value through data collection and analytics. 2018. Available at: https://www.deliveringvaluethroughdata.org/.
3. Fragidis LL, Chatzoglou PD. Implementation of a nationwide electronic health record (EHR). Int J Health Care Qual Assur 2018;31(2):116–30.
4. Mangin D, et al. Embedding "Smart" disease coding within routine electronic medical record workflow: prospective single-arm trial. JMIR Med Inform 2020;8(7):e16764.
5. Choi JS, Lee WB, Rhee PL. Cost-benefit analysis of electronic medical record system at a tertiary care hospital. Healthc Inform Res 2013;19(3):205–14.
6. Light TD, et al. Digital photography: a technique to optimize reimbursement. J Burn Care Res 2008;29(1):147–50.
7. Fung KW, et al. Using SNOMED CT-encoded problems to improve ICD-10-CM coding-A randomized controlled experiment. Int J Med Inform 2019;126:19–25.
8. Melnick ER, et al. Perceived electronic health record usability as a predictor of task load and burnout among us physicians: mediation analysis. J Med Internet Res 2020;22(12):e23382.

9. Burstin H, Leatherman S, Goldmann D. The evolution of healthcare quality measurement in the United States. J Intern Med 2016;279(2):154–9.

10. Manca DP. Do electronic medical records improve quality of care? Yes. Can Fam Physician 2015;61(10):846–7, 850-847.

11. Jasuja GK, et al. Ascertainment of testosterone prescribing practices in the VA. Med Care 2015;53(9):746–52.

12. Nabovati E, et al. Information technology interventions to improve antibiotic prescribing for patients with acute respiratory infection: a systematic review. Clin Microbiol Infect 2021;27(6):838–45.

13. Muhiyaddin R, et al. The impact of clinical decision support systems (CDSS) on physicians: a scoping review. Stud Health Technol Inform 2020;272:470–3.

14. Office of Health Policy, O.o.t.A.S.f.P.a.E.A., Report to Congress: E-health and Telemedicine. 2016.

15. Croymans, D., Hurst, I., and Han, M., Commentary: telehealth: the right care, at the right time, via the right medium. NEJM Catalyst innovations in care delivery, 2020.

16. Betts D, Korenda L, Giuliani S. Are consumers already living the future of health?. 2020. Available from. https://www2.deloitte.com/us/en/insights/industry/healthcare/consumer-health-trends.html.html.

17. Yafi FA, et al. Erectile dysfunction. Nat Rev Dis Primers 2016;2:16003.

18. Frederick LR, et al. Undertreatment of erectile dysfunction: claims analysis of 6.2 million patients. J Sex Med 2014;11(10):2546–53.

19. Handelsman DJ. Global trends in testosterone prescribing, 2000-2011: expanding the spectrum of prescription drug misuse. Med J Aust 2013;199(8):548–51.

20. Jensen PB, Jensen LJ, Brunak S. Mining electronic health records: towards better research applications and clinical care. Nat Rev Genet 2012;13(6):395–405.

21. Beesley LJ, Mukherjee B. Bias reduction and inference for electronic health record data under selection and phenotype misclassification: three case studies. medRxiv 2020.

22. Park J, et al. Prostate cancer trajectory-map: clinical decision support system for prognosis management of radical prostatectomy. Prostate Int 2021;9(1):25–30.

23. Thomas AA, et al. Extracting data from electronic medical records: validation of a natural language processing program to assess prostate biopsy results. World J Urol 2014;32(1):99–103.

24. Sheikhalishahi S, et al. Natural Language Processing of Clinical Notes on Chronic Diseases: Systematic Review. JMIR Med Inform 2019;7(2):e12239.

25. Koopman RJ, et al. Physician Information Needs and Electronic Health Records (EHRs): Time to Reengineer the Clinic Note. J Am Board Fam Med 2015;28(3):316–23.

26. Tsou AY, et al. Safe Practices for Copy and Paste in the EHR. Systematic Review, Recommendations, and Novel Model for Health IT Collaboration. Appl Clin Inform 2017;8(1):12–34.

27. Pelland KD, Baier RR, Gardner RL. It's like texting at the dinner table": A qualitative analysis of the impact of electronic health records on patient-physician interaction in hospitals. J Innov Health Inform 2017;24(2):894.

28. Farber NJ, et al. EHR use and patient satisfaction: What we learned. J Fam Pract 2015;64(11):687–96.

29. Verghese A, et al. Inadequacies of physical examination as a cause of medical errors and adverse events: a collection of vignettes. Am J Med 2015;128(12):1322–1324 e3.

30. Fortin S. Between reason, science and culture: biomedical decision-making. J Int Bioethique Ethique Sci 2015;26(4):39–56, 153-154.

31. Gremy F, Fessler JM, Bonnin M. Information systems evaluation and subjectivity. Int J Med Inform 1999;56(1–3):13–23.

32. Margalit RS, et al. Electronic medical record use and physician-patient communication: an observational study of Israeli primary care encounters. Patient Educ Couns 2006;61(1):134–41.

33. Arar NH, Wang CP, Pugh JA. Self-care communication during medical encounters: implications for future electronic medical records. Perspect Health Inf Manag 2006;3:3.

34. Gregory ME, Russo E, Singh H. Electronic health record alert-related workload as a predictor of burnout in primary care providers. Appl Clin Inform 2017;8(3):686–97.

35. Chaparro JD, et al. Reducing interruptive alert burden using quality improvement methodology. Appl Clin Inform 2020;11(1):46–58.

36. Baron JM, et al. Use of machine learning to predict clinical decision support compliance, reduce alert burden, and evaluate duplicate laboratory test ordering alerts. JAMIA Open 2021;4(1):ooab006.

37. Rayo MF, et al. Comparing the effectiveness of alerts and dynamically annotated visualizations (davs) in improving clinical decision making. Hum Factors 2015;57(6):1002–14.

38. Shanafelt TD, et al. Changes in burnout and satisfaction with work-life balance in physicians and the general US Working Population Between 2011 and 2014. Mayo Clin Proc 2015;90(12):1600–13.

39. Yan Q, et al. Exploring the relationship between electronic health records and provider burnout: A systematic review. J Am Med Inform Assoc 2021;28(5):1009–21.

40. Akbar F, et al. Physician stress during electronic health record inbox work: in situ measurement with wearable sensors. JMIR Med Inform 2021;9(4):e24014.

41. Hilliard RW, Haskell J, Gardner RL. Are specific elements of electronic health record use associated with clinician burnout more than others? J Am Med Inform Assoc 2020;27(9):1401–10.

42. Sutton DE, et al. Defining an essential clinical dataset for admission patient history to reduce nursing documentation burden. Appl Clin Inform 2020;11(3):464–73.

43. Diaz-Garelli F, et al. Workflow differences affect data accuracy in oncologic ehrs: a first step toward detangling the diagnosis data babel. JCO Clin Cancer Inform 2020;4:529–38.

44. Esserman D. From screening to ascertainment of the primary outcome using electronic health records: Challenges in the STRIDE trial. Clin Trials 2020;17(4):346–50.

45. McCormick BJ, et al. Implementation of medical scribes in an academic urology practice: an analysis of productivity, revenue, and satisfaction. World J Urol 2018;36(10):1691–7.

46. Pranaat R, et al. Use of simulation based on an electronic health records environment to evaluate the structure and accuracy of notes generated by medical scribes: proof-of-concept study. JMIR Med Inform 2017;5(3):e30.

47. Baillargeon J, et al. Trends in androgen prescribing in the United States, 2001 to 2011. JAMA Intern Med 2013;173(15):1465–6.

48. Inspections, O.o.H., Healthcare Inspection: testosterone replacement therapy initiation and Follow-up evaluation in VA male patients. 2018: Washington, DC 20420.
49. Jasuja GK, et al. Understanding the context of high- and low-testosterone prescribing facilities in the veterans health administration (VHA): a qualitative study. J Gen Intern Med 2019;34(11):2467–74.
50. Tan RS, Cook KR, Reilly WG. High estrogen in men after injectable testosterone therapy: the low T experience. Am J Mens Health 2015;9(3):229–34.
51. Naelitz B, et al. Prolactin-to-testosterone ratio predicts pituitary abnormalities in mildly hyperprolactinemic men with symptoms of hypogonadism. J Urol 2021; 205(3):871–8.
52. Pantalone KM, et al. Testosterone replacement therapy and the risk of adverse cardiovascular outcomes and mortality. Basic Clin Androl 2019;29:5.
53. Jick SS, Hagberg KW. The risk of adverse outcomes in association with use of testosterone products: a cohort study using the UK-based general practice research database. Br J Clin Pharmacol 2013;75(1):260–70.
54. Shortridge EF, et al. Symptom report and treatment experience of hypogonadal men with and without type 2 diabetes in a United States health plan. Int J Clin Pract 2015;69(7):783–90.
55. Majzoub A, Shoskes DA. A case series of the safety and efficacy of testosterone replacement therapy in renal failure and kidney transplant patients. Transl Androl Urol 2016;5(6):814–8.
56. Ford AH, et al. Prospective longitudinal study of testosterone and incident depression in older men: The Health In Men Study. Psychoneuroendocrinology 2016;64:57–65.
57. Le B, et al. Laboratory evaluation of secondary causes of bone loss in Veterans with spinal cord injury and disorders. Osteoporos Int 2019;30(11):2241–8.
58. Ford AH, et al. Sex hormones and incident dementia in older men: The health in men study. Psychoneuroendocrinology 2018;98:139–47.

Moving?

Make sure your subscription moves with you!

To notify us of your new address, find your **Clinics Account Number** (located on your mailing label above your name), and contact customer service at:

Email: journalscustomerservice-usa@elsevier.com

800-654-2452 (subscribers in the U.S. & Canada)
314-447-8871 (subscribers outside of the U.S. & Canada)

Fax number: 314-447-8029

Elsevier Health Sciences Division
Subscription Customer Service
3251 Riverport Lane
Maryland Heights, MO 63043

*To ensure uninterrupted delivery of your subscription, please notify us at least 4 weeks in advance of move.

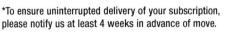

Moving?

Make sure your subscription moves with you!

To notify us of your new address, find your Clinics Account Number (located on your mailing label above your name), and contact customer service at:

Email: journalscustomerservice-usa@elsevier.com

Fax number: 314-447-8029

Elsevier Health Sciences Division
Subscription Customer Service
3251 Riverport Lane
Maryland Heights, MO 63043

To ensure uninterrupted delivery of your subscription, please notify us at least 4 weeks in advance of move.

Printed and bound by CPI Group (UK) Ltd, Croydon, CR0 4YY

08/05/2025

01864713-0003